TREE PATHOLOGY

A SHORT INTRODUCTION

TREE PATHOLOGY:

A SHORT INTRODUCTION

The Mechanisms and Control of
Pathological Stresses of Forest Trees

WILLIAM H. SMITH

Yale University

ACADEMIC PRESS • NEW YORK AND LONDON

ACADEMIC PRESS, INC.
111 Fifth Avenue, New York, New York 10003

United Kingdom Edition published by
ACADEMIC PRESS, INC. (LONDON) LTD.
Berkeley Square House, London W1X 6BA

LIBRARY OF CONGRESS CATALOG CARD NUMBER: 75-107547

PRINTED IN THE UNITED STATES OF AMERICA

To my wife and sons: Judy, Scott, and Phil,
for their enthusiasm for life
and love of the natural world.

CONTENTS

PREFACE

This book is a compendium of the significant pathological stress factors that are capable of inducing tree injury and disease; it is not a comprehensive account of the diseases of forest trees.

For numerous reasons the pathological consideration of forest trees is quite distinct from that of agricultural plants. The comparatively large size and long life span of trees coupled with their relatively low value have been of primary significance in the development of these differences. The high value of certain agricultural crops has led to a rather intensive consideration of their pathology. The significance of nematodes, viruses, bacteria, and fungi as disease-inducing agents has been well documented for several plants. In the case of forest trees, however, disease research has been less intensive, and, until recently, primary emphasis was placed on studies of fungal disease agents. Fungi are still considered the principal biotic agents of tree disease. Evidence is being accumulated, however, that indicates that nematodes, viruses, and bacteria are also significant biotic stress factors of trees. In addition, greater attention is being given to the significance of numerous abiotic stress factors.

Forest trees are long-lived, and over the course of their lives may be exposed to several stress factors including those of an abiotic as well as of a biotic nature. At any point in time the health of an individual tree or group of trees will represent the sum and perhaps interacting nature of all of the stress factors to which the tree or trees are exposed. This makes an appreciation of all potential stress factors extremely critical to those wishing to understand tree pathology.

The value of trees growing in the forest has generally been so low that efforts to control tree disease have typically been completely unjustified or of a rather inexpensive and unsophisticated nature. Recent development of new wood products and new markets coupled with the realization of aesthetic, amenity, and other values associated with forests and groups of trees has led to the application of controls previously restricted to agricultural crops and to the development of new controls specifically for tree diseases.

This book attempts to provide a comprehensive consideration of all agents capable of inducing pathological stresses of trees. Representative examples of the damage caused by each agent are discussed. Current hypotheses relating to the mechanism by which the agent causes abnormal tree physiology are reviewed. Control procedures that are currently employed in the treatment of tree disease are outlined along with those agricultural control techniques that may become appropriate for use in the treatment of tree injury and disease.

I would like to express my sincere thanks to Dr. David R. Houston and Mr. Harold G. Eno of the U. S. Forest Service, Forest Insect and Disease Laboratory, Hamden, Connecticut for their cooperation in securing photographs; to Mrs. Jacquelin Lee Steinfield of the Yale School of Forestry for manuscript typing; and to the staff of Academic Press for their efforts in the production of this work. Special gratitude is expressed to Mrs. Nancy W. Canetti of the Yale School of Forestry for her numerous efforts associated with the preparation of this book and to my students for their unbiased perspectives and constant inspiration.

TREE PATHOLOGY

A SHORT INTRODUCTION

1

INTRODUCTION

Plants throughout their lives are subject to various factors which interfere with their normal development. These factors may be conveniently termed stresses. Stress factors are extremely diverse in character and include, for example, viruses, bacteria, fungi, nematodes, arthropods, birds, mammals, as well as fire and other nonliving environmental extremes.

The science of pathology deals with those stress factors which cause injury or disease. Injury refers to abnormal physiology caused by a short-term interaction of a plant and a stress factor. Generally stress factors which cause injuries are nonliving, or abiotic. Disease, on the other hand, is characterized by abnormal physiology occasioned by an extended interaction between a plant and a stress factor. In the case of most diseases the stress factors are living or biotic entities (Table I).

Stress factors which have traditionally been considered nonpathological, for example, insects and other arthropods and fire, are treated by separate disciplines. The rather arbitrary fragmentation of stress factors into pathological, entomological, and other types is unfortunate, for the division may lead to the impression that the factors operate independently of one another. In fact, plants at any point in time are generally subjected to the concurrent influence of several stress factors. The healthfulness of the plant will be determined by the total effect of all stresses. In addition, many stress factors facilitate or enhance the significance of others. Injuries caused by fire, wind, snow, and other agents provide ingress to microbial disease agents. Some stress factors are obligately dependent on others for meaningful persistence. Certain virus and fungus disease agents, for example, have critically important insect vectors.

To those interested in the study of natural plant ecosystems, an understanding of pathological stresses is of primary significance. Disease and in-

TABLE I

PATHOLOGICAL STRESS FACTORS OF PLANTS

Cause injury		Cause disease	
Abiotic	Biotic	Abiotic	Biotic
Moisture extremes	Birds	Air pollutants	Nematodes
Temperature extremes	Mammals	Mineral defi-	Viruses
Wind		ciencies and	Bacteria
Snow		excesses	Fungi
Ice			Plants (higher)
Lightning			
Salt			
Radiation			
Pesticides			

jury agents frequently assume roles of fundamental importance in succession, diversity, adaptation, and evolution.

To those involved in managing ecosystems, especially artificial ones (for example, agricultural crops or certain forests), pathological knowledge assumes an economic as well as ecologic importance. It has been estimated, for example, that losses due to plant diseases equal 1% of the gross national product (10% of annual agricultural production) in the United States (National Academy of Sciences, 1968).

An estimate of the significance of tree diseases has been provided by the U.S. Forest Service's "growth impact" device. The concept of growth impact involves the summation of mortality and growth loss. In terms of growth impact, diseases represent the most important subtractive influence on commercial forests (Fig. 1).

A recent estimate of the annual disease impact on the forest productivity of Oregon and Washington suggested that the annual loss from disease was approximately 3133 million board feet. This amount represents roughly 13% of the total annual growth (U.S. Forest Service, 1967).

The economic significance of tree disease is not confined to commercial forests. In 1968, the City of New York spent in excess of $400,000 to remove dead trees.

This text represents an attempt to provide an introduction to the agents, mechanisms, and control of the pathological stresses of forest trees. It presupposes only an introductory exposure to general biology. Specific examples discussed generally involve forest tree species, mostly from the northeastern portion of the United States, but some are concerned with forest trees from other regions and with citrus and other fruit or nut tree species.

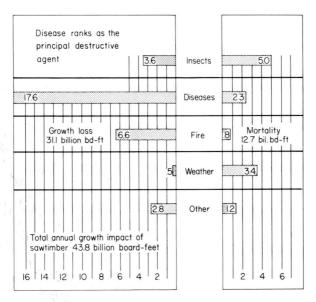

Fig. 1   Growth impact resulting to saw timber from 1952 damage on commercial forest land in the continental United States and coastal Alaska. [From U.S. Forest Service (1958). Reproduced by permission of U.S. Forest Service.]

All injury and disease agents of significance are discussed. In the case of biotic agents, their taxonomy, morphology, physiology, and ecology are reviewed.

Mechanisms of injury and disease are considered by reviewing current evidence and hypotheses.

Control possibilities utilized in mitigating disease influences of plants are discussed. The specific utility of these various procedures to forest tree disease control is considered.

This book brings together information that was previously widely scattered in numerous texts, journal articles, and research reports. In addition to the references cited at the end of each chapter, general reading lists are provided to facilitate access to additional information if desired. The "General References" citations following this chapter comprise the major publications available concerning forest tree pathology.

REFERENCES

National Academy of Sciences. (1968). Plant-disease development and control. *Natl. Acad. Sci. — Natl. Res. Council, Publi.* **1596**.

U.S. Forest Service. (1958). Timber resources for America's future. *Forest Resource Rept. U.S.* No. 14.

U.S. Forest Service. (1967). Annual losses from disease in Pacific Northwest forests. *Res. Bull., Pacific Northwest Forest Range Expt. Sta.* **PNW-20**, 1-19.

GENERAL REFERENCES

Baxter, D. V. (1952). "Pathology in Forest Practice." Wiley, New York.

Baxter, D. V. (1967). "Diseases in Forest Plantations: Thief of Time." Cranbrook Inst. Science, Bloomfield Hills, Michigan.

Boyce, J. S. (1961). "Forest Pathology." McGraw-Hill, New York.

Browne, F. G. (1968). "Pests and Diseases of Forest Plantation Trees; An Annotated List of the Principal Species Occurring in the British Commonwealth." Oxford Univ. Press (Clarendon), London and New York.

Edlin, H. L., and Nimmo, M. (1956). "Tree Injuries." Thames & Hudson, New York.

French, D. W., Kelman, A., and Cowling, E. B. (1967). "An Introduction to Forest Pathology," D. W. French, Univ. of Minnesota, St. Paul, Minn.

Gilmour, J. W. (1966). The pathology of forest trees in New Zealand. The fungal, bacterial, and algal pathogens. *Tech. Paper, New Zealand Forest Serv.* No. 48, 1-82.

Hartig, R. (1894). "The Diseases of Trees." Newnes, Ltd., London.

Hepting, G. H. (1966). Diagnosis of disease in American forest and shade trees, U.S. Forest Serv., Washington, D.C.

Hubert, E. E. (1931). "An Outline of Forest Pathology." Wiley, New York.

International Union of Forest Research Organizations. (1964). Diseases of widely planted forest trees. *FAO/IUFRO Symposium on Internationally Dangerous Forest Diseases and Insects, Oxford,* 20-30 July 1964, FAO, Rome.

Kozlowski, T. T. (1969). Tree physiology and forest pests. *J. Forestry* **67**, 118-123.

North American Forestry Commission. (1967). Important forest insects and diseases of mutual concern to Canada, the United States and Mexico, Dept. Forestry and Rural Develop., Canada, Publi. No. 1180.

Parker, J. (1965). Physiological diseases of trees and shrubs. *Advan. Fron. Plant Sci.* **12**, 97-248.

Peace, T. R. (1962). "Pathology of Trees and Shrubs." Oxford Univ. Press, London and New York.

Pirone, P. P. (1959). "Tree Maintenance." Oxford Univ. Press, London and New York.

Pirone, P. P., Dodge, B. O., and Rickett, H. W. (1960). "Diseases and Pests of Ornamental Plants." Ronald Press, New York.

Rankin, W. H. (1918). "Manual of Tree Diseases." Macmillan, New York.

Spaulding, P. (1958). Diseases of foreign forest trees growing in the United States. *U.S. Dept. Agr., Agr. Handbook* **139**, 1-118.

Spaulding, P. (1961). Foreign diseases of forest trees of the world. *U.S. Dept. Agr., Agr. Handbook* **197**, 1-361.

U.S. Forest Service. (1962). Tree diseases of eastern forests and farm woodlands. *U.S. Dept. Agr., Agr. Inform. Bull.* **254**, 1-48.

PART I

Abiotic Stress Agents

2

MOISTURE EXTREMES

I. INSUFFICIENT WATER — DROUGHT

Adequate supply of water is of critical importance for tree development. In addition to being the primary component of green tissues, frequently 90 — 95% of the fresh weight, water renders mechanical strength via cell turgor to unlignified tissue, acts in metabolic reactions both as a raw material and as a conditioner of various reactants, and assumes a fundamental role in the distribution of dissolved materials in the transpiration stream (Vaadia et al., 1961).

A. Definition

In Britain an "absolute drought" is defined as a period of 14 or more consecutive days without rain. The U.S. Weather Bureau defines "drought" as a period of 21 days or longer when the rainfall is but 30% of the average for the time and place (Parker, 1965). With respect to plant damage, Meyer et al. (1960) have suggested that a drought exists when the soil contains little or no water that is available to plants. It must be remembered, however, that within any region, considerable site-to-site variation will exist with respect to soil moisture availability, due to differences in slope, aspect, ground water, and plant cover (Parker, 1965).

B. Occurrence

Throughout U.S. history, particular years or series of years have occurred when rainfall amounts were considerably less than normal over relatively large areas. Some of the most serious droughts occurred in 1749, 1762, 1860, 1925, the 1930's, and 1957 (Parker, 1965). Pool (1939) presents a vivid description of the vegetative influence of the dry years during the early 1930's in Nebraska. The summers from 1962 through 1966 were characterized by subnormal rainfall in large areas of the U.S., particularly in the New England and Midatlantic states. This drought is presumed to have induced the mortality of extensive areas of spruce-fir forest in northern New England and of scarlet oak in scattered locations in New York (Karnig and Lyford, 1968).

C. Symptoms

1. Wilting. Loss of turgor is the most obvious symptom of water deficiency. The visible collapse, droop, or fold of leaves is frequently the first indication that a tree is under moisture stress (Table II). It must be remembered, however, that if drought conditions persist, dehydration will spread through the tree. Any *living* cell in a plant may wilt (Meyer *et al.*, 1960). Some species wilt considerably more readily than others. Black cherry and dogwood are representatives which frequently display wilting symptoms (Parker, 1965). Wilting in conifers may be less readily detected than in angiosperms.

TABLE II

THE PHYSIOLOGICAL STATES OF WILTING[a,b]

Type of wilting	Frequency	Degree of turgor loss	Visible effects	Duration
Incipient	Probably daily around mid-day, especially in summer	Slight and short-lived	None	Short. Recovery takes place when the transpiration rate falls slightly
Transient	Often, mainly on hot, dry, or windy days	More marked	Obvious drooping of leaves and perhaps of herbaceous stems	Short. Recovery takes place when transpiration is reduced, as at night
Permanent	Occasionally, chiefly during prolonged dry periods	Very severe	Marked drooping of leaves and often of herbaceous stems	Persists until soil moisture is replenished. So little water is available that deficits cannot be restored merely by reducing transpiration
Irreversible	Only in very prolonged dry periods	Complete, and permanent	Very severe drooping of softer parts, followed by withering	Permanent. Tissues have become so desiccated that virtually no water is absorbed even if supplied. Death follows

[a]From Knight (1965). Reproduced by permission of Dover Publications, Inc.
[b]Permanent and irreversible wilting might be considered "pathological" wilting.

2. Leaf discoloration and distortion. Leaves of broad-leaved trees usually become brown on the outer margin. This "marginal scorch" tends to progress inward toward the midleaf region. Frequently, leaves will curl upward. Premature autumn coloration may be expressed. Leaves of black cherry, yellow poplar, and hickory commonly turn yellow before wilting or curling. Coniferous species, on the other hand, often merely turn brown under moisture stress. An early summer drought may cause the needles to be short and to develop yellow tips. These tips later become brown as the yellow area progresses down the needle.

3. Stem cankers and cracks. Drought may be capable of causing cankers on oak stems (True and Tryon, 1956). Cambial damage due to moisture stress is frequently manifest in drought rings which contain cells of abnormal morphology (Peace, 1962). Drought cracks are frequent on numerous coniferous species. These fissures, which are typically simple splits in the trunk from bark to center, may be several feet in length. Unlike frost cracks (Chapter 3, Fig. 5), they are generally wider in the middle portion than at the top or bottom (Parker, 1965).

4. Dieback. Progressive killing of the upper portion of the crown may result when insufficient soil moisture occurs. Peace (1962) cites reference to evidence which has been presented indicating involvement of low-rainfall periods in the bark disease of European beech.

D. Mechanism of Drought Injury

The effects of water deficits on the various physiological processes of plants are diverse and have been ably reviewed by Kozlowski (1964). The mechanisms by which these abnormal physiological responses are brought about are not fully appreciated.

Henckel (1964) has outlined the reaction of plants to the drought influence. This influence is most commonly a complex of dehydration and overheating. Dehydration and overheating alter normal metabolism and submicroscopic protoplasmic structure. Severe overheating causes hydrolysis (splitting) of proteins into constituent peptides and amino acids. Ammonia, in toxic amounts, may be released during this process. Nonproteinaceous materials, for example, polysaccharides, may also be hydrolyzed. In general, during overheating and dehydration, hydrolytic reactions tend to dominate over synthetic reactions. Xerophytes (dry habitat plants) may maintain their synthetic reactions at a higher rate than mesophytes or hydrophytes (wet habitat plants).

In addition to hydrolysis, other reactions to moisture stress are thought relatively common. Dehydration increases the protoplasmic viscosity and also interferes with the process of phosphorylation. This latter phenomenon would critically reduce the plants' capacity to accumulate and transform energy. Iljin (1957) has stressed the importance of mechanical injury to protoplasm when cells rapidly lose water. Vacuoles condition the contraction and expansion of the protoplast. Large cells, with correspondingly large vacuole and cytoplasmic membranes, may be particularly liable to physical destruction as the result of rapid hydration changes. Xerophytic species typically have smaller cells than those of more moist habitats. Lichens, for example, may have a cell volume of only 50–300 μ^3. Trees, on the other hand, may have cell volumes of 2–3 million μ^3.

E. Drought Resistance

Large differences exist with respect to the capacity of individual species to withstand moisture stress (Table III).

Mechanisms which account for the differential species reaction to drought are not completely understood. Hypotheses have been reviewed by Kozlowski (1964) and Parker (1965, 1968b). The significance of various characteristics of leaves, stems, and roots in moisture retention has been ably reviewed by Parker (1968b).

In the case of leaves, regulation of stomatal opening probably plays a critical role in drought resistance. Complete winter closure of stomata in *Rhododendron, Kalmia,* and *Pinus* leaves has been demonstrated (Parker, 1968b). Other leaf characteristics which may have significance in water retention include hairs, cutin, and waxes. Premature leaf abscission may enhance drought resistance. Parker (1968b) suggests that this phenomenon is common in deciduous trees in the eastern United States. In some species this process may result in reduced growth or dieback during the following season. Parker (1965) has presented evidence that indicates certain species have the capacity to avoid irreversible physical or metabolic damage during dehydration. Excised leaves of *Juniperus virginiana,* for example, when dehydrated over 2 *M* sucrose, rehydrated more rapidly and completely than leaves of *Pinus strobus* or *Picea abies* similarly treated.

TABLE III

RELATIVE DROUGHT RESISTANCE OF SELECTED SPECIES[a]

Resistant	Intermediate	Sensitive
Ulmus parvifolia	Pinus resinosa	Acer spp.
Fraxinus pennsylvanica	Pinus strobus	Abies grandis
Pinus ponderosa		
Juniperus virginiana		

[a]From Parker (1956). Reproduced by permission of the New York Botanical Garden.

Water in large branches and stems may be available in certain species for use under moisture stress conditions. Trunk water is known to decline during a drought more so than could be accounted for by bark transpiration alone (Parker, 1956). The twig cortex of *Pinus ponderosa* is able to give up its moisture to the leaves more readily than any other pine species. The significance of this and related phenomena, however, in supplying water during droughts remains undetermined.

The ability to absorb moisture from the soil may vary from species to species, depending on the character and size of the root system. The ability of *Quercus* and *Pseudotsuga menziesii* seedlings to establish deep roots has been suggested to contribute to their ability to become successfully established (Parker, 1968b). Presumably, fibrous root systems would be more efficient accumulators of soil moisture than nonfibrous systems as they would permeate a much larger soil mass. Features other than those related to size and morphology may also be important. In a recent study, Parker (1968a) presented evidence that *Fraxinus americana* and *Quercus rubra* roots lost less water through their bark than did *Acer saccharum* roots.

F. Pathology and Drought

The pathological significance of water stress may be manifest in numerous ways. In temperate regions, successive growing seasons of below normal rainfall frequently result in a gradual decline in vigor of many tree species. If this water deficiency is associated with other stresses, for example, insect defoliation, the resulting consequences may be disasterous.

In areas with winter temperatures below freezing for extended periods, the phenomenon of "winter killing" is important in many coniferous and broad-leaved evergreen species. In this case, leaf necrosis results when transpiration, which continues at a reduced rate through the winter, exceeds the supply of liquid water in the plant. Water cannot be replenished from the soil via the stem because moisture in soil and stem are frozen. Hygen (1965), however, has recently presented some evidence which suggests that limited movement may be possible even under these frozen conditions.

Drought conditions may exert their greatest pathological significance by acting to predispose trees to damage by other destructive agents. Towers and Stambaugh (1968) have observed that the rate of penetration of *Fomes annosus* in roots of 12-year-old *Pinus taeda* 6 months after direct innoculation was enhanced by induced drought conditions.

G. Management Practices

Little can be done to avoid or mitigate drought damage in established forests. It may be wise during drought periods to avoid sudden thinnings, particularly with sensitive species. The increased exposure and consequent transpiration may be deleterious. When developing a new forest stand on dry sites, however, it would be most wise to use species which are known to possess a certain degree of drought resistance. It would further be important to avoid planting on shallow soils. In areas of frequent winter winds it might be desirable to consider the establishment of some form of shelterbelt around the new plantation.

In nursery situations, where more intensive management is possible, the danger of drought injury may be lessened by irrigation, shelter, mulching, or early spring or fall planting. In studying the effects of planting site, shade, and local seed source on emergence and survial of *Pinus strobus* seedlings, Graber (1968) found that heavy shade favorably modified the environment on a dry site and greatly increased emergence.

In other areas of high-value plants, for example ornamental plantings, wax and plastic-based emulsions have been sprayed on plants to reduce transpiration. This influence was presumed due to the fact that these materials were less permeable to water vapor than to carbon dioxide or oxygen. Recent evidence (Gale and Poljakoff-Mayber, 1967), however, suggests that these sprays may act to actually increase photosynthesis or in other indirect ways lower the transpiration/photosynthetic ratio.

II. EXCESS WATER – FLOODING

The primary causes for excessive soil moisture are site alterations, which raise the water table or cause more water to drain into an area, and flooding. The former are common near and about construction projects, for example, dams and new highways. The latter are periodically common throughout the country and especially important in the southeast because the land is relatively flat and the rainfall high. Interest in flooding phenomena has increased over the years and Stransky and Daniel (1964) list over 80 references which relate this influence to tree development.

A. Symptoms

In most species, including both conifers and angiosperms, the most characteristic initial symptom is some degree of chlorosis (chlorophyll decomposition). This is generally followed by leaf browning and ultimately abscission.

B. Mechanism of Excess Water Damage

Two broad theories have been advanced to account for the detrimental influence of excessive soil moisture. The older theory proposes the accumulation of toxic materials in flooded soils. These toxins may be humic acids, soluble salts, or alkalies. The proliferation of anaerobic microorganisms may result in fermentations which produce deleterious volatile organic acids.

Acids of this nature can cause serious damage to feeding roots. Certain flooded soils have been shown to produce methane, hydrogen sulfide, and various methyl compounds.

A more recent hypothesis for flooding injury relates to soil aeration. Aeration is the process by which gases produced or consumed under the soil surface are exchanged for gases in the aerial atmosphere (Letey, 1965). The normal condition of the soil atmosphere is given in Table IV.

Under conditions of poor aeration, oxygen cannot reach the roots and carbon dioxide cannot diffuse away. As a result, oxygen levels decline and carbon dioxide levels increase. It is not clear which of these two phenomena is responsible for root damage. Indeed, it may be both. It has been shown, however, that reduced oxygen has a more retarding influence on rate of water absorption by numerous plants than the presence of carbon dioxide in concentrations up to approximately 20% (Meyer et al., 1960).

C. Resistance to Flood Damage

It is generally assumed that species which naturally persist in poorly drained soils will be more resistant to injury caused by flooding. This generalization is supported by the examination by Hall and Smith (1955) of the tolerance of 39 Kentucky tree species to flooding during the growing season (Fig. 2).

Parker (1950), however, examined the flood tolerance of 16-inch seedlings of several dry- and moist-site southern species and found that species which grew in soils flooded for long periods were injured as quickly as species from drier sites.

Observations in an Oregon nursery following flooding conditions revealed that two-year-old seedlings of dormant *Pinus ponderosa* withstood 3 months burial under silt (1-8 in) without serious damage. Dormant two-year-old *Pseudotsuga menziesii*, however, began to lose vigor after 8 weeks in silt (Hermann and Lavender, 1967). Williston (1962) found that during the growing season *Pinus taeda* seedlings survived 12 days submergence to the root collar or complete submergence. After 21 days, however, only 50% survived and after 1 month, almost all were killed.

TABLE IV

PERCENTAGE BY VOLUME OF SOIL AND ATMOSPHERIC AIR

	O_2 (%)	CO_2 (%)	N_2 (%)
Soil	20	0.25	79
Atmosphere	20	0.02	79

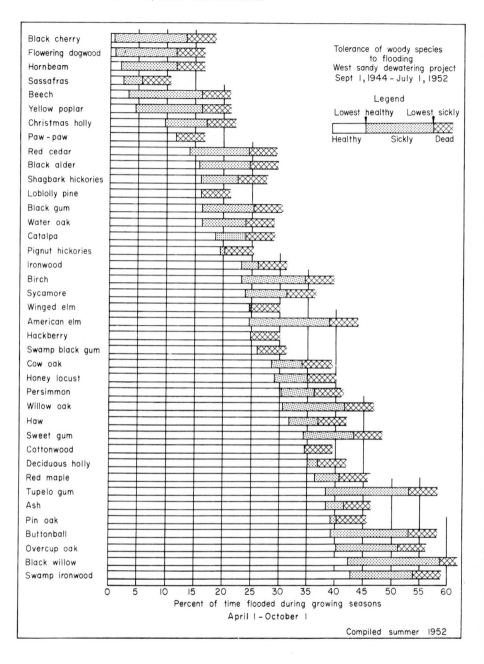

Fig. 2. Tolerance of Kentucky woody species to flooding during the growing season. [From Hall and Smith (1955). Reproduced by permission of Society of American Foresters.]

Several generalizations might be made concerning susceptibility to excess water damage. Almost all species will be injured less severely if they are subjected to short periodic flood periods rather than prolonged submergence. Considerably less damage will accrue from floods in the dormant season than during the growing season. Any tree with water over the root crown for 10–12 months will usually die regardless of the species.

D. Management Practices

In areas where floods are sufficiently frequent to be a potential threat to tree welfare, careful consideration should be given to species selection. If possible provisions should be made to permit flood water to be drained off rather than let it evaporate.

In areas of disturbance due to construction, attention should be paid the influence that grade alterations will have on drainage patterns and ultimately surrounding tree vigor. The numerous stands of dead trees which line our new roadways are mute testimony to the degree to which the influence has been ignored (Fig. 3).

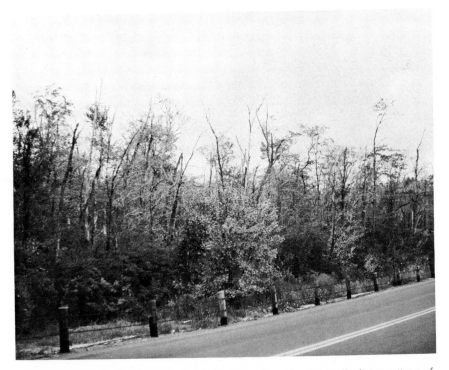

Fig. 3.   Declining stand of red maple caused by excessive soil moisture. Drainage patterns of this area were drastically altered by improvements made on the road in the foreground.

REFERENCES

Gale, J., and Poljakoff-Mayber, A. (1967). Plastic films on plants as anti-transpirants. *Science* **156**, 650-652.

Graber, R. E. (1968). Planting site, shade and local seed source: Their effects on the emergence and survival of eastern white pine seedlings. *Res. Paper, Northeast. Forest Expt. Sta.* **NE-94**, 1-12.

Hall, T. F., and Smith, G. E. (1955). Effects of flooding on woody plants, West Sandy Dewatering Project, Kentucky Reservoir. *J. Forestry* **53**, 281-285.

Henckel, D. A. (1964). Physiology of plants under drought. *Ann. Rev. Plant Physiol.* **15**, 363-386.

Hermann, R. K., and Lavender, D. P. (1967). Tolerance of coniferous seedlings to silting. *J. Forestry* **65**, 824-825.

Hygen, G. (1965). Water stress in conifers during winter. *In* "Water Stress in Plants" (B. Slavik, ed.), pp. 89-95. Junk Publ., The Hague.

Iljin, W. S. (1957). Drought resistance in plants and physiological processes. *Ann. Rev. Plant Physiol.* **8**, 257-274.

Karnig, J. J., and Lyford, W. H. (1968). Oak mortality and drought in the Hudson Highlands. *Black Rock Forest Papers* **29**, 1-13.

Knight, R. O. (1965). "The Plant in Relation to Water." Dover, New York.

Kozlowski, T. T. (1964). "Water Metabolism in Plants." Harper, New York.

Letey, J. (1965). Measuring aeration. *Proc. Am. Soc. Agr. Eng.* pp. 6-10.

Meyer, B. S., Anderson, O. B., and Böhning, R. H. (1960). "Introduction to Plant Physiology." Van Nostrand, Princeton, New Jersey.

Parker, J. (1950). The effects of flooding on the transpiration and survival of some southeastern forest tree species. *Plant Physiol.* **25**, 453-460.

Parker, J. (1956). Drought resistance in woody plants. *Botan. Rev.* **22**, 241-289.

Parker, J. (1965). Physiological diseases of trees and shrubs. *Advan. Fron. Plant Sci.* **12**, 97-248.

Parker, J. (1968a). Drought resistance of roots of white ash, sugar maple and red oak. *Res. Paper, Northeast. Forest Extp. Sta.* **NE-95**, 1-9.

Parker, J. (1968b). Drought-resistance mechanisms. *In* "Water Deficits and Plant Growth" (T. T. Kozlowski, ed.), Vol. 1, pp. 195-234. Academic Press, New York.

Peace, T. R. (1962). "Pathology of Trees and Shrubs." Oxford Univ. Press, London and New York.

Pool, R. J. (1939). Some reactions of the vegetation in the towns and cities of Nebraska to the Great Drought. *Bull. Torrey Botan. Club* **66**, 457-464.

Stransky, J. J., and Daniel, H. E. (1964). References on effects of flooding on forest trees. *Res. Note, Southeast. Forest Expt. Sta.* **12**, 1-5.

Towers, B., and Stambaugh, W. J. (1968). The influence of induced soil moisture stress upon *Fomes annosus* root rot of loblolly pine. *Phytopathology* **58**, 269-272.

True, R. P., and Tryon, E. H. (1956). Oak stem cankers initiated in the drought year 1953. *Phytopathology* **46**, 617-622.

Vaadia, Y., Raney, F. C., and Hagan, R. M. (1961). Plant water deficits and physiological processes. *Ann. Rev. Plant Physiol.* **12**, 265-292.

Williston, H. L. (1962). Loblolly seedlings survive twelve days' submergence. *J. Forestry* **60**, 412.

GENERAL REFERENCES

Ahlgren, C. E., and Hanson, R. L. (1967). Some effects of temporary flooding on coniferous trees. *J. Forestry* **55**, 647-650.

Billings, W. D. (1952). The environmental complex in relation to plant growth and distribution. *Quart. Rev. Biol.* **27**, 251-265.

Daubenmire, R. F. (1943). Soil temperature versus drought as a factor determining lower altitudinal limits of trees in the Rocky Mountains. *Botan. Gaz.* **105**, 1-13.

Day, W. R. (1954). Drought crack of conifers. *Gt. Brit. Forestry Comm., Forest Record* **26**, 1-40.

Filer, T. H., Jr., and Broadfoot, W. M. (1968). Sweetgum mycorrhizae and soil microflora survive in shallow-water impoundment. *Phytopathology* **58**, 1050. (abstr.).

Fraser, D. A. (1962). Tree growth in relation to soil moisture. *In* "Tree Growth" (T. T. Kozlowski, ed.), pp. 183-204. Ronald Press, New York.

Glinka, Z., and Reinhold, L. (1962). Rapid changes in permeability of cell membranes to water brought about by carbon dioxide and oxygen. *Plant Physiol.* **37**, 481-486.

Holmes, F. W. (1968). Injury to sugar maple from deep planting. *Phytopathology* **58**, 400 (abstr.).

Kozlowski, T. T., ed. (1968a). "Water Deficits and Plant Growth," Vol. 1. Academic Press, New York.

Kozlowski, T. T., ed. (1968b). "Water Deficits and Plant Growth," Vol. 2. Academic Press, New York.

Kramer, P. J. (1951). Causes of injury to plants resulting from flooding of the soil. *Plant Physiol.* **26**, 722-736.

Kramer, P. J., and Kozlowski, T. T. (1960). "Physiology of Trees." McGraw-Hill, New York.

Levitt, J. (1956). "The Hardiness of Plants." Academic Press, New York.

Levitt, J. (1961). Frost, drought and heat resistance. *Ann. Rev. Plant Physiol.* **2**, 245-268.

Rothacher, J. S., and Glazebrook, T. B. (1968). Flood damage in the national forests of Region 6. *Pacific Northwest Forest Range Expt. Sta.* pp. 1-20.

Slavik, B., ed. (1965). "Water Stress in Plants." Junk Publ., The Hague.

Walker, L. C., Green, L. R., and Daniels, J. M. (1961). Flooding and drainage effects on slash pine and loblolly pine seedlings. *Forest Sci.* **7**, 2-15.

Zahner, R. (1968). Water deficits and growth of trees. *In* "Water Deficits and Plant Growth" (T. T. Kozlowski, ed.), Vol. 2, pp. 191-254. Academic Press, New York.

3

TEMPERATURE EXTREMES

I. HIGH TEMPERATURE—HEAT INJURY

Plant species exhibit their most successful growth at some average, optimum range of temperatures. Species also have maxima and minima temperature ranges for growth which, if exceeded, will result in abnormal physiological responses.

The upper limit for all plant growth is apparently in the 80-90°C (176°-194°F) range where blue-green algae grow in hot springs. In the case of higher plants, however, approximately 58°C (136°F) is assumed to be the upper limit for hydrated tissue. Dry seeds may survive temperatures approaching 120°C (260°F) (Levitt, 1956). Levitt has compiled a listing of lethal high temperatures for several plant species. (Table V.)

High temperatures are more readily attained in the natural environment than is commonly realized. During the summer, for example, the south side of a pine tree may reach 55°C (130°F), viburnum leaves 44°C (110°F), and fleshy fruit 35-46°C (95-115°F) (Levitt, 1956). Soil surfaces exposed to direct insolation may exhibit temperatures in the 55-75°C (130-168°F) range and result in heat injury, especially to seedlings. Maguire (1955) presents a thorough discussion of soil surface temperatures.

A. Symptoms

1. Seedling collapse or girdling.   Seedling damage by high temperatures is very common during their first or second year. Small seedlings typically collapse while larger individuals become girdled but remain standing (Fig. 4). The latter gradually decline as flow of food materials from leaves is restricted (Peace, 1962). Occasionally, only lesions will be observed on seedlings exposed to high temperatures.

Smith and Silen (1963) have presented the progression of anatomical

TABLE V

HEAT KILLING TEMPERATURE FOR DIFFERENT PLANTS AND PLANT PARTS[a]

Plant	Heat killing temperature (°C)	Exposure time
(a) Lower plants		
Cryptogams	42–47.5	15–30 min
Ulothrix	24	—
Mastigocladus	52	—
Blue-green algae	70–75	A few hours
Thermoidium sulfureum	53	—
Thermophilic fungi	55–62	—
Hydrurus foetidus	16–20	A few hours
Sea algae	27–42	12 hr
Ceramium tenuissimum	38	8.5 min
(b) Higher plants		
(1) Herbaceous plants		
Zea mays	49–51	10 min
Citrus aurantium	50.5	15–30 min
Opuntia	>65	—
Shoots of Iris	55	—
Sempervivum arachnoideum	57–61	—
Succulents	53–54	10 hr
Potato leaves	42.5	1 hr
(2) Trees		
Pine and spruce seedlings	54–55	5 min
Cortical cells of trees	57–59	30 min

[a]From Levitt (1956). Reproduced by permission of Academic Press, Inc.

events which result in the expression of the collapse–girdle syndrome in Douglas fir. Initially, water is lost to the intercellular spaces, and cells lose their turgor. This causes a progressive collapse of epidermal and parenchymal cells of the cortex and pericycle. Collapse of phloem and xylem cells follows, and ultimately, collapse of the cambium and inner phloem cells progresses upward from the constriction.

   2. Sun scorch.   This symptom is frequently found on the south and southwest sides of relatively thin-barked trees which have suddenly been exposed to direct insolation. Injury of this nature has been documented in numerous gymnosperm and angiosperm species (Peace, 1962). Kessler and

Ohman (1967) have discussed the occurrence of a canker which develops on the south or southwest stem faces of understocked second-growth northern hardwoods. These cankers apparently develop because a fungus–insect complex prevents closure of fissures resulting from sunscald following removal of protective overstories. Sunscald injury is commonly found in roadside and ornamental plantings which are exposed to excessive heat reflected from nearby roadways or buildings. Injury of this sort is very common on beech, sycamore, and maple.

    3. Sunburn.   This symptom is common in the tropics and is characterized by leaf abscission and discoloration of twig tips.

    4. Leaf burning.   This symptom is characterized by the development of reddened or browned patches on broad-leaved species. "Brennflecken" or brown spots occur in the greenhouse when glass imperfections concentrate the rays of the sun on leaf parts (Parker, 1965). Necrosis of the distal portions of coniferous needles are commonly caused by high temperatures.

B. Mechanisms of Heat Injury

    A precise explanation of the mechanism causing heat injury is not available. Overheating, like dehydration, alters the colloidal–chemical properties of protoplasm and induces metabolic shifts which may contribute to abnormal physiology.

    High temperatures may cause denaturation of proteins. The S-S and H-H bonds are particularly susceptible to breakage at high temperatures. This is

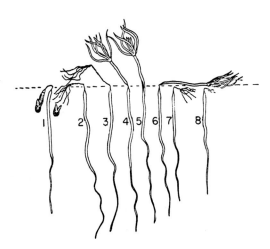

Fig. 4.   Heat killing of pine seedlings at soil level due to overheating of soil surface. Note collapse (6), girdling (4) and lesion (5) symptoms. [From Levitt (1956). Reproduced by permission of Academic Press, Inc.]

especially true when excess water exists in the cell, as free water weakens these bonds (Parker, 1965).

Protein decomposition may lead to the release of ammonia in toxic amounts. In the case of some heat-resistant plants, high temperatures have been shown to induce the accumulation of organic acids. These acids react with ammonia, forming various salts and amides, and thereby mitigate its toxic influence. Cactus metabolism, for example, characteristically results in the accumulation of organic acids (Henckel, 1964).

The destruction of protoplasmic microstructure may result in disruption of protein-lipoid complexes and plastid integrity.

An excess of respiration over photosynthesis may be occasioned at high temperatures. At elevated temperatures, the respiratory curve increases sharply while photosynthesis may decline at about 35°C (Henckel, 1964).

C. Management Practices

In the nursery, care should be taken to avoid heat injury to young coniferous seedlings. Beds should be kept dense and sandy-dark soils avoided. Shading may be required in some instances.

In older stands, consideration should be given to the potential damage which may result from sunscald following a heavy thinning or selective cutting.

D. Fire

A discussion of high temperature as a stress factor would be incomplete without mentioning the extremely important effect that fires have on trees. This subject is, of course, a discipline unto itself. The destruction of trees by excessively "hot" fires is self-evident. Pathologically, however, injuries caused by fires of sublethal temperature are also extremely important. These injuries act to reduce the overall vigor of trees and may predispose them to additional injury by insects or infection by disease agents. Basal wounds of fire origin are particularly important entrance courts for fungi capable of heartwood decay. A general discussion of fire effects is available in K. P. Davis (1959) and a review of the recent literature in Cushwa (1968).

II. LOW TEMPERATURE—COLD INJURY

Cold is an imprecise concept and not easily defined. In the United States, the term "frost" has a more specific meaning and is generally defined as occurring when the temperature is 0°C or below.

A. Definition

Frosts can be conveniently divided into two types: advective and radiation. Advective frosts result when the horizontal movement of a cold air mass brings freezing temperatures into an area. This area may be large and encompass thousands of square miles. In the case of an advective frost the vertical temperature-lapse rate is usually normal, that is temperature decreases with increasing altitude. The plant damage resulting from this type of freeze is generally quite uniform within regions of similar elevation.

A radiation frost, on the other hand, results from a temperature inversion at the surface of the earth. This results when the earth loses heat through long-wave radiation and its surface becomes colder than the adjacent air. The depth of the inversion may vary from a few inches to several hundred feet. Since cooler air has a greater density than warmer air, the inversion is stable. If the topography permits, this cooler air will be "drained" by gravity into depressions. As a result, damage due to radiation frosts is particularly common in local depressions and on lower slopes. Table VI contains a summary of these two frost types.

B. Symptoms

Considerable variation is seen in symptom expression depending on the season in which the tree is exposed to freezing temperatures.

TABLE VI

SUMMARY OF FROST TYPES AND DAMAGE TO FORESTS[a]

Characteristic	Advective frost	Radiation frost
Cause	Horizontal movement of cold air mass into a warmer area	Cooling of ground and adjacent air through loss of heat from longwave terrestrial radiation.
Condition of atmosphere	Windy, overcast, often with precipitation, including snow	Clear with still air, cloudless sky
Area involved	Large, may be hundreds of mi² and may be confined to mountain tops	Small, often only valley bottoms and lower slopes
Severity	Usually causes heavy damage if buds have broken	Variable. Damage may be very light to heavy
Elevation and damage	Damage may become heavier with increase in elevation	Damage usually greater on lower slopes and valleys
Uniformity	Degree of damage uniform within same elevation belt	Degree of damage spotty from area to area, and even within same locality
Frequency	Less common	More common
Time of occurrence	Early in spring, late in fall	First in fall, last in spring, and throughout frost danger period

[a]From Tryon and True (1964). Reproduced by permission of West Virginia Agricultural Experiment Station.

1. Spring. This season may present the greatest cold-injury threat to woody plants. Radiation frosts represent the primary danger during this period. If the frost occurs before bud break, the damage is frequently confined to the buds themselves, as they tend to be in a metabolically more advanced state than the shoots. Bud destruction will commonly be followed by the development of dormant or adventitious buds causing the trees to become bushy or develop witches'-broom fasciculations. Damage following bud break is also quite common and is caused by the lack of cold resistance characteristic of young growth. In this case, leaves and soft succulent shoots are killed and frequently turn black. Leaves killed in this manner usually do not fall as sudden death prevents abscission layer formation. Cambial damage may also occur in the spring but is usually less obvious. Injury may range from slight, in which case a frost ring is formed, to severe, which results in necrosis involving canker or dieback development, depending on the amount of tissue killed. Frost rings are formed when exposure to low temperatures results in the deposition of large, thin-walled, irregularly shaped cells in the growth ring.

Nichols (1968) concluded that the primary factor responsible for crown dieback and mortality in Pennsylvania members of the red oak group was defoliation caused by insects and spring frosts.

2. Summer. Frost damage during summer months, while unlikely, has been documented in northern areas where below-freezing temperatures occasionally occur (this would include some of the northern Midwestern and Rocky Mountain states and large areas of Canada). In this instance, injury may be expressed by shriveling and browning of leaves or, more subtly, in cambial damage.

3. Winter. Damage during the winter months, which is frequently mistaken for spring injury, may be expressed in several ways. Leaf discoloration (yellow, red, brown) is commonly noted in coniferous species. Trunk cracks are a common symptom in hardwoods damaged by low winter temperatures (Fig. 5). While the exact mechanism is unknown, the cracks are presumed due to unequal expansion and contraction of the wood during rapid freezing and subsequent thawing. During warming, the sapwood may expand more rapidly than the heartwood. It has also been found that water-saturated wood expands on freezing, but as temperature continues to lower, the wood shrinks (Parker, 1965). Differential expansion and/or shrinkage probably results in stresses causing trunk cracks. These cracks are normally radial and occur on the south, southeast, or southwest sides. Larger cracks open to the stem surface but smaller ones may be entirely internal. In the case of the former, increasing temperatures tend to close the cracks. Frequently, cracks will be reopened in subsequent winters. These fissures, until healed over with callus, may represent important infection courts for wood-decay fungi.

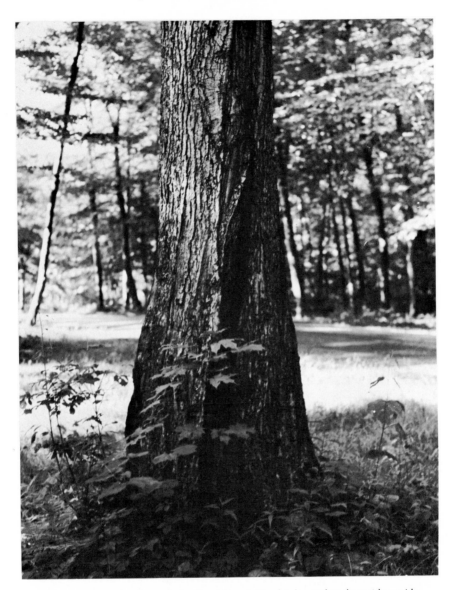

Fig. 5.   Frost crack on lower bole of a white oak. Crack is located on the southern side.

Frost lift or heave is an important winter phenomenon in nurseries. In this case the formation of ice in the nursery soil during periods of slow freezing will physically displace small seedlings. Schramm (1958) discusses this process in some detail.

4. Autumn.   Damage during this season is primarily confined to succulent shoots or tips of these shoots which have continued to be internally active beyond the point of normal growth cessation. Unusually severe autumn frosts may produce dieback of older, hardened shoots, but this is uncommon.

C. Mechanism of Low Temperature Damage

The damage to living cells is not from cold per se, but from the formation of ice. Ice may form inside the cells (intracellular) or outside the cells (extracellular). Intracellular freezing is the most rapid and most damaging of the two. It is nearly always fatal to the cell as formation of ice crystals inside the cell vacuole results in gross physical membrane destruction. Extracellular freezing is slower and more subtle in its effect. In this instance, ice formed on the external surface of the cell wall continuously grows, withdrawing water from the cell interior as the temperature declines. Cells frozen in this manner undergo a remarkable dehydration and may be injured in two ways; physical collapse and protein denaturation.

D. Resistance to Frost Injury.

Native woody plants in relatively cold regions are capable of surviving low temperatures without injury if they are properly conditioned. Some, for example eastern white pine, can be cooled to extremely low temperatures (−321°F) without injury (Parker, 1965.) The conditioning which permits survival at low temperatures is termed the hardening process.

Soon after twig growth ceases, from late August to early September, considerable changes take place in the cells of twigs, especially in deciduous trees. There is a decrease of both water content and activity in the cambium cells and an increase in both starch granules and osmotic concentration as the starch is converted to sugar. This increase in viscosity of vacuolor material is particularly noticeable in the parenchyma cells of bark and phloem. Some vacuoles become so thick as to actually gelate (common in some of the most hardy conifers). Most vacuoles, however, develop viscous, but liquid, contents (Sakai, 1966).

The actual mechanisms which permit these hardened cells to resist freezing damage are unclear but may involve one or more of the following (Parker, 1965): (1) Increase in osmotic concentration due to sugars and other materials, for example polyhydric alcohols, which may lower the freezing point in the vacuole and inhibit intracellular freezing. (2) Protein denaturation may be avoided as the sugars act to bind much of the free water and inhibit dehydration and ice formation. (3) Alteration of phospholipid content may increase membrane flexibility and avoid physical disruption. (4) Soluble protein increase may result, causing the binding of free water and thereby inhibiting ice formation. Protein changes may also be associated with increased permeability and/or cell elasticity.

E. Variation in Susceptibility to Damage among Species

It is difficult to generalize concerning variation in resistance to frost damage. Considerable variation exists within species and resistance appears to vary with season and particular plant part in question. Tryon and True (1964) have, however, rated several hardwood species with respect to their susceptibility to damage by late spring frosts. Their results appear in Table VII.

Ecologically, the temperature factor has fundamental significance in the distribution of plant communities. The limitations imposed on species distribution, however, do not result primarily from the direct injury or damage caused by low temperatures but rather may be caused by insufficient heat during the growing season for normal physiological processes (Daubenmire, 1959).

F. Management Practices

In an effort to avoid damage by autumn frosts, all activities which might encourage sustained or renewed fall growth, for example, late-season irrigation, fertilization, or pruning, should be avoided.

Little can be done silviculturally or otherwise to reduce tree injury due to advective winter frosts. Amelioration of damage caused by radiation frosts, on the other hand, may be realized. These procedures would be justified only in areas where radiation frosts pose a significant threat. If possible, a partial canopy should be left following a harvest. The denser this canopy,

TABLE VII

SUSCEPTIBILITY OF GENERA AND SPECIES OF HARDWOODS TO FOLIAGE DAMAGE BY LATE FROSTS[a]

Highly susceptible	Moderately susceptible	Less susceptible	Least susceptible
American chestnut	Magnolia	Basswood	Birch
Ash	Oak	Maple	Cherry
Beech			Elm
Black locust			Hawthorn
Sassafras			Willow
Sycamore			
Walnut			
Yellow poplar			

[a]From Tryon and True (1964). Reproduced by permission of West Virginia Agricultural Experiment Station.

the better the frost protection. Single tree selection, group selection, or shelterwood systems might be employed to provide a residual canopy. When a choice is possible, species which have the greatest apparent resistance to low-temperature damage should be planted. In extremely cold areas, conifers only should be used, particularly pines. In valleys, or depressions, slopes should be afforested first and harvested last. Trees on the slopes will prevent deep pooling of cold air in the lower regions (Peace, 1962).

In nurseries, where more intensive procedures may be justified, direct air heating or slow moving fans to prevent cold-air pooling may be employed. Any effort to produce better rooted seedlings will reduce frost lift. These might include lower planting density, fertilization, irrigation, early planting, and mulching.

REFERENCES

Cushwa, C. T. (1968). Fire: summary of literature in the United States from the mid-1920's to 1966. *Southeast. Forest Expt. Sta.* 1-117.

Daubenmire, R. F. (1959). "Plants and Environment." Wiley, New York.

Davis, K. P. (1959). "Forest Fire Control and Use," Chapter 2, pp. 31-60. McGraw-Hill, New York.

Henckel, P. A. (1964). Physiology of plants under drought. *Ann. Rev. Plant Physiol.* **15**, 363-386.

Kessler, K. J., Jr., and Ohman, J. H. (1967). Sunscald canker of sugar maple. *Phytopathology* **57**, 817 (abstr.).

Levitt, J. (1956). "The Hardiness of Plants." Academic Press, New York.

Maguire, W. P. (1955). Radiation, surface temperature, and seedling survival. *Forest Sci.* **1**, 277-284.

Nichols, J. O. (1968). Oak mortality in Pennsylvania—a ten-year study. *J. Forestry* **66**, 681-694.

Parker, J. (1965). Physiological diseases of trees and shrubs. *Advan. Fron. Plant Sci.* **12**, 97-248.

Peace, T. R. (1962). "Pathology of Trees and Shrubs." Oxford Univ. Press, London and New York.

Sakai, A. (1966). Studies of frost hardiness in woody plants. II. Effect of temperature on hardening. *Plant Physiol.* **41**, 353-359.

Schramm, W. (1958). The mechanism of frost heaving of tree seedlings. *Proc. Am. Philo. Soc.* **102**, 333-350.

Smith, F. H., and Silen, R. R. (1963). Anatomy of heat-damaged Douglas-fir seedlings. *Forest Sci.* **9**, 15-32.

Tyron, E. H., and True, R. P. (1964). Relative susceptibility of Appalachian hardwood species to spring frosts occurring after bud break. *West Va. Univ., Agr. Expt. Sta., Bull.* **503**, 1-15.

GENERAL REFERENCES

Arnold, C. I. (1958). Frost damage. *Tree Plant. Notes* **31**, 8-9.

Bailey, I. W. (1925). The "Spruce budworm" biosoenose. I. Frost rings as indicators of the chronology of specific biological events. *Botan. Gaz.* **80**, 93-101.

Bates, C. G., and Roeser, J., Jr. (1924). Relative resistance of tree seedlings to excessive heat. *U.S. Dept. Agr., Dept. Bull.* **1263**, 1-16.

Bates, C. G. (1930). The frost hardiness of geographic strains of Norway pine. *J. Forestry* **28**, 327-333.

Beckley, W. S. (1937). Frost damage to forest trees in the Northeast. M. F. Thesis, Yale School of Forestry.

Belyea, H. C., and MacAloney, H. J. (1926). Winter injury to terminal buds of Scotch pine and other conifers. *J. Forestry* **24**, 685-690.

Boyce, J. S. (1961). "Forest Pathology," McGraw-Hill, New York.

Davis, J. R., and English, H. (1969). Factors involved in the development of peach seedling cankers induced by chilling. *Phytopathology* **59**, 305-313.

Day, W. R. (1928). Damage by late frosts on Douglas fir, spruce, and other conifers. *Forestry* **2**, 19.

Day, W. R., and Peach, T. R. (1928). Frost as a cause of disease in trees. *Quart. J. Forestry* **22**, 179.

Day, W. R., and Peach, T. R. (1936). The influence of certain accessory factors on frost injury to forest trees. *Forestry* **10**, 124-132.

Day, W. R., and Peach, T. R. (1937). The influence of certain accessory factors on frost injury to forest trees. *Forestry* **11**, 13-29 and 92-103.

Goodell, B. C. (1939). Soil freezing as affected by vegetation and slope aspect. *J. Forestry* **37**, 626-629.

Haasis, F. W. (1923). Frost heaving of western yellow pine. *Ecology*, 379-390.

Harris, H. S. (1934). Frost ring formation in some winter-killed deciduous trees and shrubs. *Am. J. Botany* **21**, 485-498.

Hepting, G. H., Miller, J. H., and Campbell, W. A. (1951). Winter of 1950-51 damaging to southeastern woody vegetation. *Plant Disease Reptr.* **35**, 502-503.

Hough, A. F. (1945). Frost pocket and other microclimate in forests of the northern Allegheny plateau. *Ecology* **26**, 235-250.

Kienholz, R. (1933). Frost damage to red pine. *J. Forestry* **31**, 392-399.

Korstian, C. F., and Fetheroff, N. J. (1921). Control of stem girdle of spruce transplants caused by excessive heat. *Phytopathology* **11**, 483-560.

Levitt, J. (1941). "Frost Killing and Hardiness of Plants." Burgess, Minneapolis, Minnesota.

Mazur, P. (1969). Freezing injury in plants. *Ann. Rev. Plant Physiol.* **20**, 419-448.

Mesavage, C. (1939). Frost damage to forests in northern New Jersey. *J. Forestry* **37**, 345-346.

Nash, R. W. (1943). Winter killing of hardwoods. *J. Forestry* **41**, 841-842.

Parker, J. (1962). Seasonal changes in cold resistance and free sugars of some hardwood tree barks. *Forest Sci.* **8**, 256-262.

Parker, J. (1963). Cold resistance in woody plants. *Botan. Rev.* **29**, 123-201.

Parris, G. K. (1967). "Needle curl" of loblolly pine. *Plant Disease Reptr.* **51**, 805-806.

Portz, H. L. (1967). Frost heaving of soil and plants. I. Incidence of frost heaving of forage plants and meteorological relationships. *Agron. J.* **59**, 341-344.

Salt, R. W., and Kahn, S. (1967). Ice nucleation and propagation in spruce needles. *Can. J. Botany* **45**, 1335-1346.

Smith, A. V. (1961). "Biological Effects of Freezing and Supercooling." Williams & Wilkins, Baltimore, Maryland.

Stoekeler, J. H. (1965). Spring frost damage in young forest plantings near LaCrosse, Wisconsin. *J. Forestry* **63**, 12-14.

Strain, B. R. (1966). The effect of a late spring frost on the radial growth of variant quaking aspen biotypes. *Forest Sci.* **12**, 334-337.

Troshin, A. S., ed. (1956). "The Cell and Environmental Temperature." Pergamon Press, Oxford.

Tryon, E. H. (1943). Stem girdling of coniferous nursery stock by frost-heaved soil. *J. Forestry* **41**, 768-769.

Tryon, E. H., and True, R. P. (1966). Effect of spring freeze on radial increment of American beech at different elevations. *J. Forestry* **64**, 625-627.

Tryon, E. H., and True, R. P. (1968). Radial increment response of Appalachian hardwood species to a spring freeze. *J. Forestry* **66**, 488-591.

4

OTHER CLIMATIC STRESS AGENTS

In addition to moisture and temperature extremes, aboreal vegetation is also subject to many other climatic stress factors which locally may have pathological and ecological significance. Among the most important of these factors are wind, snow, ice and hail, and lightning.

I. WIND

The influence of wind on tree growth is very complex. Wind itself is an erratic force. The direction and velocity of wind is influenced by the configuration of topography and vegetation, proximity to water masses, and regional wind patterns.

A. Symptoms and Mechanisms of Wind Damage

1. *Windthrow.* In high winds, uprooting of trees is far more frequent than stem breakage or any other form of mechanical injury. Because trees are asymmetrical structures and are irregularly anchored in a substratum of extremely variable properties, it is difficult to make generalizations concerning windthrow. Uprooting is seldom the result of steady wind pressure, but rather of lashing to and fro. This creates stresses which are exerted in several directions. There is no general agreement as to whether trees of small or large crowns (of equal height) will be more susceptible to windthrow. It has, however, been observed that heavy pruning of young trees increases their liability to wind damage (Peace, 1962). This may be due to the pendulum effect of a top-heavy tree.

In general, the taller the tree crop, the more susceptible it is to windthrow. The depth of rootable soil is also extremely important. If root penetration is restricted by underlying strata or drainage impedence, predisposition to windthrow is enhanced.

2. Windbreak. This type of damage is usually less common than windthrow. Normally, breaks develop from initial compression failures on the leeward sides of trees rather than from tension failures on the windward sides. Trees subjected to this stress, but which do not break, may develop swellings at the stress site. Windbreakage is particularly common where there are strong eddy currents, in which case the trees are subjected to heavy buffeting from more than one direction (Peace, 1962).

Butt-rotted trees are especially liable to breakage in the lower 6 feet. Branch breakage is very common in large-crowned hardwoods. Branches are actually subject to twisting forces. The broken branch stubs act as extremely important infection courts for stem-inhabiting microbes.

3. Windbend. Displacement from the upright position, frequently caused by snow or ice deposition, is also caused by wind. Bending is more likely to influence trees with slender, pliable stems and is most serious in overstocked plantations. Even though a tree can develop quite normally in a bent condition, its utility for certain commercial processes may be reduced. Bent trees tend to develop compression wood on the leeward side and tension wood on the windward side. The properties of these reaction woods differ materially from those of normal wood. Differential shrinkage during seasoning and irregularities in veneer peeling are among the most important of these alterations (Peace, 1962).

4. Windshake. Shakes are small splits which develop in the heartwood of trees. These internal cracks may be radial, in which case they often originate at the pith and are known as star shakes or rift cracks; or they may follow the line of an annual ring and are known as ring or cup shakes. Both kinds of cracks are serious log defects in terms of commercial value (Peace, 1962). Wind, in addition to frost and drought, is thought to induce these splits. More study of this phenomenon is needed.

5. Windrock. Wind may damage young trees, particularly those with heavy tops and restricted root systems, by "rocking" them. In this instance, bark is chaffed at the root collar by abrasive contact with stones or compressed soil. Injured areas may serve to permit the entrance of root decay fungi, for example *Armillaria mellea* (Peace, 1962).

6. Dwarfing and deformation. Trees which are subject to desiccation due to consistent wind exposure are frequently unable to expand cells to normal sizes and therefore assume a dwarf posture (Daubenmire, 1959). The influence is particularly common in seacoast and timberline areas. Deformation is commonly expressed in extremely asymmetrical growth resulting when branches develop only in a leeward direction. This may result entirely from physical pressure, that is, branches developing on the windward side are actually pushed around to grow in the lee direction, or from desiccation of buds developing on the windward side.

B. Susceptibility to Wind Damage

Relative resistance to the various types of wind damage is very difficult to establish. With respect to windthrow and windbreak, however, trees possessing brittle wood are commonly more seriously affected. Alden (1939) enumerates the relative wind resistance of shade trees based on the observations made in the aftermath of the 1938 hurricane. See Fig. 6 for examples of wind damage caused by this storm.

C. Management Practices

In areas of known significant wind stress, certain precautions should be observed. Establishment of plantations in areas which will permit only shallow rooting is undesirable. All efforts which can be taken to insure healthy root systems should be encouraged. Thinnings should be carefully planned to avoid rapid exposure to increased wind stress. Since large areas of single species of uniform age are particularly susceptible to wind damage, unevenaged management may be more desirable if possible. Restricted

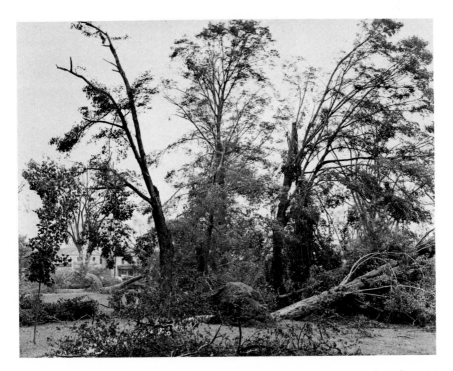

Fig. 6. Wind damage to street and ornamental trees in Connecticut resulting from the 1938 hurricane. Note windthrow and windbreak. (Photograph courtesy U.S. Forest Service.)

blocks of different species and ages provide boundaries against which damage may stop in the event of extensive windfall. The proper location of cutting boundaries was seen by Alexander (1967) to be capable of reducing windfall losses in spruce-fir and lodgepole pine forests.

In instances of high-value individuals, for example ornamental plantings, staking should be employed when establishing young trees to avoid wind-throw, windbend, and windrock.

II. SNOW

Damage caused by this agent is, of course, restricted to northern and western areas of this country but may be locally important. In general, coni-fers are much more susceptible than hardwoods. Considerable variation exists, however, in the degree of snow injury, depending on the gross morphology of the tree. Spruce, for example, have a tendency to shed a great deal of intercepted snow, while *Thuja* species have a tendency to accumulate it. Trees with asymmetric crowns also tend to be more severely damaged due to stresses established as snow accumulates on the side with greatest branch development (Curtis, 1936). Other influences, for example temperature and wind, also play significant roles in determining degree of snow damage. Temperatures near or slightly above the freezing point frequently result in wet, heavy snows, which are very damaging. In the absence of wind stress, tree branches may be able to support the added weight of accumulated snow. In the presence of winds, however, branch breakage is more common.

A. Symptoms

Snow damage is manifest in much the same way as wind injury. Stems and branches may be broken, lean may be produced, or trees may be pushed over (Fig. 7). This latter occurrence is relatively common in western conifers on steep slopes and results in what has been termed the "domino effect" as successively lower trees are toppled by ones from above.

B. Susceptibility to Snow Injury

In addition to the importance of morphological differences in determining degree of snow injury, it is apparent that other factors are operative. In a recent study conducted in the Oregon Cascades, Williams (1966) found that, in general, noble fir saplings suffered fewer snow injuries than did Douglas fir, but more than western hemlock, western white pine, and Pacific silver fir in many upper slope areas (Table VIII).

C. Management Practices

As more western-slope areas become more intensely managed, snow damage may become a more important problem. Douglas fir, found to be

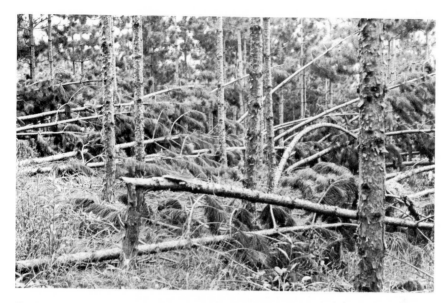

Fig. 7. New York red pine plantation exhibiting extensive snow damage from the previous winter. Note bending and breakage. (Photograph courtesy U.S. Forest Service.)

particularly susceptible to snow injury, may be a poor choice for regeneration of upper slope areas. Since heavily thinned sapling stands appear especially vulnerable to snow damage it would seem very desirable to employ frequent light thinnings, beginning at an early age, in snow-hazard areas.

Blum (1966) has suggested that, in terms of growth, quality, and stocking, a 7-year-old stand of paper and yellow birch in New Hampshire demonstrated remarkable recovery following severe snow damage. Snow may even have been beneficial by hastening the natural thinning process.

III. ICE

As in the case of snow, ice in various forms may pose a significant threat to tree welfare in certain areas. Glazed frost, freezing rain, and hail are all potentially capable of causing damage. The former two result during winter periods when there is a substantial layer of air above freezing lying over a lower layer of air below freezing. Passage of precipitation through the lower cold layer supercools it and, upon touching any solid object, the supercooled droplets turn instantly to ice. These meteorological conditions are unstable and rarely persist for extended periods of time. Hail is also a product of extremely unstable atmospheric conditions and may occur during any season.

The amount of ice damage realized is dependent on numerous factors. Winds, if present, will generally cause greater injury. Aspect is important,

TABLE VIII

TREES RATED ACCORDING TO DEGREE OF SNOW DAMAGE
OBSERVED AT LAVA LAKE[a]

Tree species	Snow damage ratings, spring, 1964	Trees studied (%)
Western white pine	None	18.2
	Very light	54.5
	Light	18.2
	Moderate	9.1
	Severe	—
Western hemlock	None	33.3
	Very light	33.3
	Light	25.0
	Moderate	8.4
	Severe	—
Pacific silver fir	None	—
	Very light	57.1
	Light	35.7
	Moderate	7.2
	Severe	—
Douglas fir	None	—
	Very light	8.3
	Light	41.7
	Moderate	25.0
	Severe	25.0
Noble fir	None	—
	Very light	45.5
	Light	54.5
	Moderate	—
	Severe	—

[a]From Williams (1966). Reproduced by permission of U.S. Forest Service.

with the greatest losses typically encountered on the northern and eastern
exposures. Normally, the taller and older a tree, the more susceptible it is to
ice damage. Older individuals have larger crowns, more internal decay
(which reduces structural strength), and less limb and bole flexibility.

A. Symptoms

Stem and branch breakage are the most serious consequences of ice deposition (Figs. 8 and 9). Lutz (1936) has described a form of ice injury that
results on young, thin-barked stems when the ice coating cracks and ice
edges cut the bark as the tree is swayed from side to side. These cracks may
serve to provide microbial ingress.

Hailstones may perforate leaves and cause small lesions on the exposed

surfaces of young soft-barked twigs. Young shoots of conifers may be severed. Broadleaved trees are, on occasion, defoliated with subsequent possibility of dieback. Hail damage is comparatively easy to diagnose, especially
in situ when the orientation of injury can be observed. Lesions are mainly on
the upper side of twigs and on one side of stems, depending on wind direction.

B. Susceptibility to Ice Damage

Considerable variation in species resistance to ice injury exists. In an Iowa
study of conifers, Goebel and Deitschman (1967) found that eastern white
pine and Scotch pine suffered by far the greatest damage. Northern white
cedar and Austrian pine were damaged much less. Norway spruce, other
Picea members, and eastern red cedar sustained practically no injury.

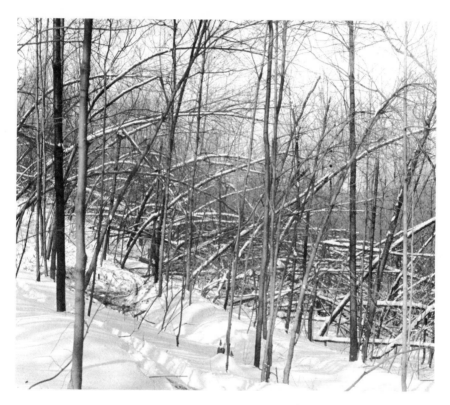

Fig. 8. Ice damage resulting from a severe glaze storm in a young Pennsylvania hardwood
stand. Bending dominated over breakage because of the relatively small size of the trees and
their consequent flexibility. (Photograph courtesy U.S. Forest Service.)

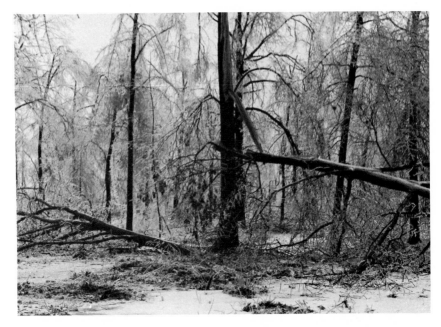

Fig. 9. Ice damage to Connecticut ornamental trees. The severe breakage of the large tree in the center of the picture resulted from an excessive weight of ice formed on the tree coupled with the relative inflexibility of the upper crown and large branches. (Photograph courtesy U.S. Forest Service.)

Downs (1938) and Croxton (1939) have both evaluated the relative susceptibility of various hardwood species and found appreciable differences (Table IX).

C. Management Practices

Silvicultural practices tending to maintain small crown sizes and eliminate individuals with large crowns, for example, "wolf trees" (trees, typically older than others in a forest, which have developed an extensive, spreading crown), are desirable. Breakage of limbs from overmature trees may damage nearby young growth. Evenaged management will tend to restrict crown size development and lessen danger of ice breakage. Species known to possess a certain amount of resistance to ice damage should be encouraged on northerly aspects and at high elevation in ice-hazard areas. The possibility that ice influence may shift the species composition in an extensively managed forest must not be overlooked. Downs (1938) has doc-

TABLE IX

SUSCEPTIBILITY OF TREES TO BREAKING BY ICE ACCUMULATION[a]

Species	Number examined	Percent injured little	Percent injured moderately	Percent badly broken
Salix babylonica	2	0	0	100
Betula alba	3	0	0	100
Betula lutea	5	0	0	100
Ulmus americana	111	6	10	84
Populus deltoides and hybrid poplars	34	9	41	50
Betula pendula	10	10	30	60
Acer saccharinum	117	11	21	68
Platanus occidentalis	6	17	33	50
Castanea dentata	11	27	46	27
Populus nigra var. italica	29	34.5	31	34.5
Pinus strobus	11	36	9	55
Prunus americana	29	38	17	45
Acer saccharum	102	41	26	33
Prunus sp. (Cherry)	26	42	16	42
Robinia pseudoacacia	11	55	9	36
Juniperus virginiana	88	55	19	26
Liriodendron tulipifera	7	57	43	0
Pyrus malus	37	73	16	11
Carya ovata	4	75	0	25
Tsuga canadensis	4	75	0	25
Acer negundo	8	75	25	0
Diospyros virginiana	21	76	24	0
Picea abies	39	77	18	5
Acer platanoides	9	77	23	0
Thuja occidentalis	29	79	14	7
Quercus alba	10	80	0	20
Salix discolor	7	86	14	0
Pinus sylvestris	7	86	14	0
Prunus sp. (Plum)	18	89	11	0
Catalpa speciosa	36	94	6	0
Pyrus communis	30	97	3	0
Juglans nigra	48	98	2	0
Pseudotsuga taxifolia	2	100	0	0
Pinus nigra	3	100	0	0
Magnolia tripetala	3	100	0	0
Gleditsia triacanthos	5	100	0	0
Ailanthus glandulosa	42	100	0	0

[a] From Croxton (1939). Reproduced by permission of the Ecological Society of America.

umented the ability of ice to shift stand composition in the direction of greater proportions of sugar maple and hemlock at the expense of black cherry in Pennsylvania.

IV. LIGHTNING

The majority of lightning bolts originate from cumulonimbus clouds which have acquired a large number of negatively charged ions on their lower surfaces. The ground under clouds of this type has a tendency to become less negative as surface electrons are repelled into the earth. Eventually, when the difference in potential between earth and cloud becomes great enough, for example as much as 10-100 million volts, the insulating capacity of the air may be breeched and electrons will migrate between cloud and earth in the form of a lightning bolt. Actually, a single bolt may consist of several discharges, all occurring within a fraction of a second. Most of the energy of the lightning bolt, perhaps 75%, is dissipated as heat. The temperature of a lightning channel may approximate 15,000°C (Parker, 1965).

Trees are frequently struck, as they project well above the ground contour. When trees are moist, they are extremely good conductors.

A. Symptoms

Expressions of lightning damage are quite variable.

1. No injury.   In this instance, the lightning passes down the tree without causing obvious harm. This is presumed to be most common when the bark is so thoroughly rain soaked that it permits the discharge to pass harmlessly down the outside of the tree. Orville (1968) has actually photographed lightning striking a European ash tree. The tree failed to display any external indication of injury.

2. Scar.   If the lightning happens to penetrate near the cambium, the bark may be torn off in a path a few inches wide down the tree. This scar may be in a spiral configuration in trees with a spiral grain. If the lightning penetrates somewhat more deeply, a jagged furrow typically results. This is not a clean fissure such as that produced by drought or frost. In some cases, the bolt may travel out along one of the roots, in which case the soil may be displaced and the roots exposed (Peace, 1962).

3. Trunk shatter.   If the discharge penetrates deeply into the stem, the moisture in the wood may be turned instantly to steam, resulting in explosive shatter of the tree bole.

B. Susceptibility to Lightning Injury

Oak, elm, poplar, and pine, which are among the most commonly struck, are also among the species most commonly found in isolated positions.

Beech, on the other hand, seems to sustain less lightning damage than one might predict. This species may owe its escape to its smooth bark which, when wet, may serve to conduct the electric current harmlessly outside the tree (Peace, 1962).

C. Management practices

High value individuals may be protected by installation of a multi-pointed lightning rod connected to the ground with a heavy copper cable.

REFERENCES

Alden, P. E. (1939). What the summer has taught us about hurricane damage. *Proc. 15th Natl. Shade Tree Cont.,* Aug. 1939, New York, N.Y., pp. 100-111.

Alexander, R. R. (1967). Windfall after clearcutting on Fool Creek—Fraser Experimental Forest, Colorado. *Res. Note, Rocky Mt. Forest Range Expt. Sta.* **RM-92**, 1-11.

Blum, B. M. (1966). Snow damage in young northern hardwoods. *J. Forestry* **64**, 16-20.

Croxton, W. C. (1939). A study of the tolerance of trees to breakage by ice accumulation. *Ecology* **20**, 71-73.

Curtis, J. D. (1936). Snow damage in plantations. *J. Forestry* **34**, 613-619.

Daubenmire, R. F. (1959). "Plants and Environment." Wiley, New York.

Downs, A. A. (1938). Glaze damage in the birch-beech-maple-hemlock type of Pennsylvania and New York. *J. Forestry* **36**, 63-70.

Goebel, C. J., and Deitschman, G. H. (1967). Ice storm damage to planted conifers in Iowa. *J. Forestry* **65**, 496-497.

Lutz, H. J. (1936). Scars resulting from glaze on woody stems. *J. Forestry* **34**, 1039-1041.

Orville, R. E. (1968). Photograph of a close lightning flash. *Science* **162**, 666-667.

Parker, J. (1965). Physiological diseases of trees and shrubs. *Advan. Fron. Plant Sci.* **12**, 97-248.

Peace, T. R. (1962). "Pathology of Trees and Shrubs." Oxford Univ. Press, London and New York.

Williams, C. B., Jr. (1966). Snow damage to coniferous seedlings and saplings. *Res. Note, Pacific Northwest. Forest Range Expt. Sta.,* **PNW-40** 1-10.

GENERAL REFERENCES

Abell, C. A. (1934). Influence of glaze storms upon hardwood forests in the southern Appalachians. *J. Forestry* **32**, 35-37.

Boyce, J. S. (1961). "Forest Pathology," McGraw-Hill, New York.

Campbell, W. A. (1937). Decay hazard resulting from ice damage to northern hardwoods. *J. Forestry* **35**, 1156–1158.

Carvell, K. L., Tryon, E. H., and True, R. P. (1957). Effects of glaze on the development of Appalachian hardwoods. *J. Forestry* **55**, 130–132.

Mergen, F. (1954). Mechanical aspects of wind-breakage and wind-firmness. *J. Forestry* **52**, 119–125.

Mergen, F., and Winer, H. I. (1952). Compression failures in the boles of living conifers. *J. Forestry* **50**, 671–679.

Meyer, B. S., Anderson, D. B., and Böhning, (1960). "Introduction to Plant Physiology." Van Nostrand, Princeton, New Jersey.

Orr, P. W. (1963). Windthrown timber survey in the Pacific Northwest, 1962. *Pacific Northwest. Forest Range Expt. Sta.*, 1–22.

Paine, L. A. (1966). Accidents caused by hazardous trees on California forest recreation sites. *Res. Note, Pacific Southwest Forest Range Expt. Sta.* **PSW-133**, 1–3.

Sartz, R. S. (1968). Hail can seriously damage eastern white pine. *J. Forestry* **66**, 353.

Spaulding, P., and Bratton, A. W. (1946). Decay following glaze storm damage in woodlands of central New York. *J. Forestry* **44**, 515–519.

Wilson, J. W. (1959). Notes on wind and its effects in artic-alpine vegetation. *J. Ecol.* **47**, 415–427.

5

MINERAL DEFICIENCIES AND EXCESSES

Normal growth and health of all higher plants is dependent on an adequate supply of 16 elements (Fritz, 1963). Of these 16, 9 are required in substantial amounts and are termed macronutrients, and 7 are required in much smaller amounts and are termed micronutrients (Table X). Carbon and oxygen are derived from atmospheric carbon dioxide, and hydrogen, from soil water. The remaining 13 are generally supplied to the plant through the soil solution. If one or more of these nutrients is absent or present in suboptimal amounts, physiological processes will be altered and abnormal metabolism may result.

An understanding of nutrient relationships is especially important in tree pathology. By reason of relative value, trees frequently are grown in areas of comparatively poor nutritional status. Correction of nutrient deficiencies is usually economically unfeasible. Appreciation of the roles of nutrient elements and an understanding of the consequences of deficiencies has developed rapidly since the turn of the century. Knowledge of tree nutrition, however, has lagged somewhat behind that of most agricultural crops.

Nutrient deficiencies are frequently most important in the nursery. Their detection and correction may also be most easily achieved in this area. Table XI includes a summary of conifer and angiosperm seedling symptoms generally displayed in reaction to the deficiency of several elements. Good photographs of deficiency symptoms of several forest trees have recently been provided by Hacskaylo et al. (1969).

The study of "deficiency diseases" is complicated by the existence of numerous experimental problems. The separation of disorders merely on the basis of symptoms is extremely frustrating. Inadequate supply of several minerals may be expressed in similar symptoms. Even if the symptoms expressed indicate the lack of a particular mineral, it can only be suggested

TABLE X

ELEMENTS ESSENTIAL FOR THE GROWTH AND DEVELOPMENT OF HIGHER PLANTS

Macronutrients	Micronutrients
Carbon	Iron
Oxygen	Boron
Hydrogen	Copper
Nitrogen	Zinc
Phosphorus	Molybdenum
Potassium	Manganese
Sulfur	Chlorine
Magnesium	
Calcium	

that this mineral is present in subnormal amounts in the plant—it may, or may not, exist in adequate quantities in the soil. Drought, for example, may induce deficiency symptoms, since the absence of available soil water restricts nutrient uptake. In extremely wet weather, transpiration may be reduced such that root absorption is abnormally restricted. Competition from other vegetation and the leaching influence of rain may also restrict nutrient uptake. Interpretation of soil analyses must also be made with considerable caution. Elements may be bound by clays and other colloids or be present in combined, insoluble forms and, hence, be unavailable to plants. Many elements, because of chemical similarity, influence the absorption of one another. Awareness of these influences is especially important in the inventory of potassium, sodium, calcium, and iron. Microbial activity of soil and its physical condition (for example, friability, penetrability, porosity, and depth) both importantly regulate the amount of nutrients absorbed by tree roots.

Perhaps one of the most accurate procedures for investigation of mineral deficiencies is to make chemical analyses of the foliage, or other tree parts, to determine nutrient levels. Even with this procedure, however, some confusion appears to exist concerning how the results should be expressed and how, when, and where the analyses should be made.

From the preceding discussion, it is readily apparent that relating specific tree disorders to nutrient inadequacies is a complex task.

I. SYMPTOMS AND METABOLIC DISTURBANCES ASSOCIATED WITH NUTRIENT DEFICIENCIES

A. Macronutrients

1. *Nitrogen (N).*   Yellowing, especially in older leaves, is very typical. Anthocyanescence (abnormal purple coloration) may develop. Normal bud

TABLE XI

SYMPTOMS OF NUTRIENT ELEMENT DEFICIENCY[a]

Element	Conifer seedlings	Hardwood seedlings
Nitrogen	Foliage uniformly pale green, yellowish, or yellow; older foliage dying in some species. Stems somewhat reddish in young seedlings. Tree leaves often short	Leaves small, uniformly faded, green or yellowish. Shoots short and spindly. In later stages, hardwood leaves may become red or purple
Phosphorus	Leaves sometimes pale, turning brown at tops. Sometimes purpling, becoming necrotic. Youngest foliage may remain green	Leaves small, bluish-green, veins purplish. Basal leaves may abcise. Shoots thin, short, upright
Potassium	Leaves short, chlorotic, often brown tipped. Yellow tipping in some species In some species, older leaves dying, younger are green	Leaves scorched or chlorotic, on tips and margins. Leaves sometimes dark bluish-green, upward curling, with speckling. Dieback. Also reddening in some species
Magnesium	Leaves yellowing and later browning at tips. Sometimes purpling. Older foliage sometimes yellower than younger. Growth not seriously affected	Basal older leaves marginal inter-veinal chlorosis and necrosis, early deciduousness. Growth near normal except where deficiency very severe. Sometimes reddening
Calcium	Young needles yellow; all needles brown or yellow on tips; no buds developed. Leaves stunted near terminal bud in some cases	Young leaves distorted, tips hooked downward, and margins curled. Margins may show some chlorosis; some spotting and brown scorching. Leafdrop; dieback. Older leaves relatively dark green
Iron	Young needles bright yellow; no top buds developed	Young leaves straw colored. Top of trees may be straw colored, with leaves marginal tip burned. Growth not seriously affected in moderate deficiency
Zinc	Inwardly folding apical needles, yellow mottling. Later bronzing and short, stiff, dark-green needles	Whitish green chlorosis with somewhat greener main veins. Rosetting, shoots long and narrow. In nut trees, nuts have kernels not ripening normally
Boron	In pines: reduced growth and necrosis in tops and growing points of roots. Young needles dead near apical bud	Young leaves often small, twisted, and somewhat corky main veins. Rosetting, dieback and sapoozing. Mottled chlorosis in some
Manganese	Paleness, retarded growth, dying. Buds turning brown; needles be-coming pale green or yellow at tips (Pinus radiata)	New leaves may be lighter green in interveinal areas, giving herringbone appearance. Spotting and necrosis may appear. Leafdrop; dieback
Copper	In pine: foliage bluish-green and tips of secondary needles dead; needles curved downward	Leaves of plum and apple whitish and soft. In peach, long and narrow leaves may be mottled green and white; irregular margins. Dieback
Molybdenum	Foliage becomes bluish in pine. No symptoms at first	In younger leaves: light-green chlorosis, but main and small veins green. Old leaves: marginal burning

[a]From Parker (1965). Reproduced by permission of the Institute for the Advancement of Science and Culture.

swelling and opening may be delayed. This latter phenomenon may be especially evident in lateral buds. A decrease in the angle between stem and leaf may be occasioned.

Limited nitrogen availability decreases the rate and amount of protein, nucleic acid, and chlorophyll syntheses. Cell division and expansion may also be retarded.

2. Phosphorus (P). Generally symptoms expressed are similar to nitrogen deficiency. Initial symptoms, however, may involve development of a very dark green leaf coloration.

Phosphorus is an integral part of the adenosine triphosphate (ATP) molecule and a component of numerous other phosphorylated compounds and, as such, is involved in practically every synthetic cell reaction. Reduced phosphate uptake will reduce ATP synthesis via photosynthetic or oxidative pathways and, consequently, generally depress anabolic processes. The structure of proteins and other organic compounds may be influenced, as phosphorus has important connective functions.

3. Potassium (K). Dieback and/or internode shortening may be expressed. A decrease in apical dominance may result in a stunted or bushy habit. Leaf necrosis or scorch may appear. Potassium is highly mobile in plants and moves readily from older to younger portions. This usually causes deficiency symptoms to appear initially in older organs.

The specific pathological effects of an inadequate potassium supply are elusive. Buffering capacity of cells or their ability to absorb other elements, for example, phosphorus, nitrogen, and iron, may be reduced. Reduced synthetic reactions, for example, in carbohydrate metabolism, may result as potassium acts as a nonspecific enzyme activator.

Sodium, which is toxic to plants at high levels, may substitute for potassium during uptake from the soil solution. This antagonistic phenomenon may be significant in the apparent damage caused to roadside trees by application of sodium chloride to reduce roadway icing (See Chapter 7, Fig. 13).

4. Sulfur (S). In general, dwarfed leaf size, yellowing, and anthocyanescence are common. Symptoms frequently develop in the younger leaves first.

Protein metabolism is impaired in the instance of sulfur inadequacy since numerous amino acids and coenzymes have this element as an integral component.

Most soils contain adequate sulfur supply and only rarely is sulfur deficiency involved in poor tree health.

5. Magnesium (Mg). Chlorosis (abnormal chlorophyll development, yellowish coloration) is the most common symptom of magnesium deficiency. Some degree of growth suppression, which is common in the case of limited supply of most macronutrients, is generally absent in the case of magnesium stress.

Since magnesium is chelated in the center of the chlorophyll molecule, the synthesis of this component is curtailed in the absence of magnesium. Reduced enzyme activity in several metabolic areas may also result as magnesium is an important nonspecific enzyme activator. Minor disturbances may also occur in ribosome structures and protein synthesis.

6. *Calcium (Ca).* Symptoms of inadequate calcium are quite varied. Young leaves in particular may show chlorosis and scorch. Root dwarfing or dieback may result. Occasionally restricted seed production may be observed. With extreme calcium stress, wilting may be evident.

Pathological disturbances resulting from calcium deficiency are incompletely understood. Possibilities which exist include: disturbed cell division or expansion; structural imperfections in chromosomes, middle lamellae membranes, or mitochondria; abnormal cell hydration or buffering capacity; and restricted enzyme activity due to lack of nonspecific activation.

B. Micronutrients

1. *Iron (Fe).* Chlorosis in young leaves is the most common symptom. Initially, this chlorosis is interveinal (between the veins).

Reduced chlorophyll development is occasioned by iron deficiency. Disturbances in the respiration process are also probable, since iron represents the principal metal in the respiratory cytochrome system.

In terms of quantity required, iron occupies an intermediate position with respect to other major and minor elements. Its occurrence in plants is in amounts sufficiently small to be considered minor, but appears to be required in the soil in quantities in excess of other minor elements. The availability of iron is critically controlled by soil pH; iron is unavailable in alkaline soils.

2. *Boron (B).* The boron deficiency syndrome includes severe root necrosis and, frequently, the death of apical meristems and stimulation of axillary bud development.

The specific role of boron is still very unclear. Pathological ramifications of the absence of this element may involve impaired cell-wall synthesis, abnormal cell division, water relations, or carbohydrate translocation. Lee and Aronoff (1967) have recently suggested that borate may act to partition metabolism between the glycolytic and pentose-shunt pathways.

3. *Copper (Cu).* Symptoms are very varied and include: dieback (death of outermost twigs), twisted, dark green leaves, tumefactions (swellings) on bark, and prolepsis (twigs which sprout from adventitious buds).

It is assumed that the most significant effect of insufficient copper would be on the several copper-containing enzymes; for example phenol oxidase, ascorbic acid oxidase, laccase, and cytochrome oxidase. In the case of these catalysts, copper acts as a specific activator.

Copper deficiencies are rarely encountered. An excess of soil copper is extremely toxic.

4. *Zinc (Zn).*   Zinc deficiency is characteristically expressed in: leaf scorch, yellowing (especially in a mottle pattern and interveinal), and dwarfing.

Pathological effects are not fully appreciated, but may involve auxin inactivations, loss of ribosome stability, or abnormal specific enzyme activation.

5. *Molybdenum (Mo).*   Typically, a bright yellow-green or pale orange interveinal mottling develops followed by necrosis of older leaves.

The incorporation of nitrogen into metabolic pathways is reduced when molybdenum is limiting. This element is essential for the enzyme nitrate reductase which mediates reduction of nitrate to nitrite.

6. *Manganese (Mn).*   In general, chlorotic and necrotic leaves result under manganese stress.

Disrupted chlorophyll formation and loss of nonspecific activation for many enzymes, especially peptidases, are assumed consequences of manganese deficiency.

Manganese and iron interact and the presence of one in high quantity will reduce the uptake and/or utilization of the other.

7. *Chlorine (Cl).*   Symptoms in this case are variable and may include dwarfed roots, wilting, chlorosis, and necrosis.

The pathological disturbances resulting from chlorine deficiency remain obscure.

C. Management Practices

Nutrient deficiencies can be corrected either by the addition of the element that is lacking or by promoting the natural availability of the element by adjustment of soil conditions, for example pH. In United States forestry practices, fertilization with macronutrients has been largely confined to nurseries and to the initial boosting of young trees at or soon after planting. Aerial applications, which are currently being evaluated, may make fertilizer applications to older trees more feasible.

In the case of microelements, their application has primarily been confined to injection and spray treatment of ornamental and certain fruit species. Application of micronutrients directly to the soil was previously undesirable as these compounds were frequently readily lost through leaching. Chelates are now available, for example in the case of iron and zinc, which permit application of these elements in stable, relatively nonleachable, organic compounds.

The primary difficulty in nutrient deficiency diseases, however, remains not in the treatment but rather in the detection. More information must be obtained which will permit accurate determination of nutrient inadequacies.

II. PATHOLOGICAL SIGNIFICANCE OF NUTRIENT EXCESS

Under certain circumstances, one or more essential elements may exist in the soil in abnormally high concentration. This may cause plant injury. Almost all elements will induce deleterious physiologic and metabolic consequences when present in the plant in excess of optimal quantities.

Considerable evidence, based on *in vitro* observations, has been presented indicating that copper, zinc, boron, and manganese are particularly phytotoxic in high concentrations. Very few data, however, are available with respect to the occurrence or significance of mineral nutrient excesses in natural forest soils.

REFERENCES

Fritz, G. J. (1963). Assimilation of minerals by higher plants. *Nature* **197**, 843–846.

Hacskaylo, J., Finn, R. F., and Vimmerstedt, J. P. (1969). Deficiency symptoms of some forest trees. *Res. Bull., Ohio Agr. Res. Develop. Center* **1015**, 1–68.

Lee, S., and Aronoff, S. (1967). Boron in plants: A biochemical role. *Science* **158**, 798–799.

Parker, J. (1965). Physiological diseases of trees and shrubs. *Advan. Fron. Plant Sci.* **12**, 97–248.

GENERAL REFERENCES

Berg, W. A., and Vogel, W. G. (1968). Manganese toxicity of legumes seeded in Kentucky strip-mine spoils. *Res. Paper, Northeast. Forest Expt. Sta.* **NE-119**, 1–12.

Bollard, E. G., and Buler, G. W. (1966). Mineral nutrition of plants. *Ann. Rev. Plant Physiol.* **17**, 77–112.

Brenchley, W. E. (1927). "Inorganic Plant Poisons and Stimulants." Cambridge Univ. Press, London and New York.

Hacskaylo, J. (1961). Deficiency symptoms of forest trees. *Proc. 7th Intern. Congr. Soil Sci., Madison, Wisc., 1960*, pp. 393–405. Elsevier, Amsterdam.

Hewitt, E. J. (1963). The essential nutrient elements: Requirements and interactions in plants. *In* "Plant Physiology" (F. C. Steward, ed.), Vol. 3, 137–360. Academic Press, New York.

Ike, A. F. (1968). Symptoms of nutrient deficiency in yellow-poplar seedlings. *Res. Note, Southeast. Forest Expt. Sta.* **SE-94**, 1-4.

Ingestad, T. (1957). Studies on the nutrition of forest tree seedlings. I. Mineral nutrition of birch. *Physiol. Plantarum* **10**, 418-439.

Ingestad, T. (1959). Studies on the nutrition of forest tree seedlings. II. Mineral nutrition of spruce. *Physiol. Plantarum* **12**, 568-593.

Krueger, K. W. (1967). Foliar mineral content of forest- and nursery-grown Douglas-fir seedlings. *Res. Paper, Pacific Northwest Forest Range Expt. Sta.* **PNW-45**, 1-12.

Loneragan, J. F. (1968). Nutrient requirements of plants. *Nature* **220**, 1307-1308.

Morris, R. F. (1951). Tree injection experiments in the study of yellow birch dieback. *Forestry Chronicle* **27**, 313-329.

Peace, T. R. (1962). "Pathology of Trees and Shrubs." Oxford Univ. Press, London and New York.

Pirone, P. P. (1951). Foliage applications of nutrients. *Proc. 27th Natl. Shade Tree Conf.,* August, 1951, Cincinnati, Ohio, pp. 23-36.

School of Foresty, Duke University. (1959). Mineral nutrition of trees. A symposium. *Bull. Duke School Forestry* **15**, 1-184.

Soil Science Society of America, Inc. (1967). "Soil Testing and Plant Analysis," Part I. Soil Testing. Soil Sci. Soc. Am., Madison, Wisconsin.

Soil Science Society of America, Inc. (1967). "Soil Testing and Plant Analysis," Part II. Plant Analysis. Soil Sci. Soc. Am., Madison, Wisconsin.

Sucoff, E. I. (1961). Potassium, magnesium, and calcium deficiency symptoms of loblolly and virginia pine seedlings. *Paper, Northeast. Forest Expt. Sta.* **164**, 1-18.

Tennessee Valley Authority. (1968). "Forest Fertilization. Theory and Practice." *Symp. Forest Fertilization, Gainesville, Fla., 1967* T.V.A., Muscle Shoals, Alabama.

Vaartaja, O. (1954). Mineral deficiences in a forest nursery. *Bi-m. Progr. Rept., Div. Forest Biol., Canada Dept. Agr.* **10(2)**, 2.

Walker, L. C. (1956). Foliage symptoms as indicators of potassium deficient soils. *Forest Sci.* **2**, 113-120.

Wilde, S. A., and Voigt, G. K. (1952). Determination of color of nursery stock foliage by means of Munsell color charts. *J. Forestry* **50**, 622-623.

6

AIR POLLUTION

Air is an extremely important natural resource vital to plants and animals. During the course of a single day, in a layer extending 25 feet above the ground, 5 billion tons of air pass above the United States. The chemical nature of this air is relatively simple, and major constituents at the earth's surface include: nitrogen (78%), oxygen (21%), and carbon dioxide, water vapor, and various other compounds (1%). For millennia this rather pleasant agglumeration of gases has, from time to time, been tinted with undesirable "natural pollutants." Examples of these natural pollutants would include volcanic dust, wind-eroded soil, pollen, microbial spores, methane from marshes, hydrogen sulfide from decaying vegetation, and hydrocarbons from coniferous species. None of these natural pollutants has apparently exerted significant deleterious influences on vegetation. The sophistication of man, however, in such areas as energy generation, goods manufacture, and waste disposal has unfortunately created some undesirable byproducts we might term "man-made" or "unnatural pollutants." These pollutants, which have been shown capable of influencing plant health, do not contaminate all 5 billion tons of United States air. Locally, however, pollution damage may accrue because the capacity of the air flowing over certain areas may not be sufficient to dilute introduced noxious materials. Unfortunately, the areas subject to potential pollution injury are increasing in size. The U.S. Public Health Service has recently estimated that more than 50% of the American population lives in areas of constant air pollution (Nelson, 1967).

Air pollution plant damage is occasioned by three broad groups of pollutant types: particulate matter, nonphotochemically produced gaseous pollutants, and photochemically produced gaseous pollutants.

I. PARTICULATE MATTER

Particulates, which may be divided into fine solids (less than 100 μ in diameter) and coarse particulates (greater than 100 μ in diameter) have been known to cause plant damage for some time. Relative to the gaseous pollutants, however, they have received only limited study and their influence in natural ecosystems is incompletely understood.

The major sources of atmospheric particulates are: (1) combustion of coal, gasoline, and fuel oil, (2) cement production, (3) lime kiln operation, (4) incineration, and (5) agricultural burning and agriculturally related activities (Wood, 1968).

In areas adjacent to roadways, lead is a primary particulate pollutant. Tetraethyl lead, which is added to gasoline to provide antiknock qualities, is given off in considerable quantity in automotive exhaust. In a study of roadside grass in Denver, 3000 ppm lead (in ash) were found near major intersections and more than 50 ppm for 500 feet downwind (Cannon and Bowles, 1962). Vegetables grown within 25 feet of roads in upstate New York and western Maryland averaged 80–115 ppm. No specific information is available on lead content of roadside trees, but in consideration of their longevity and potential for accumulation, lead may cause physiological disturbances in certain tree species.

Soot particles arising from the routine combustion of number 6 fuel oil were found to damage several greenhouse plants (P. M. Miller and Rich, 1967). These particles were found to have a very low pH (2.0) and cause necrotic spots on the leaves of intercepting vegetation.

Dusts, which are representative coarse particulates, frequently form undesirable deposits on vegetation. Naturally deposited dust from cement plants may cause chlorosis and death in both deciduous and coniferous species (Darley and Middleton, 1966).

Corn and Montgomery (1968) have proposed that particulates may interact with gaseous pollutants and cause a synergistic response. The mechanism may be one of adsorption or absorption of gases by the particle such that the gases become concentrated. When the particle is ultimately deposited in or on the plant, the high local concentration of gases may be sufficient to cause injury.

II. NONPHOTOCHEMICALLY PRODUCED GASEOUS POLLUTANTS

These pollutants are conveniently separated from other gaseous pollutants in that they generally originate at the source in a form toxic to plants, do not have photochemical processes involved in their synthesis, and most have been in existence and appreciated for several hundred years.

A. Sulfur Compounds

Numerous compounds containing sulfur are important air pollutants (sulfur dioxide, hydrogen sulfide, mercaptans). Sulfur dioxide (SO_2) is, however, by far the most important sulfur pollutant. Moreover, SO_2 is probably the most widespread and it has been the most intensively studied pollutant.

In the United States, more than 20 million tons of sulfur are discharged in the air per year, most in the form of SO_2 (Abelson, 1967). Wood (1968) has listed the following sources for SO_2 emission: (1) combustion of coal; (2) production, refining, and utilization of petroleum and natural gas; (3) manufacturing and industrial utilization of sulfuric acid and sulfur; and (4) smelting and refining of ores (especially copper, lead, zinc, and nickel). The primary United States sources of SO_2 are from coal and oil combustion. New York City ejects 600,000 tons of SO_2 annually into the air. Sulfur dioxide emission in Connecticut totals 300,085 tons per year (Hilst et al., 1967).

The bulk of the severe SO_2 damage to forests has been in the vicinity of smelters in the west and south. The influence of chronic exposure to low-level SO_2 levels in both urban and rural environments is unknown.

1. Symptoms.   In general, acute injury may occur at SO_2 concentrations above 0.50 ppm. Chronic injury may be realized at concentrations of 0.10 to 0.03 ppm for susceptible species under favorable conditions. In the instance of broad-leaved species, symptoms include irregular marginal and interveinal necrotic blotches bleached white to straw (sometimes brown). In the case of conifers, needle tips are typically necrotic, often with a banded appearance. Chlorosis of adjacent tissue is generally present (Brandt and Heck, 1967).

2. Mechanism of injury.   Sulfur dioxide enters leaves through open stomata. If stomata are closed, much higher concentrations are required for injury. After entrance, SO_2 is absorbed on the moist reactive surfaces of the spongy mesophyll and palisade cells. In this position, sulfite (SO_2^{2-}) is formed. Sulfite is very toxic to cells and will quickly kill them if present in sufficiently high concentration. At low or chronic levels, however, sulfite is slowly oxidized to sulfate (SO_4^{2-}) which has considerably less toxicity than sulfite (Thomas, 1965). It is possible, if SO_2 is not present in high concentration, that sulfite can be oxidized as rapidly as it forms in the plant.

By some mechanism incompletely understood, SO_2 has been shown capable of reducing photosynthesis in alfalfa (Thomas and Hill, 1937) and in lichens (Rao and LeBlanc, 1966).

3. Susceptibility to injury.   Conifers are particularly susceptible to SO_2, as their needles remain on the tree for several years, thereby greatly extending their exposure time beyond that of annuals and deciduous species. Sulfur dioxide concentrations are considerably higher during the winter months due to the combustion of fossil fuels. Western larch is the most sensitive conifer in the northwest followed by Douglas fir and ponderosa pine. Western red cedar, western white pine, western hemlock, Engelmann spruce, grand fir, and lodgepole pine, while occasionally severely damaged, are considerably more resistant. Northern white cedar is a particularly resistant northeastern conifer. With respect to hardwoods, elm, birch and poplar species appear intermediate in susceptibility and live oak, maple and boxelder are quite resistant (Magill et al., 1956).

4. *Amelioration.* A recent editorial in SCIENCE (Abelson, 1967) has proposed five means of meeting the SO_2 problem:

(1) Use fuels with low amounts of sulfur. (2) Discharge fumes from tall smoke stacks (greater than 200 meters). (3) Add powdered limestone to flue gas (following combustion) to convert gaseous sulfur oxides to solid forms. (4) Convert coal to gas and remove sulfur from gas prior to combustion. (5) Pass the flue gases through chemical processing plants and recover sulfur in the elemental form or as sulfuric acid.

Drummond and Wood (1967) found that eastern white pine in the vicinity of a coal-burning, electric generating station increased height growth following increase in stack height. Two years following stack elevation, increases of 3- and 1.8-fold were noted on trees at 2.5 and 10 miles distance, respectively.

B. Halogen Compounds

The most important pollutants in this group include hydrogen fluoride (HF), silicon tetrafluoride (SiF_4), hydrogen chloride (HCl) and chlorine (Cl_2). Primary sources of fluorine compounds are: (1) aluminum reduction processes, (2) manufacture of phosphate fertilizer, (3) brick plants, (4) pottery and ferroenamel works, (5) steel manufacturing plants, (6) refineries, and (7) rocket fuel combustion.

Hydrochloric acid and Cl_2 originate from refineries, glass making, incineration, and scrap burning, and accidental spillage. Combustion of polyvinyl chloride results in HCl emission. The widespread use of polyvinyl chloride in packaging will result in increased HCl air pollution as these containers are incinerated (Wood, 1968).

1. *Symptoms.* Fluoride is considered an accumulative poison of leaf tissue. Generally, leaf concentrations in the range of 50–200 ppm will result in necrosis of susceptible plants. Treshow et al. (1967) studied Douglas fir in an area where 200 acres of this species had been killed by fluoride from a phosphate reduction plant in Idaho (Fig. 10). They found that when fluoride levels reached 100–200 ppm, growth reduction (radial increment) was observed. When needle concentrations reached 500 ppm, the trees were killed. Analysis of needles collected from the ground revealed fluoride concentrations of up to 1469 ppm.

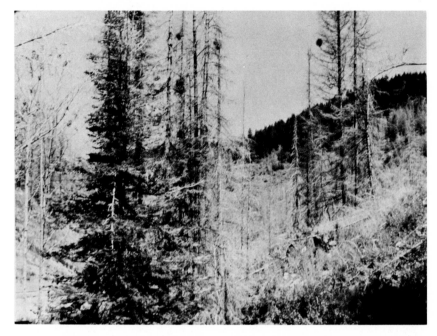

Fig. 10.   Area of Douglas fir in Idaho where mortality was caused by atmospheric fluoride. The lone healthy tree in the foreground is a white fir. (Photograph courtesy of M. Treshow, Univ. of Utah.)

Fluoride symptoms on broad leaves commonly involve necrotic or scorched leaf margins with occasional interveinal blotches. Dead and living tissue interface is generally distinct. On conifers, brown to red-brown necrotic needle tips are usually observed (Brandt and Heck, 1967).

Brennan *et al.* (1966) found that needles of shortleaf, slash, and loblolly pine were all injured by a 3-hour fumigation with 1.0 ppm chlorine.

In general, acute chlorine injury is expressed in symptoms similar to SO_2 injury. Marginal and interveinal lesions generally occur on broad-leaved species, and necrotic tips with sharp demarcation on conifers.

2. Mechanism.   Fluoride is absorbed from the air and is translocated and accumulated in leaf tips and margins. The toxicant remains in a soluble form and seems to retain the chemical properties of free inorganic fluoride (Heggestad, 1968). This excessive concentration results in the rapid death of leaf cells. The significance of fluoride in the disruption of enzyme systems and the formation of organic fluoride compounds is not fully understood. Chloride injury is presumed to involve mechanisms similar to those of fluoride.

C. Ethylene

This gas is one of a group of hydrocarbons with carbon-carbon double bonds termed olefins. Its sources include illuminating gas, certain plastic manufacturing processes, and fuel combustion, especially automobile exhaust (Heggestad, 1968).

Ethylene is a plant hormone and many of the symptoms expressed in reaction to high concentrations (0.005-0.1 ppm depending on species) are similar to typical hormonal responses. In broad-leaf species, epinasty (atypical downward leaf curvature) and/or abscission of leaves may occur. Sensitive plants may develop general chlorosis of older leaves, necrosis, and leaf abscission. More resistant plants may show only retardation of growth and possible loss of apical dominance. Coniferous symptoms generally involve needle abscission, retarded elongation of new needles, or poor cone development (Brandt and Heck, 1967).

D. Nitrogen Oxides

The most important phytotoxic nitrogen oxides are nitric oxide (NO) and nitrogen dioxide (NO_2). Numerous sources of these gases exist: (1) gasoline combustion in motor vehicles [the typical tailpipe concentration of nitric oxide is in the range of 1000-3000 ppm (Buchan and Charlson, 1968)]; (2) petroleum refining; (3) the combustion of natural gas, fuel oil, and coal; (4) the incineration of organic wastes; (5) the manufacture of nitric acid; (6) the manufacture of sulfuric acid by the chamber process; (7) the manufacture of paint, roofing, rubber, and soap; and (8) the manufacture of nylon intermediates (Wood, 1968).

In the case of NO_2, acute injury often is manifest as necrotic lesions, similar to SO_2 lesions, on broad-leaved plants at concentrations of 2-10 ppm (Brandt and Heck, 1967).

E. Miscellaneous

Several nonphotochemically produced gases have, on occasion, been observed to produce plant injury. Ammonia, whose influence may be mitigated by rain as it is very water soluble, has caused complete leaf collapse of some species. Carbon monoxide appears to damage plants only above 1000 ppm (Heggestad, 1968). Concentrations in vegetation at busy intersections are generally in the 200-500 ppm range. Mercury vapor and aldehydes may also exert detrimental influences on plant growth.

III. PHOTOCHEMICALLY PRODUCED GASEOUS POLLUTANTS

Until recently, nonphotochemically produced pollutants were thought to be responsible for most air pollution damage to plants. Approximately 20 years ago, however, a new type of pollution was recognized, especially in the Los Angeles region of California. These pollutants required alteration after release from their source by reaction with sunlight, other atmospheric materials, or both to become phytotoxic. The majority of these materials are generated in the sunlight from relatively nontoxic stack and exhaust pipe gases.

A. Ozone

This is one of the most important toxicants of this class and is a primary component of urban smog. Three major sources of ozone (O_3) exist.

The first, and perhaps the most important, involves the interaction of nitrogen oxides, hydrocarbons, and sunlight. Oxygen and nitrogen are nonreactive at normal temperatures. When exposed to elevated temperatures, for example those occurring in furnaces and automobile cylinders, nitrogen and oxygen react to form nitrogen oxide:

$$N_2 + O_2 + heat \rightarrow NO$$

In Los Angeles and San Francisco, automobiles are responsible for 70-80% of the NO formed. Nitrogen oxide is vented along with other wastes into the free air. Upon cooling, and in the presence of UV light rays (2900-3700 Å) and olefins (for example, ethylene, propylene, isobutylene), NO_2 is formed:

$$NO + O_2 + hydrocarbons + UV\ light \rightarrow NO_2$$

Under the influence of sunlight, NO_2 releases an atom of oxygen which may unite with molecular oxygen forming ozone (Daines et al., 1967):

$$NO_2 + O_2 + UV\ light \rightarrow NO + [O]$$

$$[O] + O_2 \rightarrow O_3$$

Ozone is unstable, but it may be produced at a rate faster than it can decompose.

A second potential source of ozone is the troposphere. The outer layers of the stratosphere are especially rich in this gas. Ozone may be brought to near ground level by certain circumstances including the following: jet streams, polar cold fronts, subsidence in anticyclones (Rich, 1964), and hurricanes and other violent storms (Wood, 1968).

Third, O_3 may be formed in thunderstorms during electrical discharges. Violent thunderstorms may produce sufficient O_3 to cause plant injury in local instances.

1. Symptoms.   Symptoms will appear on sensitive plant species after 4-8 hour exposure to 0.02 ppm and after 1-2 hour exposure to 0.05 ppm. Eastern white pine is an extremely sensitive indicator of ozone presence. Berry (1967) has recorded damage by 0.10 ppm O_3 in 4 hours. Sinclair and

Costonis (1968), on the other hand, have observed acute injury following exposure to 7 ppm for 4 hours or 3 ppm for 48 hours. Symptoms on broad-leaf species are *upper*-surface stipple or flecking with small irregular, collapsed areas, pigmented red-brown stipple, or bleached straw to white fleck. Frequently injury is visible *only* on upper leaf surfaces. This may be because of presence in this region of the palisade cells, which are very susceptible to damage. The most typical coniferous symptom is brown necrotic tips of needles similar to SO_2 injury, but lacking a definite separation between necrotic and healthy tissue (Brandt and Heck, 1967).

Costonis and Sinclair (1967) have presented a detailed description of ozone injury symptoms to eastern white pine. Initially, immediate collapse of mesophyll cells radiating from individual stomata located 7-20 mm from the needle sheath is observed. This collapse is externally visible as tiny silvery (water-soaked) spots. After a 6-8 hour exposure, affected areas become yellow-pink and then purple in color. Eventually, these colored areas coalesce to form chlorotic or necrotic bands. On highly susceptible trees, distal enlargement of bands occurs until tip necrosis or blight is manifest.

2. Mechanism of injury. Three hypotheses have been proposed to account for O_3 damage (Rich, 1964). The first proposes interference with mitochondrial activity. Ozone has been found to inhibit the O_2 uptake of mitochondrial preparations. The second hypothesis involves destruction of membrane permeability. Ozone may react with the double bonds of unsaturated membrane lipids. It may also destroy sulfhydryl groups and inhibit the production of new lipids. The water-soaked appearance of ozone injured leaves may result as water leaks from cells into intercellular spaces. A third hypothesis proposes an inhibition of photosynthesis. Tomlinson and Rich (1967) exposed spinach to 1 ppm O_3 for 30 minutes and inhibited CO_2 fixation by 37%. Chloroplasts from these leaves showed a normal Hill reaction, indicating that photophosphorylation was not depressed. P. R. Miller and Parmeter (1967), working with ponderosa pine seedlings, exposed them to 0.25-0.35 ppm O_3 9 hours per day and observed a 10% decrease in photosynthesis. In contrast to Tomlinson and Rich (1967), these investigators claimed that the Hill reaction did appear to be depressed. The ability of ozone to influence photosynthesis has also been observed in beans, tomato, coleus, duckweed, lime, orange, and tobacco.

3. Susceptibility to injury. Considerable variation in ozone resistance exists in agricultural crops. Tree species have not received extensive investigation in this regard. Davis and Wood (1968) have, however, recorded the reaction of 3-year-old seedlings of 22 species to exposure to 24 ppm O_3 for 8 hours (Table XII).

TABLE XII

RELATIVE SUSCEPTIBILITY OF SELECTED TREE SEEDLINGS TO OZONE INJURY[a]

Injured	Uninjured
Fraxinus americana	Abies balsamea
Larix leptolepis	A. concolor
Liriodendron tulipifera	Acer saccharum
Pinus banksiana	Betula pendula
P. nigra	Picea abies
P. rigida	P. glauca
P. strobus	P. glauca var. densata
P. virginiana	P. pungens
Quercus alba	Pinus resinosa
Tsuga canadensis	Pseudotsuga menziesii
	Thuja occidentalis
	Tilia cordata

[a]From Davis and Wood (1968). Reproduced by permission of The American Phytopathological Society.

B. Peroxyacetyl Nitrate (PAN)

The heat occurring in the cylinders of internal combustion engines cracks certain of the hydrocarbons contained in gasoline. Included among the approximately 180–200 hydrocarbons released in automobile exhaust are several olefins and aromatics. These compounds are oxidized in the presence of nitrogen oxides and light shortly after their release. Olefins are quickly oxidized, being broken at the double-bond position, and produce decomposition products rich in aldehydes. Further reaction of the aldehydes with ozone and other hydrocarbons results in the formation of numerous other compounds, for example peroxyacetyl nitrate (PAN).

$$H-\underset{\underset{H}{|}}{\overset{\overset{H}{|}}{C}}-C\overset{\displaystyle O}{\underset{\displaystyle O-O-NO_2}{\diagdown}}$$

PAN

In addition to the internal combustion engine as a source of PAN, evidence has been presented which suggests that terpenes released by coniferous vegetation may be photochemically altered in the presence of nitrogen oxides to form PAN and ozone. PAN is only one of a series of toxicants produced in a manner homologous to that outlined above. Some closely related compounds in the series may be four to eight times more toxic (Heggestad, 1968).

1. Symptoms.   Ambient concentrations of 0.02-0.05 ppm for a few hours will cause injury to sensitive species. On broad-leaf species a collapse of the tissue on the *underside* of the leaf giving a glazed, silvered, or bronzed appearance is characteristic. Conifers generally display rather unspecific needle blight symptoms with some chlorosis or bleaching (Brandt and Heck, 1967). The fact that PAN influences the lower leaf surfaces is most helpful in distinguishing it from ozone injury.

2. Mechanism and consequences of disease.   The mechanism by which PAN and its homologues cause disease in plants is not known. It may operate in a manner similar to ozone. Little work has been done on the influence of PAN on trees. Severe leaf mottle and leaf drop of ponderosa pine and Jeffrey pine in the San Bernardino Mountains of California, at altitudes up to 7000 feet, have, however, been attributed to ozone and PAN. In a recent test involving 29 tree species, Drummond and Wood (1970) concluded that none of the species was injured by exposure to PAN concentrations well in excess of that normally found in ambient air. In terms of agricultural crops, PAN and its analogs are believed to destroy several million dollars worth annually in the United States (Daines *et al.,* 1967).

IV. AIR POLLUTION IN PERSPECTIVE

In urban areas, air pollution currently presents a relatively continuous stress on tree health. In nonurban areas, atmospheric turbulence is probably still capable of dissipating air pollutants sufficiently to avoid excessive chronic injury. This flushing does not occur, however, when stagnant air masses or inversions exist.

Air pollution and its effects on vegetation are going to become worse before they improve. Sulfur dioxide, fluoride, ozone, and peroxyacetyl nitrate are among the most important phytotoxicants. These materials result from transportation, industry, and the generation of electricity. Our increases in population will require attendant expansion in these areas, with subsequent release of more pollutants, for at least the next 30 years. By 2000 AD, reductions may be realized in some emissions, but then others may be worse. Amelioration of the problem will not come easily or inexpensively. With the possible exception of Green (1967), imaginative alternatives to the use of fossil fuels have not been forthcoming. Estimates at the cost of controlling pollution over the next 30 years approximate 300 billion dollars.

Finally, we do not, even now, totally appreciate the influence of atmospheric pollutants on plant health (much less human health). We are particularly ignorant of the influence of chronic exposure to low level contamination. It may well be that this "hidden damage" (Todd, 1956) represents a truly significant cost that we pay for our modern technology.

REFERENCES

Abelson, P. H. (1967). Diminishing the role of sulfur oxides in air pollution. *Science* **157**, 1265.

Berry, C. R. (1967). An exposure chamber for forestry air pollution studies. *Phytopathology* **57**, 804 (abstr.).

Brandt, C. S., and Heck, W. W. (1967). Effects of air pollutants on vegetation. *In* "Air Pollution" (A. C. Stern, ed.), 2nd ed., Vol. 1, pp. 401–443. Academic Press, New York.

Brennan, E., Leone, I. A., and Daines, R. H. (1966). Response of pine trees to chlorine in the atmosphere. *Forest Sci.* **12**, 386–390.

Buchan, W. E., and Charlson, R. J. (1968). Urban haze: The extent of automotive contribution. *Science* **159**, 192–194.

Cannon, H. L., and Bowles, J. M. (1962). Contamination of vegetation by tetraethyl lead. *Science* **137**, 765–766.

Corn, M., and Montgomery, T. L. (1968). Atmospheric particulates: Specific surface areas and densities. *Science* **159**, 1350–1351.

Costonis, A. C., and Sinclair, W. A. (1967). Seasonal development of symptoms of ozone injury on eastern white pine. *Phytopathology* **57**, 339 (abstr.).

Daines, R. H., Brennan, E., and Leone, I. (1967). Air pollutants and plant response. *J. Forestry* **65**, 381–384.

Darley, E. F., and Middleton, J. T. (1966). Problems of air pollution in plant pathology. *Ann. Rev. Plant Pathol.* **4**, 103–118.

Davis, D. D., and Wood, F. A. (1968). Relative sensitivity of twenty-two tree species to ozone. *Phytopathology* **58**, 399 (abstr.).

Drummond, D. B., and Wood, F. A. (1967). Recovery of eastern white pine following reduction in levels of ambient air pollution. *Phytopathology* **57**, 810 (abstr.).

Drummond, D. B., and Wood, F. A. (1970). The sensitivity of twenty-nine northeastern tree species to PAN. *Phytopathology* **60**, 574.

Green, L., Jr. (1967). Energy needs versus environmental pollution. A reconciliation? *Science* **156**, 1448–1450.

Heggestad, H. E. (1968). Diseases of crops and ornamental plants incited by air pollutants. *Phytopathology* **58**, 1089–1097.

Hilst, G. R., Yocum, J. E., and Boune, N. E. (1967). The development of a simulation model for air pollution over Connecticut, Vol. I. Summary report. Travelers Res. Center, Inc., Hartford, Connecticut.

Magill, P. L., Holden, F. R., and Ackley, C. (1956). "Air Pollution Handbook." McGraw-Hill, New York.

Miller, P. M., and Rich, S. (1967). Soot damage to greenhouse plants. *Plant Disease Reptr.* **51**, 712.

Miller, P. R., and Parmeter, J. R., Jr. (1967). Effects of ozone injury to ponderosa pine. *Phytopathology* **57**, 822 (abstr.).

Nelson, B. (1967). Air pollution: The "Feds" move to abate Idaho pulp mill stench. *Science* **157**, 1018-1021.

Rao, D. N., and LeBlanc, F. (1966). Effects of sulfur dioxide on the lichen algae with special reference to chlorophyll. *Bryologist* **69**, 69-75.

Rich, S. (1964). Ozone damage to plants. *Ann. Rev. Phytopathol.* **2**, 253-266.

Sinclair, W. A., and Costonis, A. C. (1968). Factors affecting acute injury of *Pinus strobus* by ozone. *Phytopathology* **58**, 403 (abstr.).

Thomas, M. D. (1965). The effects of air pollution on plants and animals. *In* "Ecology and the Industrial Society" (G. T. Goodman, R. W. Edwards, and J. M. Lambert, eds.), pp. 11-33. Wiley, New York.

Thomas, M. D., and Hill, G. R. (1937). Relation of sulphur dioxide in the atmosphere to photosynthesis and respiration of alfalfa. *Plant Physiol.* **12**, 309-383.

Todd, G. W. (1956). "Hidden damage" to plants as caused by air pollutants. *Plant Physiol.* **31**, Suppl., p. xv.

Tomlinson, H., and Rich, S. (1967). A comparison of the effects of ozone and sulfhydryl reagents on plants. *Phytopathology* **57**, 834 (abstr.).

Treshow, M., Anderson, F. K., and Harner, F. (1967). Responses of Douglas-fir to elevated atmospheric fluorides. *Forest Sci.* **13**, 114-120.

Wood, F. A. (1968). Sources of plant-pathogenic air pollutants. *Phytopathology* **58**, 1075-1084.

GENERAL REFERENCES

Agricultural Research Council. (1967). "The Effects of Air Pollution on Plants and Soil." Agr. Res. Council, London.

Ahmadjiaa, V. (1967). "The Lichen Symbiosis." Ginn (Blaisdell), Boston, Massachusetts.

Air Conservation Commission (AAAS). (1965). "Air Conservation," *Publ. No. 80, Am. Assoc. Advance. Sci.,* Washington, D.C.

Altshuller, A. P., Cohen, I. R., and Purcell, T. C. (1967). Photooxidation of hydrocarbons in the presence of aliphatic aldehydes. *Science* **156**, 937-939.

Berry, C. R., and Hepting, G. H. (1954). Injury to eastern white pine by unidentified atmospheric constituents. *Forest Sci.* **10**, 2-13.

Berry, C. R., and Ripperton, L. A. (1963). Ozone, a possible cause of white pine emergence tipburn. *Phytopathology* **53**, 552-557.

Brandt, C. S. (1962). Effects of air pollution on plants. *In* "Air Pollution" (A. C. Stern, ed.), Vol. 1, pp. 255-281. Academic Press, New York.

Brandt, C. S., and Heck, W. (1967). Effects of air pollutants on vegetation. *In* "Air Pollution" (A. C. Stern, ed.), 2nd ed., Vol. 1, pp. 401-443. Academic Press, New York.

Brennan, E., and Davis, S. H., Jr. (1967). Air pollution damage to Austrian pine in New Jersey. *Plant Disease Reptr.* **51**, 964-967.

Brennan, E., and Leone, I. A. (1968). The response of plants to sulfur dioxide or ozone-polluted air supplied at varying flow rates. *Phytopathology* **58**, 1661-1664.

Brennan, E., Leone, I. A., and Daines, R. H. (1967). Characterization of the plant damage problem by air pollutants in New Jersey. *Plant Disease Reptr.* **51**, 850-854.

Daines, R. H., Leone, I. A., and Brennan, E. (1967). Air pollution and plant response in the Northeastern United States. *In* "Agriculture and the Quality of our Environment," *Publ. No.* 85, pp. 11-31. *Am. Assoc. Advance. Sci.*, Washington, D.C.

Darley, E. F. (1966). Studies on the effect of cement-kiln dust on vegetation. *J. Air Pollution Control Assoc.* **16**, 145-150.

Dochinger, L. S. (1968). The impact of air pollution on eastern white pine: The chlorotic dwarf disease. *J. Air Pollution Control Assoc.* **18**, 814-816.

Dugger, W. M., and Ting, I. P. (1968). The effect of peroxyacetyl nitrate on plants: Photoreductive reactions and susceptibility of bean plants to PAN. *Phytopathology* **58**, 1102-1107.

Gilbert, O. L. (1965). Lichens as indicators of air pollution in the Tyne Valley. *In* "Ecology and the Industrial Society" (G. T. Goodman, R. W. Edwards, and J. M. Lambert, eds.), pp. 35-46. Wiley, New York.

Hansbrough, J. R. (1967). Air quality and forestry. *In* "Agriculture and the Quality of Our Environment," *Publ. No.* 85, pp. 45-55. *Amer. Assoc. Advance. Sci.*, Washington, D.C.

Hepting, G. H. (1964). Damage to forests from air pollution. *J. Forestry* **62**, 630-634.

Hepting, G. H. (1966). Air pollution impacts to some important species of pine. *J. Air Pollution Control Assoc.* **16**, 63-65.

Hepting, G. H. (1968). Diseases of forest and tree crops caused by air pollutants. *Phytopathology* **58**, 1098-1101.

Hibben, C. R. (1969). Plant injury by oxidant-type pollutants in the New York City Atmosphere. *Plant Disease Reptr.* **53**, 544-548.

Johnson, K. L., Dworetzky, L. H., and Heller, A. N. (1968). Carbon monoxide and air pollution from automobile emissions in New York City. *Science* **160**, 67-68.

Lagerwerff, J. V. (1967). Heavy-metal contamination of soils. *In* "Agriculture and the Quality of Our Environment," *Publ. No.* 85, pp. 343-364. *Am. Assoc. Advance. Sci.*, Washington, D.C.

Landau, E. (1967). Economic aspects of air pollution as it relates to agriculture. In "Agriculture and the Quality of Our Environment," Publ. No. 85, pp. 113–126. Am. Assoc. Advance. Sci., Washington, D.C.

McCune, D. C., Weinstein, L. H., MacLean, D. C., and Jacobson, J. S. (1967). The concept of hidden injury to plants. In N. C. Brady, ed., "Agriculture and the Quality of Our Environment," Publ. No. 85, pp. 33–44. Am. Assoc. Advance. Sci., Washington, D.C.

Means, W. E., Jr., and Lacasse, N. L. (1969). Relative sensitivity of twelve tree species to hydrogen chloride gas. Phytopathology 59, 401 (abstr.).

Panofsky, H. A. (1969). Air pollution meteorology. Am. Scientist 57, 269–285.

Parmeter, J. R., Jr., and Miller, P. R. (1968). Studies relating to the cause of decline and death of ponderosa pine in Southern California. Plant Disease Reptr. 52, 707–711.

Rasmussen, R. A., and Went, F. W. (1965). Volatile organic material of plant origin in the atmosphere. Proc. Natl. Acad. Sci. U.S. 53, 214–224.

Rich, S., and Tomlinson, H. (1968). Effects of ozone on conidiophores and conidia of Alternaria solani. Phytopathology 58, 444–446.

Richards, B. L., Sr., Edmunds, G. F., Jr., and Taylor, O. C. (1966). Ozone needle mottle of pine. Phytopathology 56, 897 (abstr.).

Santamour, F. S., Jr. (1969). Air pollution studies on Plantanus and American elm seedlings. Plant Disease Reptr. 53, 482–484.

Scurfield, G. (1960). Air pollution and tree growth. Part I. Forestry Abstr. 21, 339–347.

Scurfield, G. (1960). Air pollution and tree growth. Part II. Forestry Abstr. 21, 517–528.

Sinclair, W. A. (1969). Polluted air: Potent new selective force in forests. J. Forestry 67, 305–309.

Smith, M. E. (1968). The influence of atmospheric dispersion on the exposure of plants to airborne pollutants. Phytopathology 58, 1085–1088.

Stephens, E. R., and Scott, W. E. (1962). Relative reactivity of various hydrocarbons in polluted atmosphere. Proc. Am. Petrol. Inst. 42, 665–670.

Stern, A. C., ed. (1968). "Air Pollution," 2nd ed., Vols. 1, 2, and 3. Academic Press, New York.

Taylor, O. C., Dugger, W. M., Jr., Thomas, M. D., and Thompson, C. R. (1961). Effect of atmospheric oxidants on apparent photosynthesis in citrus trees. Plant Physiol. 36, Suppl., p. xxvi–xxvii.

Thomas, M. D. (1961). Effects of air pollution on plants. World Health Organ., Monograph Ser. 46, 233–278.

Todd, G. W., and Arnold, W. N. (1961). An evaluation of methods used to determine injury to plant leaves by air pollutants. Botan. Gaz. 123, 151–154.

Treshow, M. (1968). The impact of air pollutants on plant populations. *Phytopathology* **58**, 1108–1113.

Went, F. W. (1955). Air pollution. *Sci. Am.* **192**, 62–72.

Went, F. W. (1960). Blue hazes in the atmosphere. *Nature* **187**, 641–643.

Wood, F. A., and Davis, D. D. (1969). The relative sensitivity of eighteen coniferous species to ozone. *Phytopathology* **59**, 1058 (abstr.).

7

MISCELLANEOUS ABIOTIC
AND LARGE ANIMAL STRESSES

In addition to the more common abiotic and biotic injury agents, several miscellaneous phenomena may cause occasional significant tree damage. Among the most important of these stresses are radiation, salt, pesticides, underground gas, insects, and animals.

I. RADIATION
Isotopes which are unstable undergo a decay process, that is, they lose mass and/or energy. Such atoms are said to be radioactive since they emit particles from their nuclei. The particles may be one or more of three varieties. Alpha particles are essentially helium nuclei and consist of two protons and two neutrons with a charge of +2. Beta particles may be electrons of very high energy content and possess a charge of -1 or high-speed electrons with a charge of $+1$, in which case they are termed positrons. Gamma particles are quanta of very high energy content and possess no charge (Bradshaw, 1966).

A. Dosage, Symptoms, and Mechanism of Radiation Damage
The unit of radiation dosage is the roentgen (r) which represents the quantity of radiation which will produce one electrostatic unit of positive or negative electricity in 1 cc of air at normal temperature and pressure. A dose of a few tenths of a roentgen per year constitutes the natural background radiation to which most plants and animals are exposed. Dental X-rays generally involve dosages in the 1-5 r range. Whole body exposure of 500-1000 r is usually fatal to man.

Pines are particularly sensitive to radiation. These species have been killed by 6 months exposure to 20–30 r per day (Woodwell, 1963). Gymnosperms are typically more sensitive than woody angiosperms. A positive correlation apparently exists between interphase chromosome volume and sensitivity (A. H. Sparrow et al., 1968). Woody species are, in general, approximately twice as sensitive as most herbaceous species, for reasons which remain unclear (R. C. Sparrow and Sparrow, 1965).

The symptoms of radiation damage are very striking and typically involve rapid and overall necrosis (Fig. 11).

The mechanism of radiation injury involves ion formation. All three particle types may possess high energy and are therefore capable of causing the ejection of electrons from molecules and atoms with which they collide. This type of interaction causes an ion pair to be formed with the remaining portion of the molecule possessing a positive charge. The term ionizing radiation stems from this ability to induce ion formation. An ion is very reactive chemically, and if a biological molecule becomes ionized in the above fashion, it may react with other compounds to form an aberrant or nonfunc-

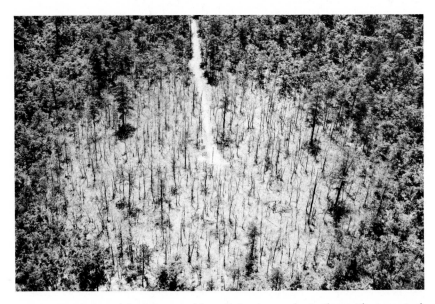

Fig. 11. Aerial view of damage caused by radiation in an oak-pine forest. The tower in the center of the photograph represents the position of a 9500 Curie ^{137}Ce gamma source which has radiated this forest for 20 hours every day since November 1961. At approximately 15 feet from the source, all trees are dead; at 300 feet, oak species survive but no living pine are present; and at 500 feet, the forest is essentially similar to unradiated areas. Exposure rates vary from several thousand roentgens per day close to the source to approximately 1.5 roentgens per day at 400 feet. (Photograph courtesy Brookhaven National Laboratory.)

tional molecule (Bradshaw, 1966). If very many critical molecules of a cell are thus taken from the supply of functional compounds, cell death may ensue.

B. Consequences

Low levels of ionizing radiation have, of course, been part of the terrestrial environment during the period in which life has evolved. Higher than background amounts, however, have resulted and may continue to result from fallout from nuclear explosions and from wastes of nuclear reactors. The detrimental influences of this radiation on vegetation has been documented.

In the event of nuclear war, or other circumstances resulting in widespread ionizing radiation, the typical North American forest would be damaged by exposures in the same range as those that approach lethal exposures in man. The ecosystems having the greatest chance for unaltered persistence in the event of widespread radiation are as follows (in decreasing order): desert, tundra, grassland, deciduous forest, and coniferous forest (Woodwell, 1963).

II. EXCESS SALT

The occurrence of salt in quantities damaging to vegetation is common in seacoast regions and along roadsides in areas of winter snow and ice.

A. Salt Spray

In regions adjacent to bodies of salt water, salt spray may be an important pathologic stress factor. Salt spray, in this context, is defined as salt water deposited by impact on vegetation. Salt spray has its beginning when waves trap air bubbles beneath the water surface. The air–water interface of these bubbles acts as a differentially permeable membrane, and salts (Table XIII) diffuse into the bubbles.

The ionic concentration of the air bubble may become very high. Eventually the bubble rises to the surface and its contained particles are ejected into the air. Evaporation of water from these particles during transportation causes them to become even more concentrated. The particles, because of their minute size, behave as aerosols and form near stable suspensions in the air. This stability permits transportation over considerable distances. The formation of salt spray is very much intensified during storm periods.

1. Symptoms. One of the most striking features of coastal vegetation which is exposed to salt spray is the frequent occurrence of plants which appear to have had portions of their aerial organs "sheared off." Asymmetrical growth habits develop due to the restriction of salt spray damage to the windward side of the plant. Other symptoms include necrotic leaves, frequently with initial scorch appearance, and twig necrosis.

TABLE XIII

MAJOR CONSTITUENTS OF SEA WATER[a]

Constituent	Concentration (Mole/liter)
H_2O	54.90
Na^+	0.470
Mg^{2+}	0.054
Ca^{2+}	0.010
K^+	0.009
Sr^{2+}	0.0001
Cl^-	0.548
SO_4^{2-}	0.0282
HCO_3^-	0.0023
Br^-	0.0008
F^-	0.00007
H_3BO_3	0.0004

[a]From Sillén (1961). Reproduced by permission of the American Association for the Advancement of Science.

2. *Mechanism.*   It is presumed that salt-spray injury is due primarily to excessive accumulation of toxic ions, especially Cl^-, from salts deposited on aerial organs. Boyce (1954) demonstrated that the heterotrophy of leaf tissue caused by exposure to salt spray did not occur until after uptake of chloride ions. Chloride, like fluoride, tends to migrate in the plant to leaf margins. It is interesting to note, however, that the chloride ions do not appear to be translocated to the leaves of the leeward side as injury is generally noted only on the windward exposure. An alternative and older hypothesis for the mechanism of salt-spray damage suggested that high osmotic pressures may result in ambient soil solutions. The soil of most maritime regions, however, is typically quite sandy and the leaching effect of rain undoubtedly minimizes soil salinity.

3. *Susceptibility.*   The hurricane that passed through New England in 1938 provided Wallace and Moss (1939) with a unique opportunity to study relative resistance to deposition of salt spray. The high wind velocity during the storm brought salt spray well inland and exposed a relatively large number of tree species. Ranking based on their observations are contained in Table XIV.

4. *Consequences.*   The potential significance of salt spray as a pathologic stress factor is very much enhanced by virtue of the ability of high-velocity storm winds to carry the spray inland. In addition to the work by Wallace and Moss (1939), Little et al. (1958) discussed foliar necrosis of loblolly pines, growing within 2 miles of Chesapeake Bay, caused during an October hurricane in 1954.

TABLE XIV

RELATIVE SUSCEPTIBILITY TO SALT SPRAY INJURY DURING THE
1938 HURRICANE[a]

Susceptible	Intermediate	Resistant
1. Conifers		
White pine	Northern white	Colorado blue
Eastern red cedar	cedar	spruce
Atlantic white cedar		Austrian pine
Hemlock		Yew
Scotch pine		
2. Hardwoods		
Norway maple		Horse chestnut
Sugar maple		
Elm		
Magnolia		
Yellow poplar		

[a]From Wallace and Moss (1939). Reproduced by permission of International
Shade Tree Conference, Inc.

Salt spray plays a fundamental role in the ecology of coastal plant communities. Martin (1959), for example, concluded that salt spray intensity, not
biotic succession, is the factor largely responsible for the existence of herbaceous, shrubby, and arborescent vegetation zones on Island Beach (a barrier
bar) in New Jersey (Fig. 12).

B. Road Salt

Increasing traffic and demand for ice-free roads has led to increased em-
ployment of sodium chloride (rock salt — NaCl) and calcium chloride ($CaCl_2$)
for efficient and economical deicing of roadways. The United States con-
sumption of salt for deicing was estimated at over 6 million tons in 1966-67.
In Canada, an additional 1.2 million tons were employed (Dickinson, 1968).
In Connecticut, 70,000 tons of rock salt, 2500 tons of $CaCl_2$, and 309,000
cubic yards of sand are used annually on approximately 4500 miles of
highway (Button and Peaslee, 1967). In 1957, the New Hampshire Highway
Department reported that it spent 1 million dollars to remove 13,997 dead
trees along 3700 miles of highway (Rich, 1968). While the cause of death
was not specified, evidence has been presented to indicate that roadside tree
mortality may in some measure be due to roadway salt applications.

1. Symptoms.   Trees only slightly damaged generally exhibit leaf scorch
and/or early autumn coloration. More severely affected individuals may

exhibit defoliation, reduced shoot growth, and dieback of twigs and branches (Fig. 13). In certain instances death may be induced.

2. *Mechanism.*   The mechanism of salt toxicity is unresolved. At least four hypotheses have been advanced to account for the detrimental influence of roadway salt (Westing, 1969). Salt may reduce soil quality. Excessive sodium, for example, may cause soil structure deterioration. Salt may increase moisture stress during drought periods. This may result as the osmotic concentration of the soil solution is raised. Salt may result in nutrient

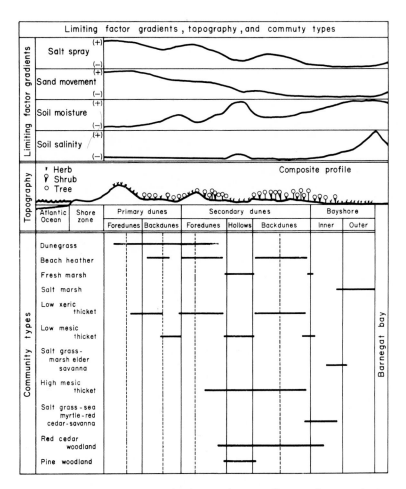

Fig. 12.   The interrelation of topography, limiting factor gradients, and community types on an Atlantic coast barrier bar. [From Martin (1959). Reproduced by permission of Ecological Society of America.]

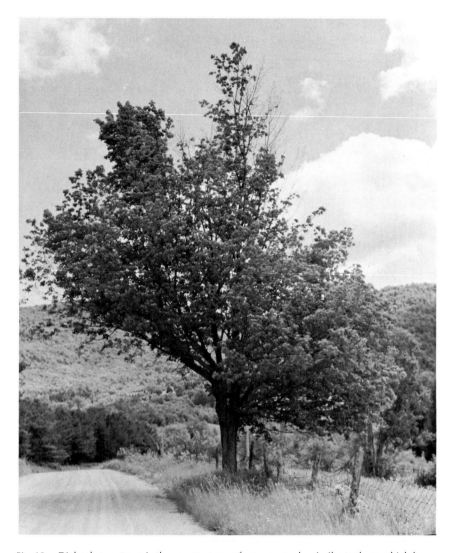

Fig. 13. Dieback symptoms in the upper crown of a sugar maple, similar to those which have been suggested to result from injury caused by winter applications of salt to roadways for snow and ice removal. (Photograph courtesy U.S. Forest Service.)

imbalances. High sodium content, for example, may lower uptake of potassium. Accumulation of sodium, chloride, and calcium ions may cause direct injury in leaves and twigs.

3. *Susceptibility.* Extensive study of relative resistance to roadway salt has not been undertaken. Rich (1968) has listed Norway maple and oak spe-

cies more tolerant than white pine, hemlock, and balsam fir. Red pine appears to be somewhat intermediate. In a study of salt damage to roadside vegetation in the Washington, D.C. area, Wester and Cohen (1968) found injury particularly prevalent on hemlock, elm, sugar maple, and linden.

4. *Discussion.*   The evidence presented relating to roadside vegetation and injury by deicing salts has been somewhat contradictory.

Holmes (1961) conducted a 7 year test of applications of NaCl and $CaCl_2$ to the bases of maple, oak, hickory, black birch, ash, and white pine and concluded that road salting would probably do little harm to these species. Holmes felt that most of the Cl^- taken up by the deciduous trees, being concentrated in the leaves, would be lost when the leaves were shed. An additional factor cited by the author which might act to mitigate the influence of salt was the fact that the frozen ground inhibits penetration and may cause harmless runoff. This same study, currently in its fourteenth year of weekly, winter salt application, has still not resulted in foliar symptoms of salt injury.

Lacasse and Rich (1964), on the other hand, conducted a study in New Hampshire to evaluate the role of NaCl in the decline of roadside sugar maples. These investigators found that the twigs, which are of course not shed, as well as the leaves contained above normal amounts of Na^+. While the injury mechanism was not known, it was proposed that Na^+ may act to antagonize the uptake or utilization of essential elements and thereby induce a nutrient imbalance. These investigators presented some striking correlations between leaf and twig Na^+ contents and symptom expression.

Holmes and Baker (1966) felt that it was an oversimplification and misconception to conclude that Lacasse and Rich had shown that roadside maple decline was due to salt injury. Even though the New Hampshire investigators were able to show a correlation between foliar ion concentrations and foliar injury, Holmes and Baker suggested that numerous roadside trees in their studies lacked excessive ion accumulation and injury symptoms. Holmes and Baker suggested that damage was probably quite variable from site to site and may depend on: amount of salt applied, timing of application (for example before or after plowing), quality and drainage of soil, aspect and slope of terrain, depth and duration of soil freezing, amount of snow runoff prior to ground thaw, and inherent susceptibility of the individual tree.

Button and Peaslee (1967), in a recent Connecticut study, selected a portion of highway where sugar maples on opposite sides of the road were in various degrees of health. Trees on the west side of the highway received more pavement drainage and displayed more leaf scorch and dieback than did trees on the east side. Sodium and chloride contents of leaves of the two groups established that the concentration of these ions increased with increasing exposure to road drainage and with increasing deterioration of tree health.

Working with Norway maple, Walton (1969) has recently presented evidence suggesting that $CaCl_2$ may be somewhat more phytotoxic than NaCl. Westing (1969), on the other hand, has proposed that the use of a calcium salt along with NaCl may lessen the damaging influences of rock salt. The calcium ion, for example, might displace the sodium ion from exchange sites in the soil. Excessive sodium in the soil is known to be detrimental to soil structure. In addition, the calcium may reduce the uptake of sodium by plant roots.

In an effort to reduce and avoid salt injury to roadside trees, new materials such as lime and gypsum should be tested for deicing, less susceptible trees such as *Quercus* spp. should be employed for roadside planting, and trees should be restricted from a 40 ft zone on either side of the paved portion of new, primary roadways.

III. PESTICIDES

The current widespread use of various chemicals to control vegetation and plant pests has resulted in numerous instances of tree damage.

A. Herbicides

Since the discovery approximately 40 years ago that indole acetic acid (IAA) is one of the principal growth-controlling factors in plants, considerable effort has been directed at finding application for related materials in vegetation control. Certain derivatives of indole acetic acid have been found to be extremely effective as growth inhibitors and herbicides. In particular, 2,4-dichlorophenoxyacetic acid (2,4-D) and its various close derivatives, for example 2,4,5-T, have had outstanding commercial success as weed and brush killers.

$$O - CH_2 - COOH$$

Cl

Cl

2, 4-D

The 2,4-D and related materials are particularly valuable because of their selective toxic action. They will, for example, kill many dicotyledonous plants without serious damage to cereals or grasses. Their application in forest practice has been largely in chemical thinning operations and in the release of coniferous species from hardwood competition. Government and utility organizations have used herbicides in restricting the growth of vegetation along roadways and power lines, respectively.

Unfortunately, these substances are sometimes carelessly applied and may be distributed to areas where they cause significant damage. Even when applied on windless days, thermal updrafts created by rising warm air may carry spray materials aloft and distribute them in undesirable areas. Root translocation may also distribute these compounds to plants unintended to receive them via root grafts.

Symptoms of herbicide damage frequently involve rapid necrosis of exposed parts. Injury induced by hormonal derivatives normally takes the form of extreme distortion of those parts of the tree which were actively growing at the time of poisoning. With greater exposure dieback may occur.

An unexplained "blight" of boxelder in the northern great plains has been attributed to careless application of 2,4-D (Phipps, 1963). Leaf necrosis of the boxelders, which are extensively employed in this region as windbreaks, resulted when 2,4-D applied aerially to crops drifted and intercepted the trees.

Fenton (1965) has described damage to a sweetgum stand thinned with frill (wound made around a tree stem in order to introduce a chemical) application of 2,4,5-T. In addition to killing unwanted trees, several crop trees were also killed apparently due to translocation of the herbicide through root grafts.

In the herbicidal treatment of roadside and right-of-way areas, it is extremely important to use low-volatile materials, to employ basal and stump sprays where possible, and avoid stem–foliar spray applications of unselective chemicals. The use of foliar roadside spray has been shown to cause tree damage as far as 300 feet back from the point of application (Niering, 1959). Nonselective stem–foliage spray applications also often exceed a height of 4 feet (Goodwin and Niering, 1962) and result in unwanted damage along roadways.

B. Fungicides and Insecticides

Damage frequently results when these compounds are applied in excessive amounts or when applied during unappropriate environmental circumstances.

Fungicides containing copper or polysulphides are particularly liable to be phytotoxic.

Insecticides are occasionally injurious because of the vehicle employed to render them soluble or aid in their application. Substances like DDT, for example, may be first dissolved in xylene or benzene and then diluted with diesel or fuel oil. Benzene, xylene, and oil (even refined light oils) can cause acute injury to plants. Organochlorine insecticides (for example, DDT) because of their considerable persistence may accumulate in trees and cause subtle physiological abnormalities.

IV. UNDERGROUND GAS

The widespread transportation and distribution of both natural and manufactured gas in underground systems has occasionally resulted in plant damage when pipe leakage has occurred. Natural gas, which is generally thought to be the less toxic of the two, contains primarily methane and ethane. Both of these gases are phytotoxic. Small impurities in the gas, however, may also contribute to the toxic effect. Manufactured gas may contain traces of hydrogen cyanide, carbon monoxide, and ethylene, all of which are quite poisonous. Effects of gas leakage are frequently extremely sudden and yellowing, wilting, and death may rapidly occur.

V. LARGE ANIMAL STRESS

Certain animals exert deleterious influences on tree health which are commonly overlooked. Storm and Halvorson (1967) have described the significant influence porcupines have on the radial growth of ponderosa pine. The feeding habits of woodpeckers and related birds cause considerable wood defect and may provide ingress routes for fungi and bacteria. The yellow-bellied sapsucker, which ranges over most of the important forest regions of North America, is known to damage at least 174 tree species (Northeastern Forest Experiment Station, 1967). Parker (1947), in an interesting discourse, reviews the damage caused to forest trees by various wild animals.

Insects, in addition to their substantial importance in direct tree damage, also are extremely important in predisposing trees to additional damage by disease agents and in acting as vectors for the transmission of these agents.

Not to be overlooked, of course, is the importance of man himself as a perpetrator of tree injury and damage.

REFERENCES

Boyce, S. G. (1954). The salt spray community. *Ecol. Monographs* **25**, 29–67.

Bradshaw, L. J. (1966). "Introduction to Molecular Biological Techniques." Prentice-Hall, Englewood Cliffs, New Jersey.

Button, E. F., and Peaslee, D. E. (1967). "The Effect of Rock Salt Upon Roadside Sugar Maples in Connecticut," *Highway Res. Record No. 161. Highway Res. Board, Natl. Acad. Sci.,* Washington, D.C.

Dickinson, W. E. (1968). Snow and ice control — a critical look at is critics. *Proc. Symp. Pollutants Roadside Environ., Univ. Conn., Feb. 29, 1968* pp. 6-14.

Fenton, R. H. (1965). Root grafts and translocation of 2,4,5-T in young sweetgum stands. *J. Forestry* **63**, 17-18.

Goodwin, R. H., and Niering, W. A. (1962). What is happening along Connecticut's roadsides? *Bull. Connecticut Arboretum* **13**, 13-19.

Holmes, F. W. (1961). Salt injury to trees. *Phytopathology* **51**, 712-718.

Holmes, F. W., and Baker, J. H. (1966). Salt injury to trees. II. Sodium and chloride in roadside sugar maples in Massachusetts. *Phytopathology* **56**, 633-636.

Lacasse, N. L., and Rich, A. E. (1964). Maple decline in New Hampshire. *Phytopathology* **54**, 1071-1075.

Little, S., Mohr, J. J., and Spicer, L. L. (1958). Salt-water storm damage to loblolly pine forests. *J. Forestry* **56**, 27-28.

Martin, W. E. (1959). The vegetation of Island Beach State Park. *Ecol. Monographs* **29**, 1-46.

Niering, W. A. (1959). A potential danger of broadcast sprays. *Bull. Connecticut Arboretum* **11**, 11-13.

Northeastern Forest Experiment Station. (1967). *Ann. Rept., Northeast Forest Expt. Sta.* pp. 1-98.

Parker, J. (1947). Damage to forest trees by wild animals in the North Temperate zone. M. F. thesis, Yale School of Forestry.

Phipps, H. M. (1963). The role of 2,4-D in the appearance of a leaf blight of some plains tree species. *Forest Sci.* **9**, 283-288.

Rich, A. E. (1968). Effect of de-icing chemicals on woody plants. *Proc. Symp. Pollutants Roadside Environ., Univ. Conn., Feb. 29, 1968* pp. 46-47.

Sillén, L. G. (1961). The physical chemistry of sea water. *In* "Oceanography," *Publ. No. 67*, pp. 549-581. *Am. Assoc. Advance. Sci.,* Washington, D.C.

Sparrow, A. H., Rogers, A. F., and Schwemmer, S. S. (1968). Radiosensitivity studies with woody plants. I. Acute gamma irradiation survival data for 28 species and predictions for 190 species. *Radiation Botany* **8**, 149-186.

Sparrow, R. C., and Sparrow, A. H. (1965). Relative radiosensitivities of woody and herbaceous spermatophytes. *Science* **147**, 1449-1451.

Storm, G. L., and Halvorson, C. H. (1967). Effect of injury by porcupines on radial growth of ponderosa pine. *J. Forestry* **65**, 740-743.

Wallace, R. H., and Moss, A. E. (1939). Salt spray damage from recent New England hurricane. *Proc. 15th Natl. Shade Tree Conf., Aug. 1939,* New York, N.Y., p. 112-119.

Walton, G. S. (1969). Phytotoxicity of NaCl and $CaCl_2$ to Norway maples. *Phytopathology* **59**, 1412-1415.

Wester, H. V., and Cohen, E. E. (1968). Salt damage to vegetation in the Washington, D.C. area during the 1966-67 winter. *Plant Disease Reptr.* **52**, 350-354.

Westing, A. H. (1969). Plants and salt in the roadside environment. *Phytopathology* **59**, 1174-1181.

Woodwell, G. M. (1963). The ecological effects of radiation. *Sci. Am.* **208**, 40-49.

GENERAL REFERENCES

Aldous, C. M., and Aldous, S. E. (1944). The snowshoe hare—a serious enemy of forest plantations. *J. Forestry* **42**, 88-94.

Baron, F. J., Stark, N., and Schubert, G. H. (1964). Effects of season and rate of application of 2,4-D and 2,4,5-T on pine seedings and mountain white-thorn in California. *J. Forestry* **62**, 472-474.

Campana, R. J. (1969). Influence of chronic gamma radiation on development of Dutch elm disease. *Phytopathology* **59**, 398 (abstr.).

Caro, J. H. (1969). Accumulation by plants of organochlorine insecticides from the soil. *Phytopathology* **59**, 1191-1197.

Crouch, G. L. (1969). Animal damage to conifers on National Forests in the Pacific Northwest region. *Res. Bull., Pacific Northwest Forest Range Expt. Sta.* **PNW-28**, 1-13.

Daines, R. H. (1952). 2,4-D as an air pollutant and its effect on various species of plants. *In* "Air Pollution," *Proc. U.S. Tech. Conf. Air Pollution, 1950,* pp. 140-143. McGraw-Hill, New York.

Egler, F. E. (1947). Effects of 2,4-D on woody plants in Connecticut. *J. Forestry* **45**, 449-452.

Fraley, L., Jr., Ragsdale, H. L., Taylor, F. G., Jr., Witherspoon, J. P., and Johnson, D. E. (1967). Response of plants to ionizing radiation. *In* "Health Physics Division Annual Progress Report for Period Ending July 31, 1967," ORNL-4168, pp. 72-78. Oak Ridge Natl. Lab., Oak Ridge, Tennessee.

Goodwin, R. H., and Niering, W. A. (1959). A roadside crisis: The use and abuse of herbicides. *Bull. Connecticut Arboretum* **11**, 1-13.

International Atomic Energy Agency. (1966). "Effects of Low Doses of Radiation on Crop Plants," Tech. Rept. Ser. No. 64. I.A.E.A., Vienna.

LaHaye, P. A., and Epstein, E. (1969). Salt toleration by plants: Enhancement with calcium. *Science* **166**, 395-396.

Lutz, H. J. (1951). Damage to trees by black bears in Alaska. *J. Forestry* **49**, 522-523.

Menzel, R. G. (1967). Airborne radionuclides and plants. *In* "Agriculture and the Quality of Our Environment," *Publ. No.* 85, pp. 57-75. Am. Assoc. Advance. Sci., Washington, D.C.

Molberg, J. M. (1960). Cautions on use of herbicides. *J. Forestry* **58**, 124.

Moss, A. E. (1940). Effect on trees of wind-driven salt water. *J. Forestry* **38**, 421–425.

Niering, W. A. (1968). The effects of pesticides. *BioScience* **18**, 869–874.

Oliver, W. W. (1968). Sapsucker damage to ponderosa pine. *J. Forestry* **66**, 842–844.

Pollard, E. C. (1969). The biological action of ionizing radiation. *Am. Scientist* **57**, 206–236.

Radwan, M. A. (1969). Chemical composition of the sapwood of four tree species in relation to feeding by the black bear. *Forest Sci.* **15**, 11–16.

Rudolf, P. O., and Watt, R. F. (1956). Chemical control of brush and trees in the Lake States. *Sta. Paper, Lake States Forest Expt. Sta.,* **41**, 1–58.

Sheets, T. J. (1967). The extent and seriousness of pesticide buildup in soils. *In* "Agriculture and the Quality of our Environment," *Publ. No. 85*, pp. 311–330. *Am. Assoc. Advance. Sci.,* Washington, D.C.

Shigo, A. L., and Kilham, L. (1968). Sapsuckers and *Fomes igniarius* var. *populinus. Res. Note, Northeast. For. Exp. Sta.,* **NE-84**, 1–2.

Sparrow, A. H., Binnington, J. P., and Pond, V. "Bibliography on the Effects of Ionizing Radiations on Plants," BNL 504. Brookhaven Natl. Lab. Upton, New York.

Staley, J. M., Altman, J., and Spotts, R. A. (1968). A sodium-linked disease of ponderosa pine in Denver, Colorado. *Plant Disease Reptr.* **52**, 908–910.

Wells, B. W., and Shunk, I. V. (1938). Salt-spray: An important factor in coastal ecology. *Bull. Torrey Botan. Club* **65**, 485–592.

Woodwell, G. M. (1967). Radiation and the patterns of nature. *Science* **156**, 461–470.

PART II

Biotic Stress Agents

8

NEMATODES

Nematodes, which are frequently referred to as thread- or eelworms, are a group of organisms which are apparently not closely related to any other group of animals. Nematodes are "wormlike" and have their organs arranged in bilateral order. Several species are predators and parasites of animals, and many are parasitic on plants. They occupy almost every conceivable habitat, including fresh water, salt water, and soil. Almost any environment with sufficient moisture and source of organic food supply will support a nematode population.

I. CLASSIFICATION

Controversy exists concerning whether nematodes should be merely given class status (Nemata, Nematoda) or phylum rank (Nemathelminthes). There is also some difference of opinion at the order level of classification. The majority of plant parasitic species, however, occur in the order Tylenchida. A few are also contained in the order Dorylaimida. Both of these orders are distinguished by the possession of a mouth spear. In the Tylenchida, the spear is a hollow cuticular structure usually with basal knobs. The spear of Dorylaimida members, on the other hand, develops subventrally from a tooth or teeth and is often asymmetrical, with basal knobs usually absent.

In total there may be in excess of 500,000 nematode species. Approximately 11,000 have been described. Of this 11,000, Nielsen (1967) suggests that approximately 2000 inhabit the soil and the rest are parasites of vertebrates or invertebrates or occur in the sea. In terms of plant disease the soil inhabitors are most important.

II. MORPHOLOGY AND ANATOMY

The typical nematode is spindle shaped, unsegmented, and bilaterally symmetrical. Plant parasitic nematodes are generally 200-2000 microns in length and 10-40 microns in width. (Figs. 14 and 15.)

a. Cuticle. The outermost layer, or cuticle, is composed of a cortex, a

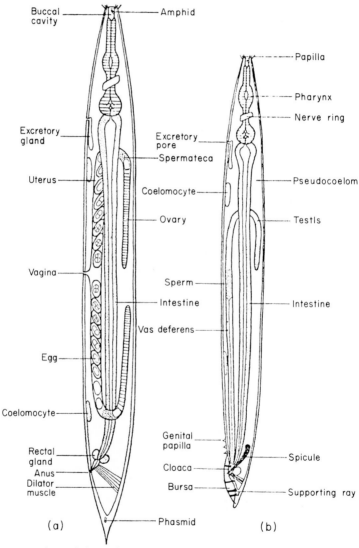

Fig. 14.   General morphology of a nematode (a) female; (b) male. [From Lee (1965). Reproduced by permission of Oliver and Boyd, Ltd.]

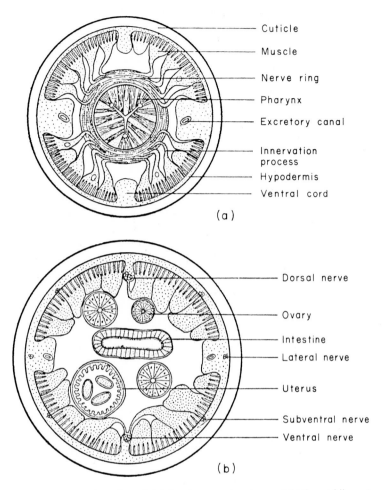

Cuticle

Muscle

Nerve ring

Pharynx

Excretory canal

Innervation process

Hypodermis

Ventral cord

(a)

Dorsal nerve

Ovary

Intestine

Lateral nerve

Uterus

Subventral nerve

Ventral nerve

(b)

Fig. 15. Transverse sections through (a) the pharyngeal region and (b) the middle region of a nematode. [From Lee (1965). Reproduced by permission of Oliver and Boyd, Ltd.]

matrix, and a fiber layer. The cortex has been shown to contain collagen and certain phenolic compounds. The matrix is made up of low molecular weight albumen-like proteins and also some fibrous proteins which resemble fibroin or elastin. Staining properties and X-ray diffraction studies suggest that the fiber layer consists of collagen. The presence of enzymes in the cuticle indicates that this region is metabolically active and not merely an inert covering.

b. Hypodermis. The hypodermis is a cellular layer beneath the cuticle that projects into the body cavity along the middorsal, midventral, and lateral lines to form four ridges, or cords, inside the body. The hypodermis contains large amounts of reserve storage materials.

c. Nervous system. The nematode nerve system is incompletely understood. It is known to consist of a circumpharyngeal nerve ring with associated ganglia. Large ventral and smaller lateral and dorsal nerves run posteriorly from the nerve ring along the cords of the hypodermis. Several nerves extend to the anterior end, where they innervate the sense organs around the mouth. In many plant parasitic nematode species, however, it has been possible to see only the nerve ring.

d. Muscle system. Body muscles consist of a single layer of elongated cells which are attached to the hypodermis. They are distributed in four longitudinal bands which run the length of the body between the hypodermis cords. There are no circular muscles. Locomotion is accomplished in three ways: serpentine movements in the dorsoventral plane, ambulatory movements on the ventral or dorsal side, and contraction–extension of the body. Active movement by the worms themselves may occasion migration of only a few feet per season. Passive movement by water, wind, or animals, however, may transport nematodes considerable distances (Agrios, 1969).

e. Alimentary system. Food is taken into the mouth, passed through the pharynx and intestine, and waste materials released through the rectum to the anus. The mouth is surrounded by "lips" that may have a sensing function. In plant parasitic nematodes, a mouth spear is present which can be protruded to penetrate tissues during feeding and/or invasion. The pharynx acts as a powerful pumping organ. This organ is also glandular and may have secretory importance. The intestine, which is essentially a straight tube, is lined by microvilli and is thought to have both absorptive and secretory functions. Very little is known concerning the absorption of food materials, but most evidence indicates that primary absorption of food is through the intestine and not through the cuticle. It is interesting to note that systems for the excretion of waste materials by nematodes are quite variable and in some species appear to be completely absent.

f. Reproductive system. In general, most species have separate sexes. In some varieties, however, parthenogenetic females occur in which case eggs develop without male fertilization. Hermaphroditic groups, in which both sexes occur in the same animal, are also known. In this instance the gonads initially produce sperm and later eggs. Males, which are frequently smaller than females, have one or two testes that produce ameoboid sperm. Females generally have one or two egg-producing ovaries. In some species of nematodes, the sex ratio is density dependent and may be controlled by nutritional factors. In large populations and under conditions of favorable nutrition, more males are generally formed than under adverse conditions. All nematodes have the same basic life cycle, involving an egg, four larval, and an adult stage. Each larval stage is separated by a moult, during which the larva undergoes certain morphological changes and grows another cuticle. Under favorable conditions a complete life cycle will span approximately 4 weeks (Agrios, 1969).

g. General anatomical. The body cavity, which is filled with fluid, is termed the pseudocoelom. In addition to the organ systems described the pseudocoleum contains large fixed cells, called coelomocytes, whose function is unknown. Hypothetical functions are: phagocytic (destroy bacteria), storage of insoluble wastes, absorptive (purification of body fluid), and/or secretory (enzyme release). The fluid which bathes all internal organs is complex and contains: proteins, fats, carbohydrates, inorganic ions, various nitrogenous compounds, and enzymes. The fact that this fluid is always under pressure, due to the tonicity of the body muscles, is of great importance in locomotion, feeding, and excretion.

III. PHYSIOLOGY

Nematodes feed upon a wide variety of foods, but most individual species are restricted to one type of food. Food is invariably "protoplasm" of one kind or other. It may be, for example, plant sap or cell contents from fungi, algae, bacteria, actinomycetes, animals, or plants. Dead organic matter of animal or plant origin is not a part of nematode diets, although it is a substratum for organisms on which nematodes feed (Nielsen, 1967). Phytophagous types may be either ectoparasites or endoparasites.

Ectoparasites feed externally upon the cells or vascular tissue of plants in a fashion similar to that of aphids. In the case of root feeding, a puncture is made by repeatedly thrusting the mouth spear at a weak area, for example, the junction of a lateral root. When penetration is accomplished, saliva is discharged through the stylet into the plant. Cellulase, chitinase, pectinase, and amylase, along with other hydrolytic enzymes, have been shown to be present in this saliva. These enzymes act to soften plant cell walls and bring about preliminary digestion. The sucking action of the pharynx then withdraws food materials from the host.

Endoparasites actually migrate into the plant and feed internally. Entrance is gained by direct penetration or through natural (lenticels and stomata) or wound openings. Once in the host, some endoparasites move around and feed on various cells and others show less movement and induce the formation of "giant cells." Giant cells result when the worms destroy several cell walls in one particular area and maintain turgor pressure through hydrolytic action.

Carbon dioxide is produced by all nematodes and is actually excreted through the general body surface. Oxygen, the uptake of which is fairly high, also travels from the external environment across the body wall to internal organs by diffusion. There is no circulatory system. Many nematode habitats are completely devoid of oxygen and, in this case, the organisms must obtain their energy requirements from fermentations. Evidence indicating the operation of anaerobic glycolysis and the aerobic tricarboxylic acid cycle has been obtained for nematode species.

IV. ECOLOGY

This discussion of ecological relationships will be in reference to plant parasitic species and will involve consideration of the soil environment, population dynamics, and the plant environment.

A. Soil Environment

The soil habitat is one of *extreme* complexity. In this brief review we will be concerned with only four major physical parameters. The low soil temperature range, over which most phytoparasitic nematodes become inactive, is approximately 5°–15°C. The optimum temperature range is between 15° and 30°C, and inactivity for most species is occasioned between 30° and 40°C. Individual nematode species may have very variable temperature relationships. Cardinal temperature ranges may vary with the age of the worm. Usually, however, the tolerance of the nematode is related to and often exceeds that of its host plant. Temperature relationships may be somewhat less important in forest soils than arable soils as the fluctuations and extremes are less in the former.

Although there is considerable variation in tolerance to dehydration and saturation among nematode species, conditions of soil moisture are of critical importance to these animals. Nematodes are entirely dependent on water for most of their activities; they characteristically live in a water film and are restricted to habitats with a saturated atmosphere. For several phytoparasitic nematodes, the relationships between the moisture characteristic and the curves for larval emergence, plant invasion, and mobility are very similar. Each species has an optimum soil moisture status for various activities. It is probable, however, that any nematode activity of the sort which involves bodily movement will be at a maximum when the soil pores are empty but where water still remains at the points of contact of soil crumbs. In general, such conditions probably occur at moisture contents slightly below field capacity (water remaining in soil after the water freely drained by gravity has been removed).

Since nematodes cannot modify soil structure, they are limited to the existing labyrinth of pore spaces. In general, light sandy soils are thought to be more favorable to many root feeding species, while closer textured soils are less favorable. The major effect of pore size on nematode activity is in its influence on soil moisture and aeration.

Aeration is an exceedingly variable aspect of any particular soil. In heavy, wet soils, anaerobic conditions may prevail. Sandy soils, however, may have atmospheres similar to the above-ground environment. There is some evidence to suggest that conditions which reduce aeration also have a tendency to decrease nematode activity. This may be due to decreased oxygen availability, increased carbon dioxide concentration, accumulation of toxic materials, or an interaction of the above.

In addition to physical aspects, the biological condition of the soil is of fundamental importance in the ecology of nematodes. The zone of maximum biotic soil activity, the rhizosphere, is of particular importance in respect to phytoparasitic species. The rhizosphere may be defined as that region of soil under the influence of plant roots. The roots are capable of modifying the soil environment in their immediate vicinity by lowering the concentration of mineral nutrients, depleting soil moisture, raising carbon dioxide tension, altering pH toward neutrality, and exuding various organic and inorganic compounds. These alterations, the latter two in particular, result in a congregation of many soil microbes and other organisms, including some nematodes, at the root-soil interface (rhizoplane) and to a certain extent in the rhizosphere proper. In this region of biotic concentration the phenomena of association, antagonism, and competition are intense and incompletely appreicated. There is considerable evidence, however, that certain root exudate components may exert a stimulatory effect on germination of the eggs of several nematode species. These exudates may also act to attract and orient larvae.

B. Population Dynamics

The study of the population dynamics of soil nematodes is in a young stage. In general, it is felt that the physical properties of the soil determine, within broad limits, the species of nematodes that can live and reproduce in any particular soil. (In the case of phytoparasitic species, however, the actual species which develop are also very closely related to the host plants growing in the region.) It is plants themselves, even in the instance of nonparasitic species, which either directly or indirectly provide the primary food supply. Population estimates for particular areas are exceedingly diverse. In general, it has been suggested that pasture or uncultivated soils may have 2–20 million worms per square meter, while arable or cultivated land may average 1–5 million per square meter. Forest soils may have the largest populations; Nielsen (1967) has suggested populations of up to 30 million worms per square meter for oak forest and up to 12 million in the humus of a birch forest.

As with all animals, numerous factors interact in a complex manner to regulate population balance. Those factors of particular importance which are said to be independent of nematode density might include soil climate and food quality. Soil climate has been previously discussed. Food quality is of extreme importance in the case of plant parasites, since some species appear quite specific in their requirements. The basic mechanisms operative in host–parasite interaction are not fully understood. Krusberg (1967) has recently reviewed the influence of host physiology on nematode populations.

More information is available relating to the significance of factors dependent upon population density to population mechanics. In this group, the two most important might be natural enemies and food quantity. Specific enemies, rather than food restrictions, are generally felt to be more important in natural soils. Natural enemies are usually thought to exert their restrictive influence prior to exhaustion of food supply. Examples of enemies which directly cause nematode mortality include: viruses, protozoa, arthropods, and fungi. Little research has been done on nematode viruses, but considerable circumstantial evidence suggests their potential importance. Numerous protozoa are known to feed on nematodes. In the case of arthropods, certain Collembola feed on nematode cysts. Certain fungi are among the most interesting, if not the most important, nematode predators. These soil fungi obtain their nutrition by catching worms in sticky or ring traps and then digesting their contents. *Arthrobotrys oligospora* is an example of a fungus which produces sticky traps. The hyphae of this fungus form an anastomosing network of loops in the soil. These loops are sticky and nematodes are held in them by an adhesive fluid secreted by the loop cells. Within 2 hours of capture, hyphae will penetrate the nematode cuticle. Ring traps produced, for example by *Dactylaria candida*, are developed when a mycelial branch forms a three-celled ring. When the nematode enters the ring the cells inflate to approximately three times their original size. In addition to these trapping fungi, other species are internal parasites of nematodes.

Increased use of various soil insecticides and soil fumigants may upset the balance of soil fauna and flora and may, in certain instances, result in increased nematode populations in reaction to reduced predator and parasite populations (Harrison, 1967).

C. Plant environment

The ecological relations of endoparasitic nematodes and their host plants is very poorly understood. Internal plant environment is primarily determined by inherent plant characteristics. Host–parasite relationships are often finely balanced and may be upset by a change in a single gene. Soil, macroclimate, and biotic factors, however, effect the plant and undoubtedly in some measure influence the parasite within.

V. NEMATODES AND TREE PATHOLOGY

Nematodes most assuredly have significance in tree disease considerably in excess of current concepts. They are directly damaging by virtue of their feeding and life cycle habits. Reduced growth resulting from mass feeding may be particularly deleterious to marginal trees. The greatest importance of nematodes to tree health, however, may be in their secondary effects. The feeding wounds caused by nematodes may provide entry courts for root infecting microbes. In addition, nematodes may function to transmit viruses from tree to tree.

Disruption of mycorrhizal relationships may be an extremely important indirect influence of nematode infection. Zak (1967) has observed *Meloidodera* sp. infecting Douglas fir mycorrhizae. Although mycorrhizae have been shown to be affected, it has only recently been demonstrated that the nematodes may feed directly on the mycorrhizal fungi. Sutherland and Fortin (1968) showed that the mycophagous nematode *Aphelenchus avenae* could feed and reproduce on seven species of ectotrophic mycorrhizal fungi grown *in vitro*. Riffle (1967) found that an undescribed *Aphelenchoides* sp. greatly reduced the diameter growth of mycelium of two mycorrhizal fungi of ponderosa pine. The author suggested that this nematode may play an indirect role in the premature mortality of low-elevation ponderosa pine following droughts in New Mexico.

On the positive side, nematodes may act to reduce the significance of certain diseases caused by the fungi upon which they feed. Klink and Barker (1968) have suggested that *Aphelenchus avenae* may be capable of controlling certain dampingoff fungi.

REFERENCES

Agrios, G. N. (1969). "Plant Pathology." Academic Press, New York.

Harrison, M. B. (1967). Influence of nematocidal treatments on nematode populations. *Phytopathology* **57**, 650-652.

Klink, J. W., and Barker, K. R. (1968). Effect of *Aphelenchus avenae* on the survival and pathogenic activity of root-rotting fungi. *Phytopathology* **58**, 228-232.

Krusberg, L. R. (1967). Influence of host physiology on nematode populations. *Phytopathology* **57**, 653-655.

Lee, D. L. (1965). "The Physiology of Nematodes." Freeman, San Francisco, California.

Nielsen, G. O. (1967). Nematoda. *In* "Soil Biology" (N. A. Burges and F. Raw, eds.), pp. 197-211. Academic Press, New York.

Riffle, J. W. (1967). Effect of an *Aphelenchoides* species on the growth of a mycorrhizal and a pseudomycorrhizal fungus. *Phytopathology* **57**, 541-544.

Sutherland, J. R., and Fortin, J. A. (1968). Effect of the nematode *Aphelenchus avenae* on some ectotrphic mycorrihizal fungi and on a red pine mycorrhizal relationship. *Phytopathology* **58**, 519-523.

Zak, B. (1967). A nematode (*Meloidodera* sp.) on Douglas-fir mycorrhizae. *Plant Disease Reptr.* **51**, 264.

GENERAL REFERENCES

Cooke, R. C., and Pramer, D. (1968). *Monacrosporium rutgeriensis* sp. n., a nematode-trapping hyphomycete. *Phytopathology* **58**, 544-545.

Crofton, H. D. (1966). "Nematodes." Hutchinson, London.

Dropkin, V. H. (1969). Cellular responses of plants to nematode infections. *Ann. Rev. Phytopathol.* **7**, 101-122.

Edmunds, J. E., and Mai, W. F. (1967). Effect of *Fusarium oxysporum* on movement of *Pratylenchus penetrans* toward alfalfa roots. *Phytopathology* **57**, 468-471.

Jenkins, W. R., and Taylor, D. P. (1967). "Plant Nematology." Reinhold, New York.

Jones, F. G. W. (1959). Ecological relationships of Nematodes. *In* "Plant Pathology, Problems and Progress 1908-1958" (C. S. Holten *et al.*, eds.), pp. 395-411. Univ. of Wisconsin Press, Madison, Wisconsin.

Miller, P. M. (1968). The susceptibility of parasitic nematodes to sub-freezing temperatures. *Plant Disease Reptr.* **52**, 768-772.

Ruehle, J. L. (1968). Nematodes in forest soils. *Symp. Forest Fertilization,* Gainesville, Fla., 1967, pp. 38-41. T.V.A., Muscle Shoals, Alabama.

Sasser, J. N., and Jenkins, W. R. (1960). "Nematology." Univ. of North Carolina Press, Chapel Hill, North Carolina.

Thorne, G. (1961). "Principles of Nematology." McGraw-Hill, New York.

Wallace, H. R. (1963). "The Biology of Plant Parasitic Nematodes." Arnold, London.

9

SPECIFIC NEMATODES, TREE HEALTH, AND CONTROL

Phytoparasitic nematodes are obligate parasites and as a result they enjoy a relatively finely balanced relationship with their hosts. The obligate dependence of the worms on plants may be due to an inability of the nematode to produce certain specific materials, for example, enzyme cofactors, vitamins, or hormones (Krusberg, 1963). Their dependence on the host for materials necessary for survival and reproduction suggests that outright killing would be inimical to their persistence. As a result, diseases resulting from nematode attack are not sudden in their effect but are gradual and typically result in a slow decline in host vigor.

Plant disease syndromes which result from nematode parasitism are very complex. Since the majority of species are root feeding, the ability of infected plants to absorb water and nutrients may be impaired. This may induce symptoms characteristic of drought and nutrient deficiency. The actual withdrawal or digestion of host protoplasm, while unimportant for vigorous plants, may be very significant for plants under additional stresses. In addition, the feeding wounds caused by worms may provide entrance for other biotic disease agents and result in symptom expression characteristic of these agents. It has also been suggested that certain biochemical interactions, as yet undetermined, may have a role in symptom expression and abnormal host physiology. This latter interaction may, for example, involve toxin production by the parasites.

I. SPECIFIC NEMATODE DISEASE AGENTS

The various genera which have been found to be significant in tree disease will be discussed. These can be conveniently divided on the basis of their general feeding habit, that is ectoparasitic, semiendoparasitic, and endoparasitic.

A. Ectoparasitic Nematodes

Species which feed externally to roots.

1. Belonolaimus (sting nematodes).   This group of migratory worms is mainly confined to the southern region of the United States. Hosts include various pines, fruit trees, strawberries, and some field crops. Attack by members of this genus may kill root tips but generally results in the formation of numerous side roots at the site of infection. Tumefaction of any sort is usually absent. *Belonolaimus gracilis* has been shown to enhance the development of a wilt disease of cotton caused by a soil fungus.

2. Paratylenchus (pin nematodes).   This genus contains nematodes frequently found on hardwood species. Members of this group typically insert their stylets into root hairs or other epidermal cells but may on occasion actually penetrate the root and feed internally. In greenhouse inoculations conducted by Sutherland (1967), *P. projectus* was found to develop better on spruce than on pine. Somerville *et al.* (1957) found pin nematodes associated with several trees with decline syndrome in many states.

3. Criconemoides (ring nematodes).   These species are sedentary and are quite short and stout. They are primarily parasites of trees and other woody plants and generally cause serious damage only in warm climates. They have been found to cause particularly important disease of pine and peach.

4. Criconema (ring nematodes).   This genus is very similar to *Criconemoides*. A peculiarity of these two genera is that their locomotion is not serpentine but rather "earthworm-like" with the body alternately lengthened and shortened.

B. Semiendoparasitic Nematodes

Semiendoparasitic genera are characterized by a tendency to feed with part of the body embedded in the root. Several species may actually spend most of their life within host roots.

1. Hoplolaimus (lance nematodes).   This genus contains members which are very important parasites of southern pines and various hardwood species. These nematodes are not root-tip feeders. They are usually found at some distance from the tip, often on roots of considerable size. These worms may feed from the outside by embedding only the anterior ends of their bodies or, if able to penetrate completely, they may enter the root. When several are feeding in a limited area, the affected root at the region of concentration may become slightly swollen, develop a spongy texture, and turn brown. Eventually, the cortex may be largely destroyed and sloughed off.

Hoplolaimus members have been isolated from several declining southern tree species (Somerville *et al.*, 1957).

2. *Helicotylenchus (spiral nematodes).* This genus is important on many southern tree species and very closely resembles *Hoplolaimus* in feeding habits.

3. *Tylenchorhynchus (stylet or stunt nematodes).* This genus, while generally not a devastating parasite, may be serious on some hardwood species. These worms seem to feed at random positions on host roots, showing no evident preference for root tips or older regions. They also feed at various depths of penetration, ranging from the epidermis to the stele. Penetration by this group generally results in very limited disruption of root tissue and discoloration, swelling, collapse, and necrosis are generally absent.

4. *Xiphinema (dagger nematodes).* Actually the members of this genus could be considered ectoparasites. They do, however, insert exceptionally long stylets into their hosts and remain in one position for extended time periods. Generally, cellular hypertrophy and a multinucleate condition of undifferentiated cortical cells develop near feeding sites. Hypertrophy and necrosis have a tendency to be most severe on root tips exposed to large populations for extended time periods. In studying areas of North Carolina where slash and loblolly pine seedling survival was frequently less than 50%, Ruehle and Sasser (1962) found *X. americanum* to be one of the predominant species associated with stunted trees. Malek (1968) has suggested that *X. americanum* may be causing stunting, dieback, and premature decline (gradual overall deterioration of health) of shelterbelt trees in South Dakota. *Xiphinema americanum* has also recently been found associated with maple trees with decline symptoms in Massachusetts (Di Sanzo and Rohde, 1969).

C. Endoparasitic Nematodes

This group contains those nematodes which feed inside the plant and which are generally thought to be the most damaging plant parasites.

1. *Meloidogyne (root-knot nematodes).* This is a cosmopolitan genus that has an extremely wide host range. Newly hatched larvae, which occur free in the soil, eventually penetrate host root tips. The males are sedentary initially but remain in the root only during larval development. Eventually, they return to the soil and live free. The females, however, remain sedentary and within the host throughout their lives. As the females mature, they become pear shaped or almost spherical due to egg production. Eggs are released from the root or very near the root surface approximately 20–30 days after the female penetrates the root as a larva.

Injury from *Meloidogyne* infection may take many forms. A certain amount of mechanical injury is occasioned when the larvae enter the host.

Generally, this is only serious when a large number of larvae enter in a limited root area. Root tumefactions or galls (swellings approximately three times the healthy root diameter) are commonly induced. These may be quite massive and impair normal root function. The specific mechanism for the formation of these abnormal swellings is not known. Numerous hypotheses to explain the disturbed hormone balance, which presumably induces gall formation, have been advanced. Nematodes, for example, may release proteolytic enzymes in their salivary secretions which may release host indolacetic acid (IAA) which is bound to cytoplasmic proteins. Alternatively, the nematode enzymes may split peptide bonds of host structural protein chains and release amino acid constituents. These amino acids could, in turn, stimulate growth directly or the tryptophane component could be metabolized by the host to IAA. A second hypothesis suggests that the nematodes may release growth-promoting substances directly in their salivary secretions. It is also possible that *Meloidogyne* species may release enzymes or other materials which are capable of destroying or inhibiting the IAA oxidase system of the host, allowing concentrations of the hormone to increase abnormally. Giant cells (or syncytia) are also formed in response to nematode infection. These are large masses of protoplasm which develop around the female worm. They usually develop from vascular parenchyma cells but may occasionally arise in the cortex. As cell walls are dissolved in giant cell formation, the cytoplasm has a tendency to become increasingly granular. It is not clear how giant cell formation is brought about. Cell wall digestion may result from cellulase secretions from the nematode stylet. Development and maintenance of syncytia appear to depend on a continuous stimulus from the nematode.

Meloidogyne members are important parasites of both hardwoods and conifers. Hendrix and Powell (1968) concluded that it was probable that *M. incognita* was parasitizing pecan (*Carya illinoensis*) roots in trees displaying symptoms of reduced growth, sparse foliage, and small leaves. These investigators demonstrated that *M. incognita* could produce typical symptoms of root-knot nematode disease and could reproduce in pecan roots. Sasser *et al.* (1966) concluded that *Meloidogyne* species could seriously damage certain *Ilex* varieties. Several important forest species are infected by *M. ovalis*. This nematode is thought to cause significant disease of sugar maple in Wisconsin and perhaps in Massachusetts. In a host range test, Riffle and Kuntz (1967) found this species capable of inducing gall formation in several species (Table XV). Donaldson (1967) has recorded the presence of *M. javanica* on slash pine seedlings in Florida.

2. *Meloidodera (citrus nematodes).*   This genus is quite similar to *Meloidogyne*; it forms similar giant cells but generally does not induce gall formation. *Meloidodera* giant cells are usually formed in either the cortex of lateral

TABLE XV

MAPLE ROOT KNOT NEMATODE DEVELOPMENT ON WOODY
PLANT SPECIES USED IN A HOST RANGE TEST[a]

Plant tested	Number plants observed	Number galls	Nematode development			
			Number third to fourth stage females	Number mature females	Number mature males	Number egg masses
Acer negundo L.	10	11	4	6	5	2
A. platanoides L.	20	59	1	52	7	2
A. rubrum L.	16	144	8	134	59	10
A. saccharum Marsh.	20	144	2	106	61	10
Betula nigra L.	12	35	5	21	12	0
B. alleghaniensis Britt.	12	42	1	39	5	3
B. papyrifera Marsh.	12	29	0	27	8	3
Catalpa speciosa Ward.	20	0	0	0	0	0
Celtis occidentalis L.	16	4	1	2	4	0
Fraxinus americana L.	20	117	16	97	29	0
F. pennsylvanica Marsh. var. lanceolata (Borkh.) Sarg.	18	103	9	97	11	0
Gleditsia triacanthos L.	20	5	1	5	1	0
Malus sp.	10	0	0	0	0	0
Prunus serotina Ehrh.	2	0	0	0	0	0
Quercus virginiana Mill.	4	0	0	0	0	0
Robinia pseudoacacia L.	10	0	0	0	0	0
Tsuga canadensis (L.). Carr.	9	0	0	0	0	0
Ulmus americana L.	20	179	22	151	74	13
U. fulva Michx.	10	0	0	0	0	0

[a]From Riffle and Kuntz (1967). Reproduced by permission of the American Phytopathological Society.

roots or in undifferentiated tissue in the meristematic regions of mycorrhizal swellings.

This genus is thought to be especially important in southern forest nurseries (Hopper, 1958; Ruehle and Sasser, 1962). *Meloidodera floridensis*, the pine cystoid nematode, causes serious disease of slash and loblolly pines. This species has also been reported to be native to New Jersey and parasitic on pitch and shortleaf pines. Zak (1967) has observed a species of *Meloidodera* infecting mycorrhizae of second-growth Douglas fir in Oregon.

3. *Heterodera (cyst nematodes).* This genus contains the true cyst-forming nematodes. The female body wall, after her death, retains all or some of the eggs. The swollen body wall develops into a relatively tough protective container for the developing eggs. The species of this group are relatively well adapted to survival in fairly cool climates, unlike many other

nematode types. They are widely distributed in temperate regions and parasitize numerous hosts. Their full significance to tree health is not appreciated.

4. *Pratylenchus (lesion nematodes).* This group may be more important on hardwood than coniferous hosts. Sutherland (1967) concluded that pines were either poor or nonhosts for *P. penetrans.* He did, however, artificially inoculate spruce with this species. *Pratylenchus vulnus* has been known for some time to be the primary cause of a root-lesion disease of walnut (Lownsbery, 1956). Recently, Lordello (1967) reported that *P. brachyurus* caused stunting, yellowing, and reduced root systems of eucalyptus seedlings and young trees in Brazil.

II. NEMATODE CONTROL

A. Biological

Certain bacteria, protozoa, fungi, and other nematodes are natural enemies. Attempts have been made to control populations of plant parasitic species by increasing the populations of a particular predator or parasite group. Attempts to bring about this increase have involved alterations in the physical soil environment, addition of certain organic amendments, and direct introduction of predator/parasite organisms. In most instances these efforts have not enjoyed success. Because there are innumerable "checks" on any floral or faunal system in the soil, it is extremely diffcult to increase certain components to greater than natural population levels. This "buffering" capacity of the soil is also important when alien populations are introduced. In this case, the introduced organism will reach a population level determined by the edaphic and biotic factors of the environment and not by the number of organisms artificially added. Greater understanding of the population dynamics of soil ecosystems may permit practical biological control.

B. Physical

These procedures are probably the most commonly used in nematode control programs.

Excellent control may be obtained by heating soil and, in some cases, infected plants and plant parts, to the thermal death point of the parasites. A temperature of 40°–55°C (104°–133°F) for a short period has proved adequate to kill most nematodes. Since most animal enzymes are inactivated after short exposure to temperatures near 50°C, death is generally explained on this basis. The heat control procedure is primarily restricted to greenhouse and nursery situations. Prescribed burning, slash burning, and wildfires may, however, result in nematode population reductions in natural forest soils.

Flooding has been employed in some instances to reduce nematode numbers. It is practical only where the necessary water is plentiful and where the land can be removed from production for fairly long periods. It is further limited in usefulness by the fact that some nematodes thrive in wet soils and the flood water itself may introduce new pests.

Other potential control procedures involve land rotation and irradiation. In agriculture, land has been left unseeded for a year or more in an attempt to kill plant parasitic species through starvation. This procedure is not appropriate for tree culture. A 160,000 r dose from a ^{60}Co source has been shown to terminate reproduction in certain nematode species examined. The practical applicability of this technique is very doubtful.

C. Chemical

Nematocides are currently restricted to use on crops with greater values than forest trees, except in special instances. These applications in forestry, however, probably will increase.

Nematocides may be applied in a solid, liquid, or gas form. The use of vaporized materials has greatly increased over the past few years. Field nematocides which have been widely used and which have a moderate cost per acre include: 1,3-dichloropropene (which frequently also contains dichloropropane and is termed "D-D"), ethylene dibromide (which is usually distributed with the volatile, oily liquid naphtha), and 1,2-dibromo-3-chloropropane (which may be diluted with naphtha or adsorbed on granules of inert carrier, for example, clay). All of these materials are volatile liquids which rapidly vaporize in the soil. They are typically applied to the soil by specially equipped tractors which deliver the liquids through tubes attached to narrow shanks 6–8 inches under the soil surface.

Certain chemicals with costs higher than those mentioned above have been employed in seedbed situations. The extremely volatile liquid chloropicrin (Cl_3CNO_2) has been reported to give excellent nematode control. Methyl bromide (CH_3Br), which is probably the most popular seedbed nematocide, is applied as an odorless gas. Both chloropicrin and methyl bromide must be introduced under a plastic cover.

Unfortunately, nematocides have been accepted without thorough investigation of their long-term effects (Harrison, 1967). Most studies have been concerned with short-term observations and have ignored longer term influences on nematode population dynamics. There is actually very little evidence that eradication (complete elimination) of a nematode population is accomplished by using a nematocide. In fact, there are numerous reports which suggest that nematode populations may increase after nematocidal treatment. These increases have all been observed after an initial decrease in population and after growing the host crop. These eventual increases may have reflected reduced competition from other nematodes, more vigorous host development and consequently a more adequate food base, or reduced natural enemy populations.

D. Genetic

Breeding for nematode resistance has only recently received attention. There is some evidence to suggest that single-gene resistance exists which would indicate that resistance may depend upon one or a few enzymes and the metabolic compounds they control.

REFERENCES

Di Sanzo, C. P., and Rohde, R. A. (1969). *Xiphinema americanum* associated with maple decline in Massachusetts. *Phytopathology* **59**, 279–284.

Donaldson, F. S., Jr. (1967). *Meloidogyne javanica* infesting *Pinus elliottii* seedlings in Florida. *Plant Disease Reptr.* **51**, 455–456.

Harrison, M. B. (1967). Influence of nematocidal treatments on nematode populations. *Phytopathology* **57**, 650–652.

Hendrix, F. F., Jr., and Powell, W. M. (1968). Nematode and *Pythium* species associated with feeder root necrosis of pecan trees in Georgia. *Plant Disease Reptr.* **52**, 334–335.

Hopper, B. E. (1958). Plant-parasitic nematodes in the soils of southern forest nurseries. *Plant Disease Reptr.* **42**, 308–314.

Krusberg, L. R. (1963). Host response to nematode infection. *Ann. Rev. Phytopathol.* **1**, 219–240.

Lordello, L. G. E. (1967). A root-lesion nematode found infesting eucalyptus trees in Brazil. *Plant Disease Reptr.* **51**, 791–792.

Lownsbery, B. F. (1956). *Pratylenchus vulnus,* primary cause of the root-lesion disease of walnuts. *Phytopathology* **46**, 376–379.

Malek, R. B. (1968). The dagger nematode, *Xiphinema americanum,* associated with decline of shelterbelt trees in South Dakota. *Plant Disease Reptr.* **52**, 795–798.

Riffle, J. W., and Kuntz, J. E. (1967). Pathogenicity and host range of *Meliodogyne ovalis. Phytopathology* **57**, 104–107.

Ruehle, J. L., and Sasser, J. N. (1962). The role of plant-parasitic nematodes in stunting of pines in southern plantations. *Phytopathology* **52**, 56–58.

Sasser, J. N., Haasis, F. A., and Cannon, T. F. (1966). Pathogenicity of *Meloidogyne species* on Ilex. *Plant Disease Reptr.* **50**, 664–668.

Somerville, A. M., Young, V. H., and Carnes, J. L. (1957). Occurrence of plant parasitic nematodes in soil and root samples from declining plants in several states. *Plant Disease Reptr.* **41**, 187–191.

Sutherland, J. R. (1967). Host range and reproduction of the nematodes *Paratylenchus projectus, Pratylenchus penetrans,* and *Tylenchus emarginatus* on some forest nursery seedlings. *Plant Disease Reptr.* **51**, 91–93.

Zak, B. (1967). A nematode (*Meloidodera sp.*) on Douglas-fir mycorrhizae. *Plant Disease Reptr.* **51**, 264.

GENERAL REFERENCES

Baker, K. F., and Snyder, W. C., eds. (1965). "Ecology of Soil-Borne Plant Pathogens." Univ. of California Press, Berkeley, California.

Christie, J. R. (1959). "Plant Nematodes. Their Bionomics and Control." Agr. Expt. Sta., University of Florida, Gainesville, Florida.

Hutchinson, M. T., and Reed, J. P. (1959). The pine cystoid nematode in New Jersey. *Plant Disease Reptr.* **43**, 801–802.

Nemec, S., and Struble, F. B. (1968). Response of certain woody ornamental plants to *Meloidogyne incognita. Phytopathology* **58**, 1700–1703.

Riffle, J. W. (1968). Plant-parasitic nematodes in marginal *Pinus ponderosa* stands in Central New Mexico. *Plant Disease Reptr.* **52**, 52–55.

Riffle, J. W., and Kuntz, J. E. (1966). Nematodes in maple blight and maple dieback areas in Wisconsin. *Plant Disease Reptr.* **50**, 677–681.

Ruehle, J. L. (1962). Plant-parasitic nematodes associated with shortleaf pine showing symptoms of littleleaf. *Plant Disease Reptr.* **46**, 710–711.

Ruehle, J. L. (1962). Histopathological studies of pine roots infected with lance and pine cystoid nematodes. *Phytopathology* **52**, 68–71.

Ruehle, J. L. (1966). Nematodes parasitic on forest trees. I. Reproduction of ectoparasites on pines. *Nematologica* **12**, 443–447.

Ruehle, J. L. (1968). Plant-parasitic nematodes associated with southern hardwood and coniferous forest trees. *Plant Disease Reptr.* **52**, 837–839.

Ruehle, J. L. (1968). Pathogenicity of sting nematode on sycamore. *Plant Disease Reptr.* **52**, 523–525.

Ruehle, J. L. (1968). Nematodes in forest soils: Classification, modes of attack, effects on tree nutrition and growth, and methods of control. *Forest Fertilization, Gainesville, Fla., 1967* pp. 38–41. T.V.A., Muscle Shoals, Alabama.

Ruehle, J. L. (1969). Forest nematology—a new field of biological research. *J. Forestry* **67**, 316–320.

Shigo, A. L., and Yelenosky, G. (1960). Nematodes inhabit soils of forest and clear-cut areas. *Res. Note, Northeast. Forest Expt. Sta.* **101**, 1–4.

Springer, J. K. (1964). Nematodes associated with plants in cultivated woody plant nurseries and uncultivated woodland areas in New Jersey. *Circ., New Jersey Dept. Agr.* **429**, 1–40.

Van Gundy, S. D. (1965). Factors in survival of nematodes. *Ann. Rev. Phytopathol.* **3**, 43–68.

10

VIRUSES

By the end of the nineteenth century, a great deal was known about the biotic agents capable of causing disease in plants and animals. Louis Pasteur and Robert Koch had shown that infectious diseases were caused by minute living organisms or "germs" and it was confidently expected that the presence of such germs could be demonstrated for all infectious maladies. The causes of certain important plant and animal diseases, however, could not be isolated by the bacteriological processes in use at the time. In plants, for example, tobacco leaves exhibited curious mottled patterns and frequently became wrinkled. Shoot elongation was commonly inhibited or retarded. This abnormality, termed tobacco mosaic disease, could not be shown to be caused by a bacterium. Animals also suffered from diseases whose causes were elusive, for example, hoof and mouth disease and rabies. Man was plagued with smallpox, yellow fever, measles, and influenza, all of which were obviously infective but not produced by "germs."

In 1892, Ivanovski showed that the mosaic symptoms of tobacco could be produced in healthy plants by rubbing their leaves with juice from infected leaves, even after this juice had been passed through a filter capable of removing particles of bacterial size. This phenomenon disturbed Ivanovski, but he did not realize the significance of his discovery and merely considered that the "bacteria" that caused tobacco mosaic disease were probably very small. In 1898, the Dutch microbiologist Beijerinck confirmed Ivanovski's work but rejected the idea of a causal bacterium. He was unclear concerning the specifics of the causal agent but suggested the concept of *contagium vivum fluidum*. Even though imprecise, this suggestion represented the first step away from the conventional bacteriological approach and the science of virology had its beginning.

For the first 30 years or so after viruses were discovered, a great amount of information was accumulated. A wide range of virus diseases were documented. Transmission methods were proposed and even some control measures were conceived. No positive information concerning the specific nature of viruses, however, was forthcoming. This is not surprising when one considers that the investigators were applying classical microbiological methods to the search for viruses. They were using microscopes which were not powerful enough to detect viruses and employed culture media upon which viruses could not grow. Gradually, however, more diverse chemical and biological methods were used to determine virus nature. In 1935-36, Stanley fractionated large volumes of infective sap from diseased tobacco plants by the methods used to isolate proteolytic enzymes. He obtained from this fractionation substantial amounts of what he called "a crystalline protein possessing the properties of tobacco mosaic virus (TMV)." The protein nature of viruses was thus finally realized. An exciting account of historical virus research is contained in "Virus Hunters" (Williams, 1959).

I. VIRUS CHARACTERISTICS

Before specifically defining viruses, several fundamental characteristics will be considered. Virus sizes vary within rather wide limits. They range from that of very small bacteria to that of very large protein molecules. Roughly, their dimensions are within the 16-475 mμ range (mμ = 10^{-6} mm). All plant viruses and the majority of animal viruses are beyond the resolution of the optical microscope.

All viruses have an extremely close affinity with living cells. Virus multiplication does not occur outside of these cells. Most viruses lack all enzymes and none have a metabolism. No virus has been cultivated on a cell-free medium. The chemical constitution of viruses is quite simple and in the very small viruses consists only of a protein and nucleic acid component. Many of these small viruses behave much like chemicals and can be crystallized. In some viruses, the nucleic acid fraction alone is presumed to be the infective unit, with the protein component serving only as a protective coating.

A variety of methods have been used to study the internal architecture of purified viruses, including: electron microscopy, X-ray diffraction, and the influence of various chemical agents (for example, enzymes). From the sum total of these and other studies, it has become very clear that, in simple viruses, each particle consists of many comparatively small protein molecules, one or occasionally a few types, covering one long, coiled up nucleic acid molecule. In plant viruses and some animal viruses, the nucleic acid is ribonucleic acid (RNA); in other animal and bacterial viruses (bacteriophages) it is usually deoxyribonucleic acid (DNA) (Table XVI). An excellent and de-

TABLE XVI

COMPOSITION OF THREE SMALL VIRUSES

Virus	Molecular weight	Percent RNA	Percent protein	Molecular weight RNA
Tobacco mosaic virus	40,000,000	6	94	2,400,000
Polio virus	10,000,000	25-30	70-75	2,500,000
Turnip yellow mosaic virus	5,000,000	40	60	2,000,000

tailed description of the biochemistry of plant viruses can be found in Markham (1959).

A suitable virus definition may be as follows: a submicroscopic, infectious, potentially pathogenic, nucleoprotein entity, unable to grow and divide and typically devoid of enzymes (no enzymes are found in viruses which cause disease in higher plants).

II. HOST-VIRUS RELATIONSHIP

Once brought into contact with the host plant by a vector or other means, the virus infection process is initiated. A plant virus cannot enter a susceptible plant unless a natural or unnatural phenomenon permits introduction directly into a plant cell. This initial contact cell may be one which is injured but it cannot be one which is killed. This implies that the virus must make intimate contact with the living substance of the cell. When TMV-RNA was inoculated onto tobacco leaves, which were then dipped immediately into a solution of RNAase sufficient to destroy the viral RNA, no reduction in disease development was observed. It appears, therefore, that the virus–living host cell union is instantaneous. This rapid union is usually called *adsorption*.

There is evidence that, immediately following adsorption, the protein of the virus particle is unravelled by some means in order to free the bound strand or core of RNA. The mechanism by which this stripping is accomplished in the living cell is not known. In the case of TMV, the protein separated from the purified TMV has been found not to be infectious or even to bring about local response when inoculated into host plants. Tobacco mosaic RNA separated from the protein, however, is fully infective. It appears that virus RNA carries within its structure the information necessary, not only for its own replication, but also for the synthesis of its protein counterpart.

The actual mechanism of viral multiplication in host cells is incompletely understood. It is generally assumed, however, that this process occurs in three stages. Initially there is a synthesis of new virus-directed enzymes. Following this, new viral nucleic acid and protein are synthesized. The third step involves assembly of the new viral precursor materials into virus particles (Tamm, 1968). Specific evidence relating to the mechanisms responsible for plant virus RNA biosynthesis is lacking (Siegel and Zaitlin, 1964). Some confusion exists in the literature concerning the actual sites of synthesis of virus particles and the temporal order in which they are formed. Some investigators suggest that the virus nucleic acid is synthesized in or on the nucleus of the host and the viral protein formed in the cytoplasm. Direct evidence in support of this suggestion, however, is lacking. It has also been suggested, and again with little supporting evidence, that viral nucleic acid synthesis may precede protein assembly. Some virologists argue that the two synthetic processes probably occur concurrently or at least overlap.

In summation of the infection process, we see that the virus' importance lies in its ability to enter a living cell and force that cell into a new, alien metabolic pathway. The cell becomes harnessed into producing primarily virus constituents instead of cell constituents. While the energy and the building materials for this synthetic work are supplied by the metabolism of the host cell, the blueprints describing the finished product, the virus, are supplied by the invading viral nucleic acid. In addition to the many unresolved biochemical questions concerning virus infection, numerous other curiosities exist specifically with respect to infection by plant viruses. With TMV, for example, for each virus particle which becomes established, 10^5-10^6 particles must be applied to the plant. With many plant viruses, there is frequently a latent period varying from approximately 20 hours to several days between infection and disease development. The length of this latent period varies with virus, host, temperature, strength of inoculum, and other factors. When a plant is infected by two unrelated viruses, the presence of one may stimulate the other. In many infections, curious crystalline, amoeboid, or fibrous inclusion bodies may be formed (Bollard and Matthews, 1966).

III. ABNORMAL PHYSIOLOGY INDUCED BY VIRUSES

The initiation of pathogenesis in microbial infections occurs primarily by the exchange of metabolites. That is, bacterial and fungal parasites may deplete metabolites of the host plant or release metabolic products toxic to the host. Pathogenesis in viral infections, on the other hand, occurs by the addition of genetic determinants to host cells. Viral infection may be more appropriately termed a genetic rather than a metabolic phenomenon (Diener, 1963). Nevertheless, these abnormal genetic consequences resulting from virus infection are ultimately expressed in disturbed physiology and, frequently, in obvious symptoms.

Plant viral diseases can be arranged in order of increasing tissue reaction to infection. In some cases, no external manifestations of disease will be evident. Physiological aberrations are so well tolerated that symptoms fail to appear. The other extreme is characterized by what have been termed "localized infections" in which the host tissue reacts so violently to the presence of the virus that the tissue is killed and the systemic spread of the virus is halted. This type of infection response is undoubtedly due to drastic metabolic changes in the host tissue. Most data implicate the polyphenol oxidase–polyphenol system in this hypersensitive reaction. Inhibition of the systemic spread of the virus may be caused by a quinone-induced death of the host cells, preventing spread, or by direct inactivation of the virus particles by accumulated polyphenol oxidation products. Intermediate between these two extremes, various external symptoms are expressed and systemic spread of the virus throughout the plant generally occurs. In this case, death of infected tissue usually does not occur.

Certain generalizations can be made regarding the disease phenomena associated with intermediate or systemic infection (Diener, 1963). Photosynthesis is typically reduced in virus-infected plants. This may be due to a decreased rate of chlorophyll synthesis or destruction of existing chlorophyll. Unlike photosynthesis, respiration is generally increased in response to virus infection. With respect to carbohydrate metabolism, a decreased photosynthetic rate coupled with enhanced respiration should result in decreased concentrations of assimilate. In some virus-infected plants this decrease is observed, but in others it is not. Very little is known about virus impact on organic acid metabolism. In nitrogen metabolism, however, protein nitrogen is frequently decreased while nonprotein nitrogen is increased. Under conditions of nitrogen stress, normal host proteins are hydrolyzed and the resulting nitrogen is apparently used for virus synthesis. The accumulation of nonprotein nitrogen may typically involve large amounts of amides. The influence of virus infection on phosphorylated compounds is very variable and poorly understood. Influences on several groups of secondary compounds have been investigated, but consistent effects have been found only with phenolic compounds. In this case, various phenolic substances are generally found to accumulate in virus-infected plant tissues. Virus effects on growth-regulating substances have been quite intensively studied. Retardation of growth, sometimes coupled with the stimulation of axillary buds, is probably the most general symptom of virus infection in plants. In contrast with some other topics dealing with the physiology of virus-infected plants, there is unanimity among workers concerning effects on growth substance metabolism. All report a virus-induced reduction in the amount of growth-promoting substances, an increase in the concentration of growth-inhibiting substances, or both.

How the invading viral nucleic acid can bring about these pathological aberrations of host-plant metabolism is still not clear. It is presumed, however, that these gross derangements are relatively late occurrences and not necessarily indicative of the initial events occurring as a consequence of infection.

IV. VIRUS TRANSMISSION

The transmission of viruses is very varied and an interesting aspect of their ecology. One of the most outstanding characteristics of viruses is their relationship with insects and other organisms on which they rely for their transportation from host to host. The study of virus vectors is extremely important in the study of virus-induced plant disease.

Four primary mechanisms for distribution might be recognized: seed, vegetative, contact, and vector transmission. Virus transmission by seed is quite rare. It is not clear why this is so, but it may be partially explained by the anatomical isolation of the embryo. All plant viruses which are systemic in their hosts are potentially capable of being transmitted through vegetative organs, such as tubers, bulbs, rhizomes, and cuttings. The latter are particularly important in the grafting or vegetative propagation of forest tree species. Contact transmission occurs commonly in infections with high virus concentration. In this case, simple mechanical rubbing, as might occur during a wind, might be sufficient to cause movement of virus particles from one plant to its neighbor. Contact transmission may be of significance in forest tree species via root contact. The rupture of a single root hair may be adequate for passage. Root grafting, which occurs when tree roots fuse, would be a very efficient means to transmit a virus from an infected tree to a healthy tree.

The most important means of virus spread, however, is through vectors. These vectors may include fungi, nematodes, birds and other large animals, and insects. Insects are probably the most significant vectors of plant viruses. Most insect vectors belong to the order Hemiptera which includes all those insects with sucking mouthparts, for example leafhoppers, thrips, and aphids. The majority of plant viruses are transmitted by aphids. Viruses carried by aphids fall into two groups: nonpersistent and persistent. The nonpersistent viruses are rapidly lost by the insect, usually after one feeding on a susceptible plant. There is presumed to be no biological relationship between the nonpersistent virus and the aphid. In the case of persistent viruses, on the other hand, the viruses are retained for long periods by the insect, frequently for a lifetime. It is not known whether or not the viruses actually multiply in the aphid. In certain leafhopper-transmitted viruses, the virus can be passed from generation to generation via the egg.

V. VIRUSES AS PATHOGENS

Since 1898, more than 400 plant viruses have been described and named. The total number of diseases caused by these agents has not been determined. Very little information is available on tree viruses, and the influence of these infective agents on tree health is without question very much more important than is currently realized.

It is interesting to note that almost all forms of plant life suffer from the effects of virus infection, including fungi and bacteria. Viruses which infect bacteria are termed bacteriophages and typically consist of a polyhedral head, generally between 50-100 mμ in cross section and a short thinner tail. The "head" has an outer coat of protein which encloses a core of DNA. The "tail" consists of protein only and has a hollow core. During adsorption, the tail becomes attached to the wall of the bacterium and a small perforation is enzymatically made in the wall. Virus DNA is then injected from the head through the tail into the cytoplasm of the bacterial cell. Once inside the bacterium, the phage nucleic acid provides the genetic information for the synthesis of more phage nucleic acid and phage protein. The use of bacterial viruses in the control of bacterial diseases has been attempted, with little success.

Algae and ferns appear to have few virus pathogens. This probably reflects a lack of sufficient research. In trees, documented viruses are most common in angiosperms and only recently have they been reported in gymnosperms. This disparity may reflect the relative amount of investigation conducted on these two groups.

REFERENCES

Bollard, E. G., and Matthews, R. E. F. (1966). The physiology of parasitic disease. In "Plant Physiology" (F. C. Steward, ed.), Vol. 4B, pp. 417-550. Academic Press, New York.

Diener, T. O. (1963). Physiology of virus-infected plant. Ann. Rev. Phytopathol. 1, 197-218.

Markham, R. (1959). The biochemistry of plant viruses. In "The Viruses" (F. M. Burnet and W. M. Stanley, eds.), Vol. 2, pp. 33-125. Academic Press, New York.

Siegel, A., and Zaitlin, M. (1964). Infection process in plant virus diseases. Ann. Rev. Phytopathol. 2, 179-202.

Tamm, I. (1968). The replication of viruses. Am. Scientist 56, 189-206.

Williams, G. (1959). "Virus Hunters." Knopf, New York.

GENERAL REFERENCES

Beemster, A. B. R., and Dijkstra, J. eds. (1966). "Viruses of Plants." Proc. Intern. Conf. Plant Viruses, Wageningen, 1965 Wiley, New York.

Bowden, F. C. (1964). "Plant Viruses and Virus Diseases." Ronald Press, New York.

Broadbent, L., and Martini, C. (1959). The spread of plant viruses. *Advan. Virus Res.* **6**, 93–135.

Burnet, F. M., and Stanley, W. M., eds. (1959). "The Viruses," Vols. 1, 2, and 3. Academic Press, New York.

Corbett, M. K., and Sisler, H. D., eds. (1964). "Plant Virology." Univ. of Florida Press, Gainesville, Florida.

Esau, K. (1968). "Viruses in Plant Hosts." Univ. of Wisconsin Press, Madison, Wisconsin.

Fraenkel-Conrat, H. (1964). "Design and Function at the Threshold of Life: The Viruses." Academic Press, New York.

Hanon, N., ed. (1964). "Selected Papers on Virology." Prentice-Hall, Englewood Cliffs, New Jersey.

Haselkorn, R. (1966). Physical and chemical properties of plant viruses. *Ann. Rev. Plant Physiol.* **17**, 137–154.

Hewitt, W. B., and Groogan, R. G. (1967). Unusual vectors of plant viruses. *Ann. Rev. Microbiol.* **21**, 205–224.

Hooper, G. R., and Schneider, H. (1969). The anatomy of tumors induced on citrus by citrus vein-enation virus. *Am. J. Botany* **56**, 238–247.

Lwoff, A. (1966). Interaction among virus, cell and organism. *Science* **152**, 1216–1220.

Maramorosch, K., ed. (1969). "Viruses, Vectors, and Vegetation." Wiley, New York.

Mundry, K. W. (1963). Plant virus-host cell relations. *Ann. Rev. Phytopathol.* **1**, 173–196.

Porter, C. A. (1959). Biochemistry of plant virus infection. *Advan. Virus Res.* **6**, 75–91.

Smith, K. M. (1957). "A Textbook of Plant Virus Diseases." Churchill, London.

Smith, K. M. (1963). "Viruses." Cambridge Univ. Press, London and New York.

Smith, K. M. (1968). "Plant Viruses." Methuen, London.

Weidel, W. (1959). "Virus." Univ. of Michigan Press, Ann Arbor, Michigan.

Zeitoun, F. M., and Wilson, E. E. (1969). The relation of bacteriophage to the walnut-tree pathogens, *Erwinia nigrifluens* and *Erwinia rubrifaciens*. Phytopathology **59**, 756–761.

11

SPECIFIC FOREST TREE VIRUS DISORDERS

The biological and economic significance of virus diseases of several agricultural crops is very well documented. The study of virus-induced maladies of forest trees, however, is in its infancy. There have been only approximately 55 virus diseases described which influence forest species of commercial importance. There is much evidence to suggest that this figure is a gross underestimation of the importance of viruses as disease agents. This hiatus of knowledge is especially meaningful when one realizes that virus diseases are most serious in perennial crops. Once infected by a virus, a woody plant will continue to remain infected throughout its life.

Since viruses are strict obligate parasites, they characteristically cause a very gradual deterioration in host vigor, rather than rapid necrosis. Species which are adapted to plantation culture, especially those vegetatively propagated, are frequently severely damaged because vegetative propagation perpetuates the viruses and favors their widespread distribution. Many virus diseases, for example many found on *Prunus* species, fail to produce symptoms on wild tree hosts. Some cause symptoms only in the early stages of infection. As a result, intercontinental spread of viruses of this type through shipment of infected stock or scion materials represents an important threat to indigenous tree hosts where the viruses may be capable of causing important and more severe diseases.

In addition to the paucity of data available with respect to the number of virus tree diseases, the information available on those which have been described primarily concerns only symptoms. Unfortunately, symptoms of virus diseases appear even more variable than the external manifestations of other plant disorders. The same virus may produce different symptoms on different hosts, and different viruses may produce like symptoms on the same host. When a single host is infected by more than one virus, unique symptoms may appear. Strains of the same virus may also induce different symptoms on identical hosts. The period of latent infection, the time between infection and symptom expression, is very variable in diseases caused by certain viruses. Diagnosis is additionally complicated by the fact that viruses cannot be grown on artificial media and observation with the ordinary light microscope is impossible.

There is no official or uniform procedural system of nomenclature for viruses. Cataloging, as a consequence, has been primarily based on the host symptoms expressed and on the manner in which the virus moves in the host. Bollard and Matthews (1966), for example, have recognized four general virus types. The first are those which generally invade both parenchyma and phloem tissues. The intrahost movement of these viruses tends to be quite slow until they reach the phloem. This type of virus is currently felt to be the most common virus agent of plant disease. These viruses apparently have the general effect of destroying chlorophyll nonuniformly in leaf tissues or preventing its uniform formation such that the most common symptom is a "mosaic" or "mottle" leaf pattern. The second virus type is restricted to parenchyma tissue and spreads very slowly from cell to cell. Movement is presumably made through plasmodesmata which are extremely fine cytoplasmic threads passing through the cellulose walls of living plant cells and which form a link between cytoplasm of adjacent cells. The third virus type moves only in the phloem. These are generally placed in the phloem by an insect with sucking mouth parts, particularly aphids, leafhoppers, mealy bugs, or white flies. This group generally exhibits a very brief latent period and moves rapidly in the host. The last virus type is confined to the xylem. This latter group is generally felt to be the least important group of phytoparasites. The symptoms induced by these last three groups include: yellowing, dwarfing, resinosis, gummosis, fasciculation, curling, spot, and infrequently, overall necrosis.

In an effort to permit a general appreciation of the nature of virus tree infections, a selected group will be discussed in the following paragraphs. This is not intended to be a comprehensive list, but rather a representative one. More complete inventories are available (Seliskar, 1966; Schmelzer *et al.*, 1966; Smith, 1957). The proof that a particular disease is virus induced has characteristically involved the experimental transmission of the virus agent. For all the diseases which follow, this has been accomplished.

I. GYMNOSPERMS

Only one virus disease of conifers has been documented. This disorder, termed spruce virosis, occurs in Norway spruce (*Picea abies*) in Czechoslovakia. Symptoms include slight mottling of foliage in early stages to complete yellowing in advanced stages. On seedlings, symptoms during the first year after infection typically include asymmetrical growth, with depressed terminals and thickened lateral shoots. In the second year, multiple development of terminal buds causes the twigs to assume a "bushy" appearance. Natural transmission is presumed to be by aphids. Experimentally, the virus has been transmitted by two aphid species (Seliskar, 1966). Cech *et al.* (1961) have reported graft transmission experimentally. These investigators also found rod-shaped particles in twig exudates of diseased spruce. The particles varied from 200–3000 mμ in length and were approximately 49 mμ in diameter. The hexagonal structure of the particles coupled with the fact that they were found only in trees expressing symptoms support the suggestion that the disease is virus induced.

Viruslike disorders have been observed on several other conifers, especially members of the *Pinus* genus (Schmelzer, 1966; Seliskar, 1966). In the near future, many of these diseases may be proved to be virus caused. The lack of research on gymnosperm viruses is probably in large measure responsible for the few virus diseases which have been documented in this group.

II. ANGIOSPERMS

The discussion of virus diseases of this group will be organized on the basis of genera. The genera discussed will be those which contain trees of particular commercial or ecological interest. This list is *not* comprehensive but rather intended to be representative.

1. Acer.   Maple variegation is an important virus disease of boxelder (*A. negundo*) and planetree maple (*A. pseudoplatanus*), which enjoys worldwide distribution. Mosaic or mottling symptoms are typical. Naturally infected red maple (*A. rubrum*) with peach rosette have been observed in Georgia. Peach rosette is caused by a systemic virus which causes severe stunting and dense green foliage.

Numerous other suspected virus disorders of maple have been studied. In the northern Sierras and throughout the coastal mountains of northern California, a disease of bigleaf maple (*A. macrocarpa*) with viruslike symptoms has been reported. Viruses have been considered as a possible cause of leaf curl of Norway maple (*A. plantanoides*), an important ornamental. An unexplained necrosis of sugar maple termed "maple blight" has resulted in severe damage and mortality in Wisconsin. Attempts to link a virus with this particular malady, however, have not been successful.

2. Betula.   Birch line pattern is a virus disease of yellow birch (*B. alleghaniensis*) found in Canada. Symptoms are a line pattern on infected leaves.

In recent years dieback of yellow birch and paper birch (*B. papyrifera*) in New England and in neighboring parts of Canada has attracted a great deal of attention. The gradual deterioration of diseased individuals stimulated the thought that a virus agent might be involved. It remains unproven, however, if a virus is or is not involved.

3. *Carya.*   Pecan bunch disease is one of the most economically important tree virus diseases. The virus is believed to have initially infected the wild native pecan (*C. illinoensis*) and water pecan (*C. aquatica*) and subsequently spread to the cultivated varieties. The disease is most significant in alluvial river bottoms in Mississippi, Louisiana, Oklahoma, and Texas.

The most characteristic symptom is fasciculation or development of witches' brooms on branches and shoots. Lateral buds in these brooms are stimulated to grow, forming long, thin sprouts about the center of the broom. Initially, fasciculation or "bunching" is confined to a single branch or small portion of the tree. Eventually, in advanced stages, systemic infection results and bunching spreads throughout the crown. Nut production may be severely curtailed. In late stages, branches die back. A phenomenon helpful in diagnosis involves foliation of diseased branches and shoots in the spring as much as 2 weeks prematurely. Symptoms similar to those described have been observed on shagbark hickory (*C. ovata*) in West Virginia.

Pecan rosette is another virus disease of *Carya*. Both viruses may infect the same host simultaneously. In the rosette disease, the affected leaves have a tendency to be chlorotic between the veins giving the leaf a striped appearance while bunch symptoms generally entail uniform chlorosis over the entire leaf.

4. *Fraxinus.*   Several virus diseases have been identified in this genus. Ash infectious variegation has been observed in Europe on white ash (*F. americana*), European ash (*F. excelsior*), and green ash (*F. pennsylvanica*). Leaves of infected trees have a yellow mosaic and some may be malformed.

Ash necrotic leaf curl has been studied in Italy where it occurs on flowering ash (*F. ornus*) and European ash. Bleaching of the midrib which eventually spreads to the lateral veins (a process termed "vein clearing") is usually followed by the development of necrotic spots which cause leaf deformation.

Ash witches' broom is a virus disease of Arizona ash (*F. berlandieriana*) in Louisiana. The fasciculations of infected trees have a tendency to retain their foliage late in the fall, long after healthy leaves are shed. In nursery situations, young trees die 3 or 4 years following infection.

White ash is an ecologically extremely interesting tree in that it has both the characteristics of a pioneer and climax species. It is an especially important component of the hardwood forests of the northeastern United States. This tree also has considerable commercial importance in several areas throughout its wide distribution in the country. During the 1930's, an unexplained dying of many white ash trees was observed along roadsides and hedgerows in New York. This malady, now commonly termed "ash dieback," was of little concern to foresters until the late 1950's when it was observed to be also present in valuable commercial forest stands. A recent survey made by the New York Conservation Department in 18 eastern counties of the state revealed that approximately 70% of the woodland ash trees were dead or dying. The dieback symptoms have been detected to a limited extent in green ash but never in black ash (*F. nigra*). Some of the symptoms characteristic of ash dieback, such as chlorotic, dwarfed foliage, and spindly epicormic branches (branches that develop from adventitious buds along the trunk of a tree), are suggestive of a virus disease agent.

Ross (1966) made a reasonably comprehensive effort to elucidate the cause of ash dieback. This effort included attempts to show a virus agent. His procedures are illustrative of the kinds of methods which are commonly employed to analyze for suspected viruses. He employed grafting, serologic studies, and indicator plants. Control grafts from healthy scions (twigs grafted onto stock of another plant) produced 1-4 inches of terminal growth in 6 months. Foliage of the healthy scions was a normal green color, but slightly dwarfed due to grafting shock. Grafts made from diseased scions to healthy rootstocks produced only from 0-1.5 inches of terminal growth but had foliage color and size similar to healthy scions. Ross concluded that none of the grafts showed signs of transmission of virus symptoms. Growth recovery, which occurred in some of the diseased scions, would further suggest that the disease is not of virus origin. Hibben (1966) has presented evidence which somewhat contradicts Ross's findings. Hibben excised buds and bark patches from white ash with dieback and abnormal foliar symptoms and grafted these onto 1-3 year old trees of several species in the Oleaceae and Rosaceae families (315 trees, total). Unfortunately, less than 1% of the graft attempts resulted in permanent union between scion and stock. On the successful grafts, however, a variety of foliar symptoms, for example chlorotic lesions, line patterns, mottle, reddish flecks, ringspots, and leaf deformations, developed. The author claimed that verification of graft transmission was achieved for 3 out of 45 white ash seedlings that received graft inocula. Hibben (1968) has recently shown transmission of a virus from declining white ash to periwinkle by using the parasitic dodder plant.

The second method employed by Ross to determine virus presence was serologic studies. Serology is the study of serum and serum reactions. It is very much concerned with two classes of protein molecules, termed antigens and antibodies. Antigens are substances which, when placed in animal blood streams, will produce new or altered proteins. Virus proteins are one kind of antigen. Antibodies are proteins of varying character produced in the blood in response to foreign proteins and less frequently to complex lipids and carbohydrates. Antigen-antibody reactions are usually quite specific; that is, a particular antigen will elicit the production of a particular antibody. This specificity is commonly manifested in the production of a precipitate when a specific antibody and its inducer antigen are brought into contact with one another. This reaction can be conveniently observed in agar in a Petri dish and is frequently used to test for virus presence. Virus protein is antigenic and usually results in the formation of specific antibodies. Antisera (sera containing these specific antibodies) are prepared and reacted with plant or animal extracts to test for virus presence. In rough outline, antisera production involves the following steps. Purified virus is obtained and injected into test animals, usually rabbits or chickens. After approximately 1 month, the animals are bled, the blood is coagulated, and the serum (containing the antibodies) is squeezed out and frozen. The serum is then reacted with material suspected to contain inducer virus and presence or absence of precipitate noted.

In Ross's investigation, antisera were produced by injecting rabbits with leaf sap of diseased trees. The leaf extracts were then reacted with the rabbit antisera. Only one leaf sap produced precipitate with its own antiserum. The same leaf sap antiserum, however, reacted positively with all other leaf sap antigens, including those from healthy leaves. This suggests that the precipitations were formed in response to nonspecific proteinaceous material in all the leaf saps instead of virus material.

Ross's third method was the use of indicator plants. Certain plant species, for example bean, cucumber, and tobacco, react to several plant viruses by developing localized, hypersensitive symptoms, usually including necrotic spots. These plants are frequently inoculated with material suspected to contain virus particles and observed for localized necrotic lesions. The inoculation of cucumbers with the leaf sap of diseased ash failed to produce visible cucumber symptoms.

Even though grafting, serologic techniques, and indicator plants provided no evidence for the presence of viruses in ash dieback trees, it is still possible that a virus is associated with the malady but is not amenable to detection by the procedures employed. In the serology experiments, insufficient antigen may have been used in each injection, or injections may not have extended over a sufficiently long time period. In the case of grafting and indicator studies, the virus may be dependent upon other agencies, such as insects or nematodes, for transmission or require a specific host or condition for development.

5. *Juglans.* Walnut bunch is an important virus disease of black walnut (*J. nigra*), butternut (*J. cinerea*), and Japanese walnut (*J. sieboldiana*) in the eastern United States. Its symptoms are very similar to those of pecan bunch, and both diseases may be caused by the same virus. The cosmopolitan dis-

tribution of this disease in the eastern United States and its capacity to reduce yield and growth suggest that this problem may be more important in
forest stands than is generally realized.

6. *Prunus.*   This genus is characterized by several important virus disorders. These are summarized in Table XVII.

7. *Robinia.*   This genus has two important virus problems. In Europe,
black locust (*R. pseudoacacia*) and clammy locust (*R. viscosa*) are frequently
damaged by black locust mosaic. This disease results in reduced growth and
is expressed as a leaf mosaic. Schmelzer (1963) in a study of suitable indicator plants for this virus found that 76 of the 107 plants he employed developed symptoms. The second locust disease is found in Europe and in the
United States. It is termed black locust witches' broom (Fig. 16). Vein
clearing (degradation of chlorophyll in, or adjacent to, vein tissue) is generally expressed in early stages followed by premature leaf fall. Eventually
brooming of stump and root sprouts, roots, and branches develops. This disease is serious because of its widespread occurrence.

8. *Santalum.*   This genus is importantly influenced by two virus diseases
in India. *Santalum album* exhibits sandal leaf-curl mosaic which causes
mature leaves to have interveinal mosaic and slight curl. Eventually, this disease results in severe leaf and fruit distortion and premature shed.

TABLE XVII

VIRUS DISEASES OF *PRUNUS* SPECIES

Disease	*Hosts*	*Distribution*
Necrotic ring spot	*Prunus cerasus, P. virginiana* naturally; *P. pennsylvanica* and several cultivated spp. artificially	Canada, United States
Ring spot	Several species including *P. virginiana*	United States
Rusty mottle	*Prunus avium, P. cerasus* natur- ally; several other spp. artificially	Western United States
Sour cherry yellows	*Prunus cerasus* naturally and others artificially	Canada, United States
Sweet cherry buckskin	*Prunus avium* naturally; *P. virginiana* var. *demissa* artificially	California
Western X disease	*Prunus persica, P. avium, P. cerasus, P. virginiana* var. *demissa* naturally; *P. virginiana* artificially	Western Canada, United States
X disease	Various species	Canada, eastern United States

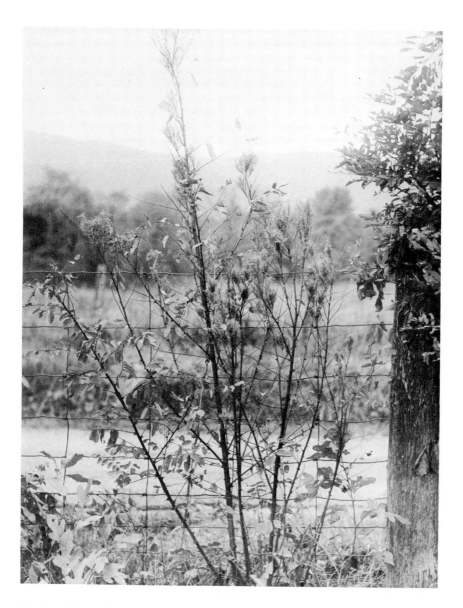

Fig. 16. Witches' broom disease of black locust. This malady is induced by a virus and most characteristically expressed by the production of tight clusters of twigs. Stump sprout in the above picture possesses typical "witches' brooms" on the upper portion of the sprouts. (Photograph courtesy U.S. Forest Service.)

leaves to have interveinal mosaic and slight curl. Eventually, this disease results in severe leaf and fruit distortion and premature shed.

Spike disease of sandal, however, is more important than the leaf-curl mosaic, although the symptoms are similar. Spike disease is considered by many to be commercially the most important forest tree virus disorder. Large numbers of sandal trees have been killed by this virus and the sandalwood oil industry is threatened.

9. *Ulmus.* This internationally important genus has four well-documented virus diseases.

Elm mosaic has been found in Europe, Canada, and the United States on American elm (*U. americana*), English elm (*U. campestris*), Wych elm (*U. glabra*), and Siberian elm (*U. pumila*). Symptoms vary widely from mild to severe but usually involve some degree of dwarfing of infected branches. In a greenhouse study, Bretz (1950) planted seed collected from mosaic-infected trees. After 3 months, approximately 3% of the seedlings developed mosaic symptoms, which suggested seed transmission of the causal virus. Another relatively uncommon transmission route was studied by Callahan (1957). This investigator made pollinations between healthy and virus-diseased parents. An average of 30.5% of the 1523 seedlings obtained from crosses between healthy pistils and infected pollen was virus infected.

Phloem necrosis of elm is confined to the United States and found primarily in the midwestern and central states. In some communities, the disease has reached epiphytotic proportions and killed 50–75 percent of the elms. This disease has been economically the most important forest tree virus in the United States. All-age elms (American and winged elm, *U. alata*) may be infected. Trees usually exhibit symptoms from 6 months to 1 year after infection and usually die within 2 years. Initial symptoms include death of some of the fibrous roots and premature leaf drop at the uppermost branch tips. Eventually, foliage becomes yellow and substantial defoliation may occur as larger roots are destroyed. A typical discoloration, found in the phloem and cambium extending from the trunk to the branches, precedes the death of the larger roots. The cambium becomes yellow, while the phloem becomes first yellow, but ultimately brown. A characteristic odor of wintergreen is associated with the discolored phloem. The causal virus, which is restricted to the phloem, has been characterized as a rod-shaped particle. Natural transmission is presumed to be most importantly accomplished by the leafhopper, *Scaphoideus luteolus.*

The remaining *Ulmus* virus diseases are much less important than the two previously discussed, as they appear confined to the United States and are found only in American elm. Elm scorch is apparently caused by a virus confined to the xylem and causes marginal leaf necrosis. Elm zonate canker is an interesting disease in that one of the symptoms expressed is a stem canker. Severely cankered branches may exhibit dieback.

REFERENCES

Bollard, E. G., and Matthews, R. E. F. (1966). The physiology of parasitic disease. *In* "Plant Physiology" (F. C. Steward, ed.), Vol. 4B, pp. 417-550. Academic Press, New York.

Bretz, T. W. (1950). Seed transmission of the elm mosaic virus. *Phytopathology* **40**, 3-4 (abstr.).

Callahan, K. L. (1957). Pollen transmission of elm mosaic virus. *Phytopathology* **47**, 5 (abstr.).

Cech, M., Kralik, O., and Blattny, C. (1961). Rod shaped particles associated with virosis of spruce. *Phytopathology* **51**, 183-185.

Hibben, C. R. (1966). Graft transmission of a ringspot-like virus from white ash. *Plant Disease Reptr.* **50**, 905-906.

Hibben, C. R. (1968). Transmission by dodder of a yellows-type virus from declining white ash. *Phytopathology* **58**, 399 (abstr.).

Ross, E. W. (1966). Ash dieback. *Tech. Publ., N.Y. State Coll. Forestry* **88**, 1-80.

Schmelzer, K. (1963). Untersuchungen an Viren der Zier-und Wildgehölze. *Phytopathol. Z.* **46**, 235-268.

Schmelzer, K., Schmidt, H. E., and Schmidt, H. B. (1966). Viroses and virussuspect phenomena found with forest tree species. *Arch. Forstw.* **15**, 107-120.

Seliskar, C. E. (1966). Virus and viruslike disorders of forest trees. *FAO/IUFRO Symposium on Internationally Dangerous Forest Diseases and Insects, Oxford, 1964* Vol. I, Meeting V, p. 1-44, FAO, Rome.

Smith, K. M. (1957). "A Textbook of Plant Virus Diseases." Churchill, London.

GENERAL REFERENCES

Atanasoff, D. (1935). Old and new virus diseases of trees and shrubs. *Phytopathol. Z.* **8**, 196-223.

Callahan, K. L., and More, J. D. (1957). *Prunus* host range of elm mosaic virus. *Phytopathology* **47**, 4 (abstr.).

Davis, R. E., Whitcomb, R. F., and Steere, R. L. (1968). Remission of aster yellows disease by antibiotics. *Science* **161**, 793-794.

Kristensen, H. R. (1960). Virussygdomme hos Forstplanter. *Dansk Skovforen. Tidsskr.* **45**, 155-166.

McLean, D. M. (1944). Histo-pathologic changes in the phloem of American elm affected with the virus causing phloem necrosis. *Phytopathology* **34**, 818-826.

Peterson, G. W. (1966). Western X-disease virus of chokecherry: Transmission and seed effects. *Plant Disease Reptr.* **50**, 659-660.

Swingle, R. V., and Bretz, T. W. (1950). Zonate canker, a virus disease of American elm. *Phytopathology* **40**, 1018-1022.

12

BACTERIA

Bacteria might be defined as microscopic, unicellular plants containing no chlorophyll, which reproduce by binary fission. A more detailed examination of the components of this definition may enable a better appreciation of this extremely important group of phytoparasites.

Bacteria are microscopic; most fall in the narrow range of sizes from 0.2 to 1.5 μ in diameter (1 mm $=$ 1000 μ). This dimension places bacteria at the upper fringe of the size of colloidal matter. When suspended in a liquid, therefore, they will exhibit Brownian movement, scatter light by Tyndall effect and increase the viscosity of the suspending medium. Bacteria may also act as electrically charged colloidal particles, they migrate in an electric field and exhibit a tendency to agglutinate.

Individual bacteria are unicellular. Billions of cells may grow closely together in chains or in colonies, but every cell remains intact and none become interrelated or interorganized.

Bacteria are generally considered to be members of the plant kingdom. Until approximately 1830, most living things were rather clearly plants or animals. As exploration of the microbial world developed, however, it became apparent that various microbial groups were not easily fitted into the plant or animal kingdoms. Biologists of the nineteenth century solved this problem in an arbitrary fashion by splitting the major microbial groups between the two kingdoms. Protozoa were generally regarded as animals, as they were mostly motile and nonphotosynthetic. Algae were quite clearly plants as they were photosynthetic. Fungi and bacteria were less easily categorized. Fungi, unlike most plants, were nonphotosynthetic, but also, unlike most animals, primarily immotile. Bacteria were similarly perplexing, but

TABLE XVIII

ORGANIZATION OF THE PLANT, ANIMAL, AND PROTISTA GROUPS[a]

Characteristics	Plants	Animals
Multicellular, showing extensive tissue differentiation	Seed plants Ferns Liverworts	Vertebrates Invertebrates
	Protists	
Unicellular, coenocytic, or multicellular; without tissue differentiation	Algae Protozoa Fungi Bacteria	

[a]From Stanier et al. (1963). Reproduced by permission of Prentice Hall, Inc.

were generally considered plants for four primary reasons (Lamanna and Mallette, 1965). First, as a group, free-living bacteria have plantlike synthetic capacities. From relatively simple substrates, they are capable of forming complex molecules of protoplasm. Second, food materials must penetrate bacteria in a soluble form in order to be assimilated. Animals, however, bring solid foods inside their bodies for digestion as well as assimilation. Third, bacteria multiply by binary fission along the transverse axis. With some exceptions, animal cells divide by binary fission along the longitudinal axis. Fourth, most species of bacteria possess a morphologically differentiated rigid cell wall outside the confines of the plasma membrane and cytoplasm, while most animals do not.

All biologists were not satisfied with this arbitrary placement. In 1866, the German zoologist Haeckel proposed establishment of a third kingdom termed the protista. Algae, fungi, protozoa, and bacteria were all proposed as members for the protista kingdom. The distinguishing feature of the protista from higher plants and animals is their relatively simple biological organization (Table XVIII).

Finally, bacteria are characterized by a lack of chlorophyll (none contain chloroplasts) and by reproduction by simple binary fission. An important distinction to bear in mind relating to bacterial growth is that growth in this instance refers to increases in numbers of cells and not to increases in the dimensions of individual cells.

I. CLASSIFICATION

Generally, bacteria are grouped in the class Schizomycetes, which is in turn divided into 10 orders:

Chlamydobacteriales
Hyphomicrobiales
Caryophanales
Actinomycetales
Bettiatoales
Myxobacterales
Spirochaltales
Mycoplasmatales
Pseudomonadales
Eubacteriales

Only the last two orders contain important (known) bacterial plant pathogens:

	Eubacteriales		Pseudomonadales
Corynebacteriaceae	Enterobacteriaceae	Rhizobiaceae	Pseudomonadaceae
Corynebacterium	*Erwinia*	*Agrobacterium*	*Xanthomonas*
			Pseudomonas

These five genera contain the most important species of plant parasites. All of these bacteria are rod shaped and none produce spores.

II. ANATOMY AND PHYSIOLOGY

Figure 17 contains a schematic representation of bacterial structure. The various anatomical features are discussed below in more detail.

a. Slime layer. The capsule or slime layer is an accumulation of viscid material around the external surface of the cell wall of bacteria. This layer is generally considered to be a nonliving secretion or excretion that lacks an active metabolic role. No disturbance in metabolism or viability is realized when this covering is removed.

b. Cell wall. The cell walls of bacteria (20-25% of the organisms' volume and 20-35% of their dry weight) is complex and variable. Staining characteristics of bacteria differ according to the constitution of their cell walls. There are, for example, consistent and major differences between the bacteria which react positively and negatively to the Gram stain, with respect to macromolecular compounds incorporated in the cell wall. The Gram reaction has proved to be one of the fundamental phenomena of bacteriology. The stain procedure involves an initial application of crystal violet (a basic dye) followed by an application of iodine. At this point all bacteria will be stained blue. The third step involves treatment with alcohol, after which some bacteria retain the crystal violet-iodine complex and remain blue (gram positive) and some become completely decolorized (gram negative). There is an intermediate bacterial group termed the gram variables. The response of an organism to the Gram stain, however, is very interestingly cor-

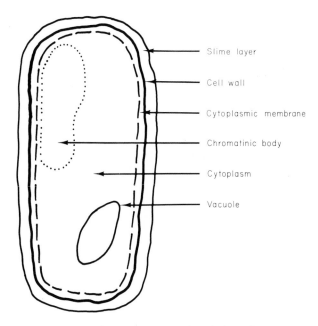

Slime layer

Cell wall

Cytoplasmic membrane

Chromatinic body

Cytoplasm

Vacuole

Fig. 17. Schematic representation of a bacterium.

related with many other physiological and biochemical characteristics (Table XIX).

The rigid structure of all bacterial walls is provided by a mucopeptide. This mucopeptide is a polymer of repeating units of hexosamine-muramic acid-peptide. Generally, gram positive bacteria also contain large amounts of proteins, lipids, and polysaccharides.

TABLE XIX

REPORTED DIFFERENCES BETWEEN GRAM POSITIVE AND GRAM NEGATIVE BACTERIA[a]

Characteristic	Gram positive	Gram negative
Cell wall thickness	Greater	Less
Cell wall ruptured by heat	No	Yes
Amino acids in cell wall	Few kinds	Numerous kinds
Separation of plasma membrane from cell wall	Difficult	Relatively easy
Hexoseamine content of cell wall	More	Less
Lipides in cell wall	None or low	Present

TABLE XIX

REPORTED DIFFERENCES BETWEEN GRAM POSITIVE AND GRAM
NEGATIVE BACTERIA[a] (Continued)

Characteristic	Gram positive	Gram negative
Mesosomes	Present	Absent
Ornithine transaminase	Present	Absent
Magnesium content	Greater	Less
Excretion of putrescine	Slight or none	Present
Digestion by gastric juice	Resistant	Less resistant
Digestion of killed organisms by trypsin or pepsin	Resistant	Not resistant
Resistance to strong alkali (1% KOH)	Not dissolved	Dissolved
Solubility of lipides in fat solvents	Resistant	Less resistant
pH of optimal growth	Relatively high	At acidic values
Apparent isoelectric point by staining (pH)	2-3	About 4-5
Amounts of acid and basic dyes retained at apparent isoelectric point	Greater	Less
Susceptibility to acriflavine dyes	Marked	Less marked
Bacteriostatic effect of triphenyl-methane dyes	Very susceptible	More resistant
Inhibition by sodium azide	Resistant	Less resistant
Permeability to dye in living state	More permeable	Less permeable
Bacteriostatic action of iodine	More susceptible	Less susceptible
Autolysis	Less common	More commonly noted
Lysis by specific complement fixation	Not readily apparent	Often observed
Lysozyme lysis	Very susceptible	Less so
Nature of toxins produced	Exotoxins	Endotoxins and antigens of Boivin type
Nutrient requirements	Generally complex, none autotrophic	Relatively simpler, many species autotrophic
Susceptibility to penicillin	Greater	Less
Susceptibility to low surface tension	Greater	Less
Susceptibility to anionic detergents	Very susceptible	Much less; susceptible only in acid media
Bacteriostatic action of tellurites	More resistant	More sensitive
Acid fastness	Some species	None
Rupture by sudden changes in pressure and supersonic energy	More resistant	Least resistant
Optical density changes of suspensions with increasing solute concentration	None or little	Extinction increases

[a]From Lamanna and Mallette (1965). Reproduced by permission of Williams and Wilkins Co.

The cell wall function, unlike the function of nematode cuticle, appears to be purely mechanical; it confers rigidity, ductility, and elasticity to the bacterial cell. It apparently has little or no role in permeability regulation or other metabolic activity. A crucial importance of the mucocomplex in maintaining normal cell wall structure has recently been shown with respect to antibiotic action. The popular antibiotic penicillin is an exceptionally effective antibacterial agent. This material specifically prevents the incorporation of subunits of the mucocomplex into bacterial cell walls. As cells grow in the presence of penicillin (penicillin is toxic only for growing bacteria), the newly synthesized regions of the wall are deprived of their tensile strength because of the absence of the mucocomplex, and bizarre, distorted cells are produced by the bulging of protoplasm. Eventually, osmotic disintegration of the cell occurs.

c. Cytoplasmic membrane. This membrane, which consists largely of protein and lipid, is located next to the inner surface of the cell wall and separates the wall from the cytoplasm. The function of the membrane is unknown but, some indirect evidence suggests that it contains permeases and it may function in the active transport of substrates into the cell. It has also been suggested that this region may have a function similar to mitochondria. The membrane contains several enzymes, among them several that participate in respiratory metabolism.

d. Cytoplasm. This term is generally applied to all the granular or protoplasmic material within the cytoplasmic membrane. Unlike fungi, bacteria do not exhibit protoplasmic streaming. Since this mechanism for enhancing diffusion is absent, it may be that kinetic motion of the molecules is sufficient, in small organisms, to distribute metabolites. The cytoplasm contains several metabolically active bodies, for example ribosomes and chromatophores, and several metabolically inactive bodies or inclusions, for example organic polymers and volutin. Ribosomes, which range in length from 100–200 Å, (1 Å = one ten thousandth of a micron), may be very numerous, approximately 10,000 per bacterium. On a dry weight basis, these bodies contain approximately equal amounts of protein and ribonucleic acid. It is presumed that they play important and fundamental roles in protein synthesis. Chromatophores, which occur in photosynthetic bacteria, are much less complex structurally than chloroplasts. They contain various red and purple pigments, but no chlorophyll. Inclusions are thought to act primarily in a reserve capacity. β-Hydroxybutyric acid and starchlike polymers of glucose are important carbon and energy reserves. Volutin, which is a polymerized inorganic metaphosphate, serves as a phosphate reserve.

e. Vacuoles. These fluid-containing cavaties enclosed by membranes have been noted in bacteria. Presumably, they function in a reserve or storage capacity.

f. Chromatinic body. The existence in bacteria of a separable morphological entity equivalent to the nucleus of higher plants and animals has been much debated. Bacterial cytoplasm contains so much RNA that basic dyes generally failed to reveal DNA and typically stained the entire cell. This led to the suggestion that the entire cell was the nucleus. Eventually, however, with acid and enzymatic hydrolysis, RNA could be destroyed and basic dyes were able to reveal DNA. Even though this DNA lacks the morphological characteristics of true nuclei, the specialized role in heredity is presumed similar to that of other organisms. Until the more precise nature of bacterial mitoses and bacterial chromosomes are appreciated, microbiologists prefer the term chromatinic bodies rather than nuclei.

Two additional structures, which are lacking or rare in plant parasitic bacterial species, are flagella and endospores. Flagella are long filamentous appendages of cytoplasmic origin which provide locomotive capacity to free swimming bacteria. Some bacteria are able to form highly resistant resting structures within their cells, termed endospores. These structures which usually possess exceptional thermal resistance (up to 70°-80°C) give rise to additional vegetative cells upon germination.

III. ECOLOGY

A. Occurrence

Bacteria are found practically everywhere they are sought. In general, bacterial species are quite cosmopolitan and rarely endemic to particular geographic locations. The kinds found in polar zones are similar to those found in more temperate regions. This is in part due to the fact that bacteria have existed for eons of time and wind, ocean currents, and migratory animals have effectively distributed them around the world. There are, of course, differences in the exact species found in specific locations and differences in relative numbers (Lamanna and Mallette, 1965). In the case of parasitic species, it is self-evident that their distribution will be coincident with the normal habitat of their host species.

In general, the kinds of bacteria found in the air are marine and soil types which are spore formers. Few of these are capable of causing plant disease as phytoparasites are not spore formers. Bacteria are tremendously abundant in the soil. The number per gram of soil ranges from one million (or less) to several billions. Two billion cells per gram might be considered a representative value for bacterial soil populations.

B. Dispersal

Bacterial distribution mechanisms are extremely diverse. In a forest, three primary dispersal procedures might be recognized. Water moves bacteria through both the air and the soil. Rain brings down airborne cells and may wash bacteria down stems and branches and over leaves. Wind acts to move bacteria directly, but more importantly indirectly, by moving objects with bacteria attached. Bacteria are also transported by vectors. Vectors are many and include insects, nematodes, and larger animals, for example birds and squirrels. All these procedures are passive. Some phytoparasitic bacteria are motile and may be capable of moving limited distances in water in an active fashion.

C. Host Infection

In general, bacterial cells must rapidly find an environment favorable to their proliferation or they will perish. The absolute requirements of such an environment are a high relative humidity and an adequate nutritional substrate (Goodman et al., 1967). Even in the presence of a suitable environment, entrance into a host plant can only be accomplished passively through natural openings or wounds. Several natural openings provide suitable bacterial entrance courts. Stomates are pores in the epidermal covering of plants, particularly leaves, through which gas exchange takes place. Stomates may occur at a frequency of 50–300 per mm^2. The average phytoparasitic bacterium is approximately 1.0μ wide and 1.5μ long. Stomates may have an area of approximately $90 \mu^2$. The relative humidity of the stomatal cavity is high, generally approximately 100%. Lenticels are also important natural entrance courts. These are small raised pores, usually elliptical in shape, which develop on woody stems and roots when the epidermis is replaced with cork tissue. Lenticels become packed with loosely arranged cells that allow gas exchange. Other natural openings of minor importance include: nectaries, hydathodes, and glandular hairs. Nectaries are glands which secrete sugary fluid in flowers of several insect-pollinated species. Hydathodes are water excreting glands which occur on the edges or tips of leaves of many species.

Wounds are also extremely important portals of bacterial entry. Timing is important here, however, as the bacterium must reach the wound when it is fresh, before healing is initiated, and while leakage of the cellular contents provides high humidity and substrate materials. Infection through a wound, however, permits the bacteria to bypass the degradation of internal cutinized cell walls. Cutin is a complex mixture of oxidation and condensation products of fatty acids, which characteristically covers the exterior cell walls of internal stomate and lenticel cells. Wounds are more common than might be supposed and include, for example, breakage of root hairs or trichomes, other mechanical root and stem wounds—low temperature, ice, abrasion, nematode wounds, insect wounds—bark beetles, aphids.

D. Development in Host

Once the bacterial pathogen has entered the plant, multiplication occurs, almost without exception in the intercellular spaces of the host tissue. Bacteria obtain nutrients by degrading the intercellular cement and cell wall materials. This degradation and possibly ultimate death of host tissue is accomplished by the release of toxins.

Numerous plant pathogens, particularly bacteria and fungi, are known to be capable of degrading host tissues and cells, and of causing abnormal physiology by releasing various metabolites once inside the plant. Included among these metabolites are enzymes, plant growth regulators, and a large number of miscellaneous and unrelated organic compounds. In plant disease, the term toxin is generally applied to the members of this latter group. Toxins which have been studied include certain polysaccharides, polypeptides, and several low molecular weight organic compounds.

Unlike viruses, bacteria cause disease at the metabolic level via toxin release rather than at the genetic level. Bacteria, also unlike viruses, are typically not obligate parasites and are quite able to persist and even flourish if the host plant is killed. As a result, bacteria are extremely important agents of plant disease. Bacterial tree diseases are incompletely appreciated.

REFERENCES

Goodman, R. N., Király, Z., and Zaitlin, M. (1967). "The Biochemistry and Physiology of Infectious Plant Disease." Van Nostrand, Princeton, New Jersey.

Lamanna, C., and Mallette, M. F. (1965). "Basic Bacteriology." Williams & Wilkins, Baltimore, Maryland.

Stanier, R. Y., Doudoroff, M., and Adelberg, E. A. (1963). "The Microbial World." Prentice-Hall, Englewood Cliffs, New Jersey.

GENERAL REFERENCES

Bernheimer, A. W. (1968). Cytolytic toxins of bacterial origin. Science **159**, 847-851.

Breed, R. S., Murray, E. G. D., and Smith, N. R. (1957). "Bergey's Manual of Determinative Bacteriology," 7th. ed. Williams & Wilkins, Baltimore, Maryland.

Gray, T. R. G., and Parkinson, D., eds. (1968). "The Ecology of Soil Bacteria." Liverpool Univ. Press, Liverpool.

Hawker, L. E., Linton, A. H., Folkes, B. F., and Carlile, M. J. (1967). "An Introduction to the Biology of Micro-organisms." Arnold, London.

Johnson, B. T., Goodman, R. N., and Goldberg, H. S. (1967). Conversion of DDT to DDD by pathogenic and saprophytic bacteria associated with plants. Science **157**, 560-561.

Owens, L. D. (1969). Toxins in plant disease: Structure and mode of action. *Science* **165**, 18-25.

Skerman, V. B. D. (1967). "A Guide to the Identification of the Genera of Bacteria." Williams & Wilkins, Baltimore, Maryland.

Sistrom, W. R. (1966). "Microbial Life." Holt, New York.

Umbreit, W. W. (1962). "Modern Microbiology." Freeman, San Francisco, California.

Whittaker, R. H. (1969). New Concepts of kingdoms of organisms. *Science* **163**, 150-160.

13

SPECIFIC BACTERIA AND TREE DISEASE

Bacteria influence tree health in numerous ways. They are important direct agents of several tree diseases. They also, however, are significant in various indirect manners. Bacteria appear to be intimately associated with a curious tree malady called wetwood. Evidence suggesting that bacteria have an important role in decay and discoloration processes is increasing.

I. BACTERIA AS DIRECT DISEASE AGENTS

Approximately 200 species of bacteria are known to cause plant disease. Generally, these parasites belong to one of five genera. Based on the symptoms usually produced, these genera might be separated as follows.

1. Soft Rots	*Pseudomonas* spp.
Erwinia spp.	*Xanthomonas* spp.
2. Wilts (Vascular Diseases)	4. Tumefactions
Xanthomonas spp.	*Agrobacterium* spp.
Corynebacterium spp.	*Pseudomonas* spp.
Erwinia spp.	*Xanthomonas* spp.
Pseudomonas spp.	
	5. Spots (Local Lesions)
3. Blights	*Pseudomonas* spp.
Erwinia spp.	*Xanthomonas* spp.

Important fruit-tree species, for example, *Citrus, Malus, Prunus,* and *Pyrus,* have received relatively intensive study with respect to bacterial diseases. Numerous economically important diseases induced by bacteria are known in these groups. There is, unfortunately, very limited knowledge available with respect to bacterial diseases of forest trees. As with viruses, even the information which is available is largely concerned only with host symptom expresssion and geographic distribution of the disease. A selected group of important bacterial diseases will be discussed to present represent- ative etiological patterns and disease syndromes. This list is *not* comprehen- sive.

1. Poplar dieback and canker. This disease, which is currently unknown in the United States but important in Britain, Holland, and France, is caused by *Pseudomonas syringae* f. *populea* (Sabet and Dowson, 1952). Cankers varying from 1 to 15 cm in length are the primary symptom of the disease and develop on minor and major branches and, occasionally, on the trunk. Two canker types are generally distinguished. Closed cankers develop in the current year of infection, generally take the form of a rough, knotted in- tumesence, and vary in size from 2-3 cm to 10-12 cm in diameter. The second canker type, usually referred to as open canker, is an elongated, pe- rennial lesion with a raised rim and exposed wood typically 12-15 cm in length. Both canker types are characterized by exudation or gummosis (leakage of fairly viscous sap) during wet weather in the spring. Excessively cankered shoots frequently exhibit dieback during the early summer.

The gum which is released from the cankers in early spring contains bac- terial cells. This gum along with bacteria is washed along shoots by spring rains. When this material reaches developing buds, bacteria are thought to reenter the host, perhaps through bud scars. Shoots which develop from these buds are frequently quickly killed. Young twigs, even though lignified, are frequently killed after bacteria are washed into cracks or lenticels. Older branches, after infection, commonly exhibit the cankers previously de- scribed.

Little research has been done on the specific mechanisms of infection and disease development. Analysis of the gum released, however, has revealed the presence of several sugar compounds with amino groups and traces of pectic enzymes. This material also has been suggested to contain "toxic" substances whose specific nature is unknown. The gum is a particularly fa- vorable medium for bacterial development.

2. European ash canker. This disease of European ash species is caused by *Pseudomonas savastonoi* f. *fraxini*. The disease is insignificant in the United States, although white ash is very susceptible to infection by the bac- terium.

In the early stages of this disease, small cracks with thickened edges ap- pear in the bark of green shoots. Eventually both bark and wood are stimu- lated to abnormal development, resulting in elongated cavities bounded by irregular callus development. These lesions persist for many years.

Causal bacteria are presumed to enter through leaf scars and occasionally through wounds, for example those caused by hailstones. Bacterial development is concentrated in the soft parenchyma of the cortex. Even though the wood itself does not appear to be invaded, toxins released by the bacteria are presumed responsible for its abnormal development.

3. Walnut blight. This is a serious disease of black walnut, butternut, and other members of the *Juglans* genus, caused by *Xanthomonas juglandis*. It is of considerable economic importance in California, Europe, Australia, and New Zealand. The most conspicuous symptom is small irregularly shaped black spots on the leaves and petioles. Young fruits may become spotted and as they mature may develop larger black spots. Internally, the edible portion may be partly or wholly destroyed. Young fruits are occasionally killed outright. A less conspicuous symptom is elongated black streaks which may occur on young shoots.

The pathogen is presumed to enter the leaves through stomates and the shoots via lenticels and wounds. Pockets of bacteria develop below the infection sites and erupt to the surface during wet weather. The vascular bundles of host trees do not appear to be invaded. The bacteria are confined to parenchymatous tissue. Rain is the chief means of distribution for the bacteria. As the organisms ooze out from blackened lesions on shoots, leaves, and petioles during rain, they are washed and splashed to new areas. In California it has also been shown that the bacterium infects male catkins (Ark, 1944). Some of these catkins are killed but others survive and produce contaminated pollen. Such pollen may infect young female flowers and either kill them or ultimately cause apical infection of developing nuts. Contaminated pollen may also be responsible for leaf spotting.

4. Walnut phloem canker. This is another important *Juglans* disease which has received recent attention. The disease, which is caused by *Erwinia rubrifaciens*, is especially serious on Persian walnut (*J. regia*) in the Sacramento Valley in California (Wilson *et al.*, 1967). A primary symptom is irregularly shaped, dark necrotic areas in the outer bark of branches and stems of mature trees. During the summer a dark, watery substance escapes from the cankers and is distributed over the surface of the bark.

Schaad and Wilson (1968) have studied the localization and movement of the bacterium in the host. At the terminal margins of necrotic cavities the bacteria were found only in sieve tubes. In the xylem, the bacteria were located in axial and lateral parenchyma (rays) and in vessel members. Bacteria appeared to move faster in the xylem than in the phleom and may have moved intracellularly over long distances in the xylem. Lateral movement from xylem to phloem was slow.

5. Live oak drippy nut. This malady, caused by *Erwinia quercina*, has been observed on California live oak (*Quercus agrifolia*) and interior live oak (*Q. wistezenii*) in the interior valleys of central and northern California

during the past several years (Hildebrand and Schroth, 1967). Symptoms include discoloration and excessive oozing from nuts. Ingress for the bacterium into the nut is primarily through ovipositor punctures made by insects such as cynipid wasps.

6. Crown gall. *Agrobacterium tumefaciens* is the cause of this extremely important plant disease. The bacterium has a very broad host range, affecting plants belonging to at least 142 genera present in 61 widely separated botanical families. Various angiosperms are commonly infected. Infection of gymnosperms occurs less abundantly in nature. Incense cedar (*Libocedrus decurrens*) and several members of the Taxaceae, Taxodiaceae, and Pinaceae families are susceptible.

Primary symptoms of *A. tumefaciens* infection are tumefactions of roots, root collars, stems, or branches. Galls vary in size from that of a pea to that of a basketball. They are generally small on tree roots, but much larger on the root collar or crown. On herbaceous stems the galls are generally soft, and on woody stems they are always hard.

II. MECHANISM OF CROWN GALL FORMATION

The similarities between crown galls and animal cancers have stimulated extensive research and study on the mechanisms involved in gall development. As a result, more is known of the etiology of crown gall than any other bacterial disease of plants.

The genesis of crown-gall tumor cells from normal cells may be divided into three major periods (Klein, 1954). These periods are designated the transformation period, the duplication period, and the organization and differentiation period (Fig. 18).

The transformation period includes four phases which have been designated preinduction, induction, promotion, and completion. The preinduction phase is initiated by the wounding of host tissues with or without the simultaneous introduction of *A. tumefaciens*. With a few questionable exceptions, no reports of tumor induction in the absence of prior wounding

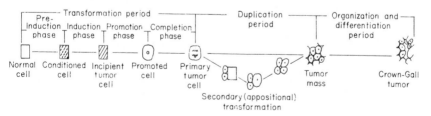

Fig. 18. Diagramatic scheme of the development of a crown-gall tumor. [From Klein (1954). Reproduced by permission of Brookhaven National Laboratory.]

have been documented. The application of bacteria to the surface of intact plants is wholly ineffective in initiating infection. The wound is not necessary for the bacteria to enter cells, that is, once the bacteria are in the plant, as the organisms are intercellular. It has been found that the wound requires an "activation" or "conditioning" period before the bacteria can act. Bacteria applied prior to or considerably after wounding are incapable of initiating infection. Since it is not the wound itself or the injured cells which are the agents of conditioning, investigators looked for products released or produced by wound tissue. They concluded that the major consequence of wounding is the release from wounded cells of materials required for the "conditioning" of the cells later to be transformed into tumor cells. Healing tissues apparently cease to release the "conditioning" substance. If a "conditioned" cell is not immediately acted upon by a tumor-inducing agent, it will lose its predisposition toward becoming a tumor cell and become a callus cell.

During the induction phase, it has been established that a tumor-inducing agent or principle (usually designated TIP) acts on conditioned cells during the 10-24 hour period following the preinduction phase to initiate tumor cells. The exact nature of TIP is unknown. Three hypotheses have been advanced relating to the character of TIP. The first suggests that it may be a metabolic by-product or toxin of A. tumefaciens. The second suggests that it may be a bacterially modified host cell material. The third, and most recent, suggests that it may be a virus, that is, a bacteriophage of A. tumefaciens. Evidence has been presented which indicates that phage particles are located in conditioned cells. If this last hypothesis is verified, then the bacterium may be merely functioning as a vector.

During the promotion phase, the "incipient tumor" cells are acted upon by auxin (IAA). The increased amount of auxin which is observed may result from: (1) bacterial synthesis, (2) enhanced host capacity for synthesis, or (3) loss of degrative capacity. The auxin is presumed to function in promoting the incipient tumor cells and alters them into enlarged "promoted cells." When the primary tumor cells commence their first division the completion phase is fulfilled and the transformation period is terminated. A review of these steps is presented in Fig. 19.

During the duplication period, the tumor develops apparently without stimulus from the bacterium. Apparently, the tumor cells acquire a capacity for autonomous growth as a result of the permanent activation of a series of growth-substance synthesizing systems. Once the cellular transformation has been accomplished, the pathogen is presumed to no longer play a role in the continued development of the disease. The altered host cells become pathogenic because they have acquired a capacity to synthesize greater than

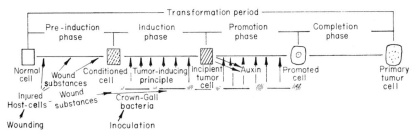

Fig. 19. Diagramatic representation of the phases of the transformation period of crown-gall tumor development, and of the sources and interrelations of the known etiological agents active during this period. [From Klein (1954). Reproduced by permission of Brookhaven National Laboratory.]

regulatory amounts of growth- promoting substances or are altered in such a way that proper hormone balance cannot be maintained.

During the final phase of crown-gall development, the tumor may undergo a certain amount of organization and differentiation. This tendency may also be hormonally influenced.

III. WETWOOD

The state of knowledge about the differences between sapwood and heartwood and the transition from one to the other is very incomplete. It has been assumed that heartwood formation coincides with the natural death of the parenchyma due to its age or distance from the cambium. Both heartwood and sapwood of healthy trees are thought of as practically free from microorganisms, except for the heart-rotting fungi or local infections (Hartley et al., 1961).

In many tree species, however, the character of the interior wood is quite different from the normal tree wood character. Most elms, willows, and true poplars have interior wood that is obviously wetter than the adjacent sapwood (Hartley et al., 1961). The "wetwood" is usually in the outermost heartwood, but in young trees may occupy the entire center. In cottonwood (Populus spp.), wetwood is commonly initially found in 2-year-old seedlings. In true firs (Abies spp.), a wet zone is common but less marked than that present in most true "wetwood" species. In several other genera, including Betula, Acer, Liriodendron, and Quercus, interior zones with similar pronounced high moisture regions have been found (Hartley et al., 1961).

The most outstanding character of wetwood is its high moisture content. Moisture levels of wetwood typically exceed those of both heartwood and sapwood. Excessive moisture, however, is not the only distinguishing trait of wetwood. Increased gas content has frequently been associated with wet-wood. In cottonwood, Lombardy poplar, and American elm, deep borer holes not only often yield an immediate flow of liquid, but also commonly exhibit gas release. In a study on Lombardy poplar, gas pressure in wetwood increased at an approximately uniform rate from 8 lbs/in.^{2} in late May to 35 lbs/in.^{2} in early August (Hartley et al., 1961). The principal gas involved is thought to be methane (CH_4). Because of the low oxygen content of the heartwood, the production of a reduction product such as methane is not surprising. Differences in pH between wetwood and normal wood have also been observed in various tree species. Fresh sapwood of both conifers and hardwoods is typically mildly acid, having a pH of 5-6. Dried sapwood is frequently more acid, with a pH usually below 5 and frequently as low as 4. Normal (uninfected) heartwood is typically more acid than sapwood. Gen-erally, it can be suggested that uninfected sapwood or heartwood usually has a pH below 7. Wetwood, on the other hand, usually exhibits a pH in excess of 7. Mineral content of wetwood is also frequently higher than normal wood. This may be due in part to precipitation of materials, for ex-ample calcium salts, in the presence of the higher pH.

Three major hypotheses have been advanced to explain wetwood forma-tion (Hartley et al., 1961). The first suggests that the parenchymatous ele-ments at the inner limit of the sapwood die of senesence or from impaired communication with the cambium. The wetwood condition is ultimately produced as a result of the action of the trees' own enzymes on the contents of these moribund cells. The second and third hypotheses involve bacterial participation in the process leading to wetwood formation. In the second theory, the parenchyma cells are presumed to die as described previously, but all subsequent degradations are mainly due to the activity of saprophytic bacteria. Numerous bacteria have been shown to be associated with wet-wood. In the third hypothesis, it is proposed that the death of the paren-chyma cells is caused or hastened by weakly parasitic bacteria. These bac-teria may or may not have been present in the normal wood; in any case, they are presumed capable of infection only after the wood cells have be-come senescent. This latter hypothesis has been the one generally accepted as explaining wetwood formation in elm and poplar species.

The pathological significance of wetwood is thought to be great in some species. Premature mortality of Lombardy poplar (trees frequently die before age 20) seems to be associated with wetwood. Wetwood has been suggested as a possible factor in the unexplained mortality frequently observed in balsam fir. Frost cracks in London planes have been suggested to be partially the result of increased freezing stresses due to excessive interior water con-tents. In a secondary manner, wetwood conditions may promote decay of the heartwood by providing more suitable moisture conditions for fungal growth or by prolonging susceptibility by lengthening the time required for the wood to dry (Hartley et al., 1961).

IV. INDIRECT BACTERIAL EFFECTS

In addition to their direct effects, bacteria are important to tree health and wood utilization in various indirect and secondary fashions. There is evidence being accumulated that bacteria may play a significant role in heartrot, wood decay, and discoloration. With respect to the succession of organisms in wood, for example, it has been suggested that decayed and discolored tissues are first infected by bacteria and nondecay fungi and later infected by decay fungi (Chapter 16). Bacteria may also interact with other disease agents and result in compound stresses. Esser et al. (1968), for example, observed several instances where root-knot nematodes were infesting crown-gall tissues of silver maple, peach, willow, and weeping willow. On the positive side of biological interactions, Jewell and Campana (1968) have suggested that three bacterial isolates from healthy elm twigs were capable of inhibiting the in vitro growth of Ceratocystis ulmi, the causal agent of Dutch elm disease.

Bacteria are also frequently damaging in the processing of forest products. Ponded logs are frequently invaded by bacteria that ultimately adversely effect veneer cutting or preservative adsorption (Knuth and McCoy, 1962). Bacteria also are frequently involved in costly slime formation in pulp and paper manufacturing mills.

REFERENCES

Ark, P. A. (1944). Pollen as a source of walnut bacterial blight infection. Phytopathology **34**, 330-334.

Esser, R. P., Martinez, A. P., and Langdon, K. R. (1968). Simultaneous occurrence of root-knot nematode and crown gall bacteria. Plant Disease Reptr. **52**, 550-553.

Hartley, C., Davidson, R. W., and Crandall, B. S. (1961). Wetwood, bacteria, and increased pH in trees. Rept., Forest Prod. Lab. **2215**, 1-34.

Hildebrand, D. C., and Schroth, M. N. (1967). A new species of Erwinia causing the drippy nut disease of live oaks. Phytopathology **57**, 250-253.

Jewell, T. R., and Campana, R. J. (1968). Antagonism of bacteria from elm to Ceratocystis ulmi in vitro. Phytopathology **58**, 400 (abstr.).

Klein, R. M. (1954). Mechanisms of crown-gall induction. Brookhaven Symp. Biol. **6**, 97-114.

Knuth, D. T., and McCoy, E. (1962). Bacterial deterioration of pine logs in pond storage. Forest Prod. J. **12**, 437-442.

Sabet, K. A., and Dowson, W. J. (1952). Studies in the bacterial die-back and canker disease of poplar. I. The disease and its cause. *Ann. Appl. Biol.* **39**, 609-616.

Schaad, N. W., and Wilson, E. E. (1968). Pathological anatomy of the phloem canker disease of Persian walnut. *Phytopathology* **58**, 1066 (abstr.).

Wilson, E. E., Zeitoun, F. M., and Fredrickson, D. L. (1967). Bacterial phloem canker, a new disease of persian walnut trees. *Phytopathology* **57**, 618-621.

GENERAL REFERENCES

Bollard, E. G., and Matthews, R. E. F. (1966). The physiology of parasitic disease. *In* "Plant Physiology" (F. C. Steward, ed.), Vol. 4B, p. 417-550. Academic Press, New York.

Braus, A. C. (1952). Plant cancer. *Sci. Am.* **186**, 66-72.

Cole, J. R. (1969). Control of crown gall, *Agrobacterium tumefaciens* on pecans. *Plant Disease Reptr.* **53**, 712-713.

Colwell, R. R., Moffett, M. L., and Sutton, M. D. (1968). Computer analysis of relationships among phytopathogenic bacteria. *Phytopathology* **58**, 1207-1215.

Crosse, J. E. (1966). Epidemiological relations of the pseudomonad pathogens of deciduous fruit trees. *Ann. Rev. Phytopathol.* **4**, 291-310.

Crosse, J. E. (1968). The importance and problems of determing relationships among plant-pathogenic bacteria. *Phytopathology* **58**, 1203-1206.

Davis, J. R., and English, H. (1969). Factors related to the development of bacterial canker in peach. *Phytopathology* **59**, 588-595.

Dochinger, L. S. (1969). Agrobacterium gall of hybrid poplar trees in Iowa. *Phytopathology* **59**, 1024 (abstr.).

Dowson, W. J. (1957). "Plant Diseases Due to Bacteria." Cambridge Univ. Press, London and New York.

Klement, Z. (1968). Pathogenicity factors in regard to relationships of phytopathogenic bacteria. *Phytopathology* **58**, 1218-1221.

Marx, D. H., and Bryon, W. C. (1969). Effect of soil bacteria on the mode of infection of pine roots by *Phytophthora cinnamomi. Phytopathology* **59**, 614-619.

Smith, E. F. (1920). "Bacterial Diseases of Plants." Saunders, Philadelphia, Pennsylvania.

Toole, E. R. (1968). Wetwood in cottonwood. *Plant Disease Reptr.* **52**, 822-823.

Ward, J. C., Kuntz, J. E., and McCoy, E. M. (1969). Bacteria associated with "shake" in broadleaf trees. *Phytopathology* **59**, 1056 (abstr.).

14

FUNGI: INTRODUCTION AND CLASSIFICATION

I. INTRODUCTION

Fungi are among the largest categories of microorganisms. This group contains more complex morphological forms, more diverse life cycles, and more species than any other microbial group, with the possible exception of the algae. There are more than 4000 genera of fungi and probably in excess of 100,000 species. Fungi are extremely cosmopolitan and exist in aerial, soil, water, animal, and plant habitats.

Some aquatic fungi, which are presumed to have been the first to evolve, have characteristics similar to flagellate protozoa. In adaptation to their most common habitat—the soil—however, fungi have acquired a peculiar and distinctive biological organization. A characteristic feature of this organization is the vegetative structure known as the mycelium, possessed by most fungi. The mycelium consists of a multinucleate (coenocytic) mass of cytoplasm enclosed within a rigid, much-branched system of tubes. The diameter of these tubes is typically in the $1-5$ μ range. Their walls are composed primarily of the polysaccharide chitin. This polysaccharide has N-acetylglucosamine as the repeating unit.

A mycelium is generally the result of the germination and outgrowth of a single reproductive cell or spore. Spores may arise directly from vegetative structures and not involve a sexual process, in which case they are termed asexual spores. Spores which involve a sexual process in their development, of course, are termed sexual spores. Following germination, a long thread or hypha emerges from the fungal spore. This hypha repeatedly branches as it elongates to form a ramifying system of hyphae which constitute the mycelium. Fungal growth and asexual spore production is typically localized in the hyphal tips. As the hyphae extend, the cytoplasm of the extending extremities is generally quite granular in appearance and characterized by active protoplasmic streaming. Older hyphal regions, in contrast, are frequently highly vacuolated, quite inactive, and may even lack cytoplasmic contents. Uninucleate or multinucleate spores are generally pinched off at the tips of the hyphae. In the presence of a suitable substrate (food base), the fungus mycelium may develop until it reaches macroscopic proportions. Although the habitats of most fungi, preclude casual observation of these organisms in nature, numerous fungi produce fruiting or spore-bearing structures which extend above the soil or out from a tree and are readily seen. Popular names applied to the former structures are mushrooms or toadstools and to the latter, conks or brackets.

All fungi are heterotrophic organisms, which means they must obtain organic food substances from their environment in order to synthesize most of their own organic constituents and to obtain their energy requirements. Compared to animals, which are strong heterotrophs, fungi have considerable synthetic capacity. Most fungi, given a preformed carbohydrate, are able to synthesize their own protein by utilizing inorganic and organic sources of nitrogen and various mineral elements. Fungi which obtain their organic food materials from dead tissues are termed saprophytes. Most fungi are saprophytes free-living in soil or water. Those fungi which have living tissues as their organic food sources are labeled parasites. Parasites strictly dependent on a living source (host) for food materials are classified as obligate parasites, while those characterized by a general saprophytic persistence, but occasional parasitic behavior, are termed facultative parasites. Facultative and obligate parasites are important plant pathogens when their activities result in, or contribute to, abnormal host physiology.

II. CLASSIFICATION

Fungi, like bacteria, are not conveniently placed in either the plant or animal kingdom. They are similar to higher plants in that they have definite cell walls, are usually nonmotile, and possess considerable synthetic capacity. They are dissimilar from plants, however, as they are devoid of chlorophyll, irritable (that is, they may respond to touch or light stimuli), and are characterized by cell walls with chitin rather than cellulose and occasionally by motile reproductive cells. Even though they may best be classified in some third kingdom, for example the protista, fungi are generally located in the plant kingdom.

The division containing fungi is termed Mycota. The Mycota is divided into two subdivisions, Myxomycotina and Eumycotina. The former subdivision contains the single class Myxomycetes or "slime molds." Slime molds are an extremely curious group of organisms whose primary distinguishing character is the absence of definite cell walls in their amoeboid, animal-like bodies. The vegetative or somatic structure of the Myxomycetes is a free-living plasmodium. Members of this subdivision feed on microorganisms and none are important agents of plant disease.

The subdivision Eumycotina contains the "true fungi." Organisms included in this category are, with few exceptions, provided with cell walls and are typically filamentous, although some unicellular types occur. Depending on the taxonomist, the Eumycotina are divided usually into four or eight classes. In the interest of brevity, we will consider the subdivision as encompassing four classes: Phycomycetes, Ascomycetes, Basidiomycetes, and Deuteromycetes.

A. Phycomycetes

Despite the *very* considerable differences extant in this class, all Phycomycetes share two characteristics that readily distinguish them from the remaining three classes. First, their asexual spores are always borne endogenously; that is, they are formed inside a saclike structure. This structure is termed a zoosporangium in aquatic Phycomycetes and a sporangium in terrestrial types. In other fungal classes, asexual spores are always borne exogenously, generally being formed free at the tips of hyphae. The second distinguishing character of the Phycomycetes is that their mycelium is nonseptate, that is, has no cross walls, except in regions where a specialized structure, for example a sporangium, is formed. In other fungal classes, distinct cross walls occur at regular intervals along the hyphae. It should be noted, however, that the cross walls in non-Phycomycetes have central pores such that cytoplasmic continuity in septate fungi is equivalent to that in the nonseptate Phycomycetes. Unlike other classes of fungi, Phycomycetes are named without regard to whether a sexual stage is known or unknown.

The Phycomycetes class contains approximately 245 genera and in excess of 1300 species. Many of the lower orders are wholly or almost wholly aquatic and are known collectively as aquatic Phycomycetes or "water molds." Many of these fungi show resemblances to protozoa in that they produce motile spores (zoospores) or motile haploid reproductive cells (gametes) furnished with flagella and may produce a vegetative structure which is not a characteristic mycelium. A representative aquatic Phycomycete is the chytrid (Fig. 20). Aquatic Phycomycetes commonly occur as saprophytes on the surface of decaying plant or animal materials in ponds and streams. Some are parasites, however, and attack algae, protozoa, or the roots of higher aquatic plants.

The Phycomycetes class also includes a group known as the terrestrial Phycomycetes which are inhabitants of soil. Two representative and important orders include the Mucorales and the Peronosporales. The Mucorales

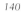

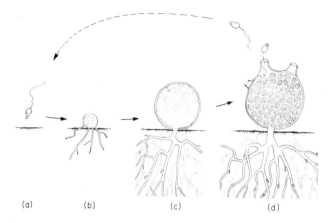

(a)   (b)   (c)   (d)

Fig. 20. The life cycle of a primitive fungus, a chytrid. The flagellated zoospore (a) settles down on a solid surface. As development begins (b), a branching system of rhizoids is formed, anchoring the fungus to the surface. Growth results in the formation of a spherical zoosporangium, which cleaves internally to produce many zoospores (c). The zoosporangium ruptures to liberate a fresh crop of zoospores (d). [From Stanier *et al.* (1963). Reproduced by permission of Prentice Hall, Inc.]

are mostly saprophytic although a few are parasitic on other fungi. The common black bread mold, *Rhizopus,* is a member of the Mucorales order (Fig. 21). The Peronosporales is pathologically an extremely important order. Many members are parasites, some obligate, of higher plants. *Pythium debaryanum* causes dampingoff in numerous tree seedlings. *Phytophthora infestans,* which causes an important potato disease called late blight, is not only pathologically important but also historically significant. During the early and midnineteenth century, potatoes were the main staple of Irish peasants. During the period 1845–1860, excessive potato destruction was occasioned by *P. infestans,* resulting in the starvation of millions of persons. The famine brought many Irish immigrants to the United States. In response to the potato failure, England also repealed her "Corn Laws," which ultimately brought free trade to Europe. Other *Phytophthora* species cause important dampingoff and root diseases of numerous economically important plants. *Phytophthora cinnamomi,* for example, causes littleleaf disease of shortleaf pine.

B. Ascomycetes

This class may comprise the largest group of fungi. Estimates of species numbers range from 15,000 to 45,000. The distinguishing feature of all Ascomycetes is that, following zygote (fertilized ovum) formation, there is an immediate reduction division which results typically in the formation of four or eight haploid sexual spores, termed ascospores. The structure containing ascospores is termed the ascus (Fig. 22). While eight ascospores are typically formed within the ascus, the number may vary from 1 to 1000.

Other characteristics of Ascomycetes include: a sepate mycelium, exogenously produced asexual spores, and complete absence of any type of flagellated cell. The vegetative mycelium of Ascomycetes is characteristically high in chitin content and has a tendency to be profusely branched. Reproduction in the Ascomycetes is very commonly by asexual spores or conidia. The conidia, however, may be very inconspicuous. Frequently, only asexual reproduction is observed in artificial culture with sexual reproduction occasioned only on natural substrates.

The classification of the Ascomycetes is based on the sexual reproductive structures. Specifically, the nature of the ascocarp, which is the structure containing the asci, determines the placement of Ascomycetes. In the subclass Hemiascomycetes, ascocarps are not formed and asci are borne free. The order Taphrinales is a pathologically important order of this subclass. This order contains many fruit tree parasites. The order Endomycetales, while not terribly significant pathologically, is an economically important group as it contains the "true yeasts." Yeast is a rather general, indefinite

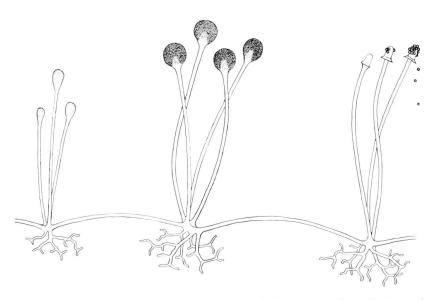

Fig. 21. The vegetative stage of *Rhizopus*, a terrestrial Phycomycete. [From Stanier *et al.* (1963). Reproduced by permission of Prentice Hall, Inc.]

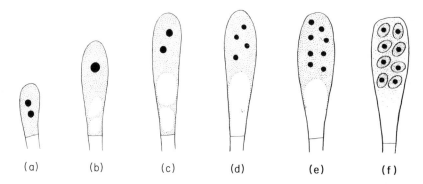

Fig. 22. Successive stages in the formation of an ascus. (a) Binucleate fusion cell; (b) nuclear fusion zygote; (c)-(e) nuclear divisions; (f) ascospores within the ascus. [From Stanier et al. (1963). Reproduced by permission of Prentice Hall, Inc.]

term and refers to a growth form characterized by unicellular development without production of a true mycelium, rather than a specific group of organisms. The "true yeasts" always exhibit this unicellular growth habit and asexually reproduce by budding. Sexual reproduction is accomplished by ascospores borne in free asci. Yeasts are noted for their ability to ferment carbohydrates, resulting in the formation of alcohol and carbon dioxide.

The subclass Euascomycetes contains those Ascomycetes whose asci are borne in ascocarps. Depending on the nature of the ascocarp, this subclass can conveniently be divided into three series (Fig. 23): (1) Plectomycetes, ascocarp in the form of a cleistothecium; (2) Pyrenomycetes, ascocarp in the form of a perithecium; and (3) Discomycetes, ascocarp in the form of an apothecium.

The series Plectomycetes contains numerous important fungi. The *Aspergillus* and *Penicillium* genera are both located in this series. The latter genus is the source of the antibiotic penicillin. An extremely significant pathological genus *Ceratocystis* is also placed in this series. *Ceratocystis fagacearum* is the cause of oak wilt, *C. ulmi* is the agent of Dutch elm disease, and *C. minor* induces blue stain in wood.

The Pyrenomycetes series also encompasses numerous fungi of economic, ecologic, and pathologic significance. *Claviceps purpurea,* which causes ergot disease of rye, results in an important human disease, St. Anthony's Fire, when this rye is ingested. This disease was more frequent during the Middle Ages than it is now. It is interesting to note that one type of a-sexual spore, the sclerotium, produced by this fungus, contains an alkaloid which yields lysergic acid diethylamide (LSD). *Neurospora* species also are members of this series and have been extensively utilized in genetic research; they are popularly referred to as the *Drosophila* of the fungus world. The Erysiphaceae and the Chaetomiaceae are two other important Pyreno-mycetes families. The former family contains the "powdery mildews" whose mycelia may cover plant leaves with a detrimental powdery coating under certain environmental conditions. The latter group includes a number of cellulose-destroying fungi, important in the destruction of paper and certain fabrics. Several Pyrenomycetes are notable as causes of tree diseases.

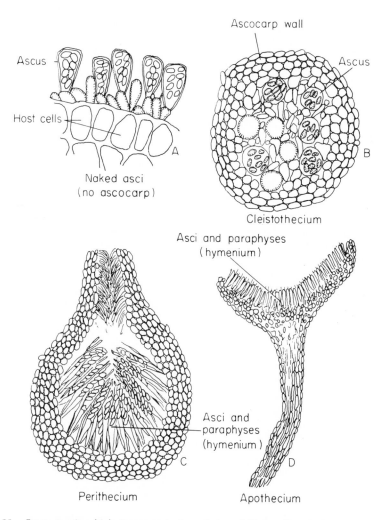

Fig. 23. Four ways in which Ascomycetes bear their asci [From Alexopoulos (1962). Reproduced by permission of John Wiley and Sons, Inc.]

The genera *Hypoxylon* and *Nectria* contain numerous species which cause important hardwood canker diseases. *Gnomonia* members are involved in the production of several leaf maladies of the anthracnose type. Perhaps the most infamous Pyrenomycete, however, is *Endothia parasitica,* the causal agent of chestnut blight.

The last series, Discomycetes, contains relatively few important plant pathogens. The order Helotiales, however, contains several species which cause needle casts of several conifers. *Rhytisma acerinum* is a member of this order and is responsible for a leaf disease of maple designated "tar spot." The Tuberales (truffles) and Morchella (morels) members of this series, however, are prized by epicures as the finest of fungus foods.

C. Basidiomycetes

This class, presumed to be the most advanced of all fungal classes, is estimated to encompass approximately 550 genera and about 15,000 species. It is an extremely important class with respect to plant and animal disease, nutrient cycling, and food and drug supply. In addition to a septate mycelium and asexual spores borne exogenously, most Basidiomycetes are characterized by possessing the following structures: (1) a three phase (or stage) mycelium, (2) clamp connections, (3) basidia and (4) dolipore septa.

The three phase mycelium consists of primary, secondary and tertiary stages. The primary mycelium usually develops from the germination of sexual spores, termed basidiospores. This mycelium may be initially multinucleate, since the nuclei repeatedly divide as the germ tube elongates. Septa are soon formed, however, and the mycelium is divided into uninucleate cells. The secondary mycelium originates when the protoplasts of two uninucleate cells fuse. This process is termed plasmogamy. Following plasmogamy, the nuclei do *not* fuse but rather divide conjugately and thereby form a mycelium with binucleate cells. The tertiary mycelium is formed when highly specialized and organized mycelial structures are formed. Examples of these structures include mushroom and conk fruiting bodies. The cells of tertiary mycelium remain binucleate.

Clamp connections are presumed to have evolved to insure that the new cells formed by the secondary and tertiary mycelia will have two nuclei similar in character to those of the parent cell. The hyphal protrusion or clamp which develops persists and may be useful in identifying the Basidiomycetes (Fig. 24).

The basidium originates as a terminal cell of a binucleate hypha and is separated from the rest of the hypha by a septum over which a clamp connection is generally found. The two nuclei within the basidium fuse, a process termed karyogamy, and a zygote is formed. This zygote immediately undergoes meiosis and gives rise to four haploid nuclei. Four slender projec-

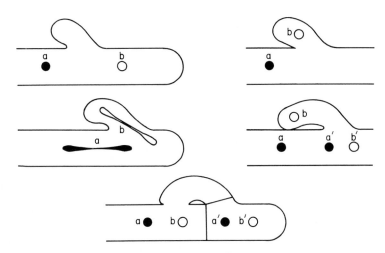

Fig. 24. Cell division of a hyphal tip of a Basidiomycete, illustrating the manner in which the clamp connection permits the daughter cell to have the same nuclear constitution as the parent cell. [From Alexopoulos (1962). Reproduced by permission of John Wiley and Sons, Inc.]

tions, known as sterigma, push out at the top of the basidium. The four nuclei migrate into the expanding sterigma and ultimately form four basidiospores on the tops of each sterigma (Fig. 25).

Unlike the Ascomycetes' simple septa, some Basidiomycetes appear to have a barrel-shaped pore with both ends covered by "caps," termed the dolipore septum (Fig. 26).

Asexual reproduction is accomplished in the Basidiomycetes class by budding, fragmentation of the mycelium, and the production of conidia.

The Basidiomycetes are generally divided into two subclasses, the Heterobasidiomycetes and the Homobasidiomycetes. The character of the ba-

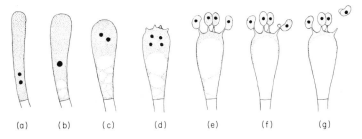

(a)   (b)   (c)   (d)   (e)   (f)   (g)

Fig. 25. Successive stages in basidium formation and basidiospore discharge. (a) Binucleate cell; (b) nuclear fusion; (c), (d) nuclear division; (e) formation of basidiospores; (f), (g) basidiospore discharge. [From Stanier *et al.* (1963). Reproduced by permission of Prentice Hall, Inc.]

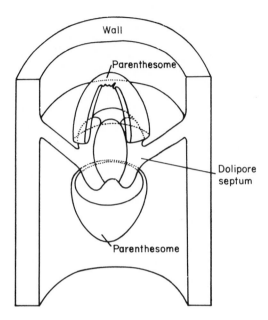

Fig. 26. Cross-sectional and three-dimensional diagramatic views of a dolipore septum [From Moore (1965). Reproduced by permission of Academic Press, Inc.]

sidium is used to distinguish these two groups. In the Heterobasidiomycetes, the basidium is usually either septate or deeply divided. Three orders are generally recognized in this subclass. The order Tremellales contains those fungi popularly termed "jelly fungi." Their economic and pathologic significance is relatively low. Many, however, may play important ecological roles as decay organisms. The remaining two orders are extremely important in plant disease. The order Ustilaginales contains the "smut fungi" which are normally parasitic on plants. Even though not obligate parasites, this group of fungi cause millions of dollars worth of loss to crops annually. Cereals are most severely damaged. The order Uredinales contains the "rust fungi" which are extremely interesting and damaging obligate plant parasites. These fungi are typically quite specific in their host infection and many require two widely unrelated hosts in order to complete their life cycles. Rust fungi are capable of causing disease in a great number of plant species. Numerous devastating tree rust diseases are known including, for example, white pine blister rust caused by *Cronartium ribicola* and juniper-apple rust caused by *Gymnosporangium juniperi-virginianae* (Chapter 17).

The members of the subclass Homobasidiomycetes have a simple basidium which is not septate or deeply divided. Two series are recognized in this subclass. The first is the series Hymenomycetes, containing those fungi which bear basidia in an exposed manner, for example, on gills or in pores of fruiting bodies. The orders Polyporales and Agaricales contain numerous fungi of economic, ecological, and pathological import. The former contains the genera *Poria, Polyporus,* and *Fomes,* all of which contain numerous species that are extremely important agents of tree disease. The latter order contains, for example, *Armillaria mellea,* an important tree root parasite; *Boletus* spp., important ectotrophic mycorrhizal components; and *Agaricus campestris bisporus,* the common edible table mushroom.

The second Homobasidiomycetes series, the Gasteromycetes, have their basidia enclosed until maturity. The members of this category are relatively unimportant pathologically.

D. Deuteromycetes

The Deuteromycetes, or *Fungi Imperfecti*, class is not strictly a class, but is rather a "form class." It is a miscellaneous assemblage of fungi which are known to have septate mycelia but which do not have a sexual or perfect stage and which reproduce only by asexual conidia or other vegetative means. Since the classification of nonphycomycetous fungi is based on the character of the sexual stage, a class had to be created for those fungi failing to produce in a sexual manner. Presumably, these "sexless" fungi are conidial (asexual) stages of Ascomycetes or, more rarely, Basidiomycetes whose sexual stages have not yet been discovered or no longer exist.

Many Deuteromycetes are exceedingly important plant parasites. Four orders are recognized in this class. The Sphaeropsidales produce their conidia in flask-shaped structures (somewhat similar to perithecia) termed pycnidia. *Phyllosticta acericola* is a member of this order; it produces a leaf spot disease of maple.

In the Melanconiales order, the conidia are borne in erupent structures embedded in plant tissue, termed acervuli (Fig. 27). Several Melanconiales members cause anthracnose-type leaf diseases.

The fungi of the order Moniliales bear their conidia free of any enclosing structure. This is the largest order of the Deuteromycetes and encompasses over 10,000 species. Several human diseases which affect the pulmonary and central nervous systems have agents classified in this order. Numerous agents of important plant diseases are contained in this group. *Fusarium* spp. cause important dampingoff and older-seedling mortality as well as canker diseases in several tree species. *Verticillium* spp. are the causal agents of important tree wilt maladies.

All Deuteromycete fungi which do not produce spores of any kind are

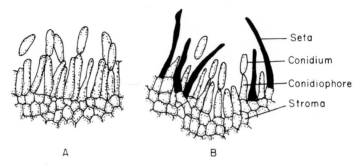

Fig. 27.   Acervuli. (A) *Gloeosporium* sp; (B) *Colletotrichum lindemuthianum*. [From Alexopoulos (1962). Reproduced by permission of John Wiley and Sons, Inc.]

placed in the order Mycelia Sterilia. These fungi reproduce exclusively by nonspore vegetative means. *Rhizoctonia*, a common soil fungus, causes dampingoff and root destruction of several plant species.

Figure 28 presents an organizational review of the classification of fungi as presented in this chapter.

Division Mycota
　Subdivision Myxomycotina
　Subdivision Eumycotina
　　Class Phycomycetes
　　　Order Mucorales
　　　　Genus *Rhizopus*
　　　Order Peronosporales
　　　　Genus *Pythium*
　　　　Genus *Phytophthora*
　Class Ascomycetes
　　Subclass Hemiascomycetes
　　　Order Taphrinales
　　　Order Endomycetales
　　Subclass Euascomycetes
　　　Series Plectomycetes
　　　　Genus *Aspergillus*
　　　　Genus *Penicillium*
　　　　Genus *Ceratocystis*
　　　Series Pyrenomycetes
　　　　Genus *Claviceps*
　　　　Genus *Neurospora*
　　　　Genus *Gnomonia*
　　　　Genus *Nectria*
　　　　Genus *Hypoxylon*
　　　　Genus *Endothia*
　　　Series Discomycetes
　　　　Genus *Rhytisma*

Class Basidiomycetes
　Subclass Heterobasidiomycetes
　　Order Tremellales
　　Order Ustilaginales
　　Order Uredinales
　　　Genus *Cronartium*
　　　Genus *Gymnosporangium*
　Subclass Homobasidiomycetes
　　Series Hymenomycetes
　　　Order Polyporales
　　　　Genus *Poria*
　　　　Genus *Polyporus*
　　　　Genus *Fomes*
　　　Order Agaricales
　　　　Genus *Armillaria*
　　　　Genus *Agaricus*
　　　　Genus *Boletus*
　　Series Gasteromycetes
Form Class Deuteromycetes
　　Form Order Sphaeropsidales
　　　Genus *Phyllosticta*
　　Form Order Melanconiales
　　Form Order Moniliales
　　　Genus *Fusarium*
　　　Genus *Verticillium*
　　Form Order Mycelia Sterilia
　　　Genus *Rhizoctonia*

Fig. 28.   Systematic review of genera discussed in Chapter 14.

REFERENCES

Alexopoulos, C. J. (1962). "Introductory Mycology." Wiley, New York.

Moore, R. T. (1965). The ultrastructure of fungal cells. *In* "The Fungi" (G. C. Ainsworth and A. S. Sussman, eds.), Vol. 1, pp. 95–118. Academic Press, New York.

Stanier, R. Y., Doudoroff, M., and Adelberg, E. A. (1963). "Microbial World." Prentice-Hall, Englewood Cliffs, New Jersey.

GENERAL REFERENCES

Ainsworth, G. C. (1961). "Dictionary of the Fungi." Commonwealth Mycol. Inst., Kent, England.

Ainsworth, G. C., and Sussman, A. S., eds. (1965). "The Fungi," Vol. 1. Academic Press, New York.

Ainsworth, G. C., and Sussman, A. S., eds. (1966). "The Fungi," Vol. 2. Academic Press, New York.

Benjamin, C. R., Haynes, W. C., and Hesseltine, C. W. (1964). Micro-organisms. *U.S. Dept. Agr., Misc. Publ.* **955**, 1–36.

Bessey, E. A. (1950). "Morphology and Taxonomy of Fungi." Blakiston, Philadelphia, Pennsylvania.

Christensen, C. M. (1965). "The Molds and Man." Univ. of Minnesota Press, Minneapolis, Minnesota.

Emerson, R. (1969). Environments of men and molds—another look at the emperor's new clothes. *Plant Sci. Bull.* **15**, 1–8.

Funder, S. (1961). "Practical Mycology." Hafner, New York.

Gray, W. D. (1959). "The Relation of Fungi to Human Affairs." Holt, New York.

Hawker, L. E. (1966). "Fungi." Hutchinson, London.

Hawker, L. E., Linton, A. H., Folkes, B. F., and Carlile, M. J. (1960). "An Introduction to the Biology of Micro-organisms." Arnold, London.

Langeron, M. (1965). "Outline of Mycology." Thomas, Springfield, Illinois.

Large, E. C. (1962). "The Advance of the Fungi." Dover, New York.

15

FUNGI: PHYSIOLOGY AND ECOLOGY

I. PHYSIOLOGY

The physiology of fungi is a very broad and complex area. We will consider only fungus nutrition, reproduction, and physical environment.

A. Nutrition

Most fungi require the following in aqueous solution or suspension in order for growth to occur: an energy source, a carbon source, a nitrogen source, certain inorganic ions, and specific organic growth factors.

1. Energy source. All living organisms require a source of energy for synthetic capacity. All chemosynthetic organisms require energy sources in the form of hydrogen donors, that is, oxidizable substrates. Hydrogen acceptors are also required in these energy-yielding oxidation–reduction reactions. For aerobic organisms (most plant pathogens), gaseous oxygen (O_2) acts as the hydrogen acceptor. In the case of anaerobes, inorganic compounds (sulfate, nitrate, carbonate) or certain organic materials serve this function (Gawetz *et al.*, 1966). Carbon sources frequently function as energy sources as well as suppliers of carbon.

2. Carbon source. Fungi require a source of carbon for the synthesis of the numerous protoplasmic constituents which contain this element. Unlike higher plants, fungi use organic carbon sources instead of carbon dioxide. Almost all fungi have the capacity to use glucose as a carbon source. Other suppliers of carbon utilizable by many fungi include sucrose, maltose, starch, and cellulose.

3. Nitrogen source. Numerous cellular constituents, principally proteins, contain nitrogen. Fungal nitrogen sources are quite varied and may be organic or inorganic in nature. All fungi can use one or more organic suppliers

of nitrogen, for example, peptones, amino acids, or amides. In some instances, carbon may also be supplied by these compounds. Numerous fungi are capable of utilizing inorganic salts containing nitrogen. These salts may contain nitrate (NO_3^-), nitrite (NO_2^-) or ammonium (NH_4^+). A few fungi may be able to obtain nitrogen via the direct utilization of molecular nitrogen (N_2).

4. Inorganic ions. Fungi require certain inorganic nutrients in relatively large quantities, and others in lesser amounts. The former include potassium, phosphorus (as phosphate), magnesium, and sulfur (usually as sulfate). Calcium, which is apparently not essential for all fungi, is also required in relatively large amounts. The inorganic nutrients needed in trace quantitites include iron, zinc, copper, manganese, and molybdenum. Other inorganic nutrients found in the mycelium of numerous fungi, and apparantly required by many, include sodium, boron, and cobalt.

5. Organic growth factors. Fungi exhibit considerable variation with respect to this class of nutrients. Some have no apparent growth factor requirement, while others will not grow unless supplies of certain organic materials are present. Most of these organic materials are required in very small quantities, and most are vitamins. Many fungi lack the capacity to synthesize thiamine and biotin and are therefore dependent on external supplies for growth and development.

Fungal plant pathogens obtain these five types of nutrients by parasitizing one or more higher plants. The acquisition of the required food materials from host plants is incompletely understood. Most information has come from the *in vitro* study of facultative parasites (Wheeler, 1968). In these, the fungi are assumed to kill host cells and then persist essentially saprophytically on host cell contents. Necrosis of host cells may be caused by enzymes which destroy the middle lamellae or cell walls or by other more specific chemicals or toxins. Enzymes may actually be considered toxins, as Ludwig (1960) has defined toxins as "a product of a microorganism or a microorganism-host interaction which acts directly on living host protoplasts to influence either the course of disease development or symptom expression." This is a broad definition and many investigators exclude enzymes, as well as plant growth regulators, from the toxin concept. Toxins, in this more narrow sense include only certain polypeptides, polysaccharides, and other miscellaneous organic metabolites. Once the cells are killed, fungal enzymes are presumed to degrade the complex cellular components into readily utilizable carbon and nitrogen sources. In the case of obligate parasites, less is known concerning the nature of nutrient acquisition, but most assimilation appears to be through specialized hyphae, termed haustoria, which are introduced into living host cells.

B. Reproduction

Among the most interesting and complex aspects of fungus physiology are their varied reproductive mechanisms. Reproductive facility is one of the primary reasons that fungi are such successful plant parasites. Both sexual and asexual reproduction occur.

1. Asexual.   Asexual reproduction, also referred to as somatic or vegetative reproduction, does not involve the union of nuclei, sex cells, or sex organs. In fungi, it is thought that asexual reproduction is more important than sexual reproduction for two primary reasons. Asexual reproduction typically results in the production of more individuals, that is more asexual than sexual propagative units are generally formed. Asexual cycles are characteristically repeated several times during the year, whereas sexual cycles may be confined to a single or a few occurrences throughout the year.

Four primary types of asexual reproduction are recognized: fragmentation, fission, budding, and spore production. Fragmentation refers to the fractionation of the cells of individual hyphae. These fragmented cells are termed oidia or arthrospores. If these cells become enveloped in a thick wall prior to separation, they are termed chlamydospores. Fragmentation may also occur by the physical tearing of mycelial parts caused by external forces. Fission refers to the simple splitting of a cell into two daughter cells. It is very characteristic of some yeast fungi. Budding refers to the formation of a small bud on the parent fungus cell. Following a mitotic division, one nucleus migrates into this bud and a daughter cell is formed. Some species form chains of buds. The majority of yeasts reproduce asexually by budding, but this process also occurs in many other fungi at certain life cycle phases. Spore production is the most common means of asexual reproduction. An infinite variety of spores, in terms of color and morphology, are produced. In the Phycomycetes, asexual spores are termed sporangiospores and are borne *enclosed* in vessels termed sporangia. If motile, sporangiospores are designated zoospores and if nonmotile, aplanospores. In the nonphycomycetous classes, asexual spores are designated conidia and are borne free at the tips or on the sides of hyphae.

2. Sexual.   Sexual reproduction is characterized by processes leading to the union of two haploid nuclei. In the sexual cycles of the true fungi, three processes occur in a regular sequence and usually at specified points in the life cycle — plasmogamy, karyogamy, and meiosis.

Plasmogamy refers to the bringing together of two haploid nuclei in the protoplasm of a single cell. Fungi exhibit five principal manners of accomplishing plasmogamy: planogametic copulation, gametangial contact, gametangial copulation, spermatization, and somatogamy. Planogametic copulation refers to the fusion of naked sex cells (gametes). Gametangial contact involves a transfer of nuclei from one sex organ (gametangium) to another.

In gametangial copulation, the entire contents of two contacting gametangia fuse. Spermatization involves the fertilization of female gametangia with minute male structures termed spermatia. In those fungi which do not produce sex organs, plasmogamy is accomplished by simple fusion of two somatic cells (somatogamy).

Karyogamy occurs when the two haploid nuclei brought together in plasmogamy fuse to form a diploid, zygote nucleus. When plasmogamy and karyogamy are separated by time, more than one nucleus exists in a single cell for that time period. This phenomenon is termed heterokaryosis. The cell containing two differing nuclei is termed a dicaryon. Dicaryons of differing nuclear constitution may exhibit varying physiological or morphological characteristics.

The final stage of the sexual cycle is meiotic division, which restores the haploid condition to the four resulting daughter nuclei.

A distinctive feature of some fungal sexual reproduction is the need for sexual compatibility between mating types. Some species are homothallic; each mycelial mass, or thallus, is self-fertile. Other species are heterothallic, in which case each thallus is self-sterile and requires the aid of another "compatible" thallus for sexual reproduction. Bipolar (two mating types, two individuals) heterothallic species differ from their compatible mating types by only a single factor. If each nucleus of one mating type carries the gene A, then each nucleus of the compatible mating type must carry gene a. In tetrapolar (four mating types, two individuals) heterothallic species, however, compatibility is somewhat more complex. Compatibility in this case is governed by two pairs of factors, for example Aa and Bb located on different chromosomes. In this case only thalli whose nuclei carry opposite genes of both pairs Aa and Bb are compatible. The zygote in this case would have the genotype $AaBb$.

Even though sexual reproduction may be quantitatively less important than asexual reproduction, the former conveys unique selective advantage to organisms possessing sexual cycles. These cycles provide for recombination of genetic material. This recombination results in greater genetic variability. This variability is the raw material of natural selection and provides the genetic flexibility necessary to adapt to changing circumstances.

Organisms lacking sexuality do not have this adaptive mechanism and may be more subject to extinction. This observation is in apparent contradiction to the persistence of Deuteromycetes (fungi lacking sexual cycles). One possible explanation is the existence of a process termed the parasexual cycle. This is a cycle in which plasmogamy, karyogamy, and haploidization occur, but *not* at specified times or at specified points in the life cycle. Plasmogamy occurs when the chance anastomosis of two hyphal filaments result in the cytoplasmic fusion of two somatic cells. Karyogamy is realized when two nuclei spontaneously fuse. This fusion occurs very infrequently; perhaps only one in one million nuclei will fuse with another. During the mitotic multiplication of the diploid nucleus resulting from spontaneous fusion, mitotic crossing over may occur. Mitotic crossing over may occur at a frequency of approximately one in 500 divisions. The final step in the parasexual cycle involves the haploidization, by some unknown mechanism, of the newly recombined diploid nucleus. Even though diploid nuclei are quite stable, evidence that haploidization occurs has been presented. This process may involve a series of mitoses in which chromosomes are gradually lost. If the existence of parasexuality is widespread in the Deuteromycetes class, they may possess the same potential for adaptation that characterizes sexual fungi.

C. Physical Environment

Growth and development of fungi are critically controlled by the nature of their physical environment. Many fungi have a recognized optimum, minimum, and maximum temperature for growth as determined by in vitro study. Most fungi have their minimum located in the 2°-5°C range, their optimum in the 22°-27°C range, and their maximum in the 35°-40°C range (Ingold, 1967). In nature, temperature relations are considerably more complex because of diurnal variation and, even more importantly, of seasonal fluctuation.

The pH of the substratum also exerts an important influence on fungus physiology. Unlike bacteria, most fungi develop best under acid conditions. The in vitro optimum for most species is within the pH range from 5 to 6.5. Many fungi exhibit a relatively broad range of pH tolerance but few develop below pH 3 or above pH 9 (Ingold, 1967).

As in the case of all living organisms, water is an absolute fungal requirement. Mycelial growth is restricted to regions of free water or those possessing a nearly saturated atmosphere. All food materials enter the hyphal filaments in solution. Degree of hydration may influence size of hyphae, degree of branching, spore production, and type of reproduction (Park, 1968).

Fungal growth is also critically controlled by oxygen supply. In contrast to bacteria, very few fungi can grow anaerobically. While able to tolerate a relatively wide range of oxygen tensions, most fungi are strict aerobes.

II. ECOLOGY

The ecological relationships of fungi encompass very broad areas. General microbial and fungus ecology have been the subject of several recent books (Ainsworth and Sussman, 1968; Brock, 1966; Garrett, 1956;

Robinson, 1967). Ecological considerations discussed in this chapter will pertain primarily to those fungi parasitic on plants. Only a few selected concepts will be discussed.

A. Soil Inhabiting and Root Inhabiting Fungi

Since soil is the primary habitat of terrestrial fungi, including plant parasites, two main ecological groups of fungi are recognized, based on their typical location in soil ecosystems. Strictly saprophytic fungi are considered soil inhabiting or root inhabiting. The former are capable of growing freely through the soil and utilizing a wide variety of nonliving organic materials for food. The latter generally have a limited capacity to "compete" with other soil microbes and as a consequence exhibit little growth through soil. They may even be confined to a particular kind of dead organic substrate. Parasitic fungi can be similarly classified as soil-inhabiting pathogens and root-inhabiting pathogens. General characteristics of the first group include: facultative parasitism (that is, they can grow quite successfully saprophytically if necessary), broad host range, infection of immature tissues, and relatively primitive evolutionary placement. Root-inhabiting pathogens are primarily restricted to growth within specific hosts, may infect mature host tissue, and are considered evolutionarily more advanced.

An example of soil-inhabiting pathogens would be the several species of *Pythium* and *Rhizoctonia* which cause dampingoff of numerous tree seedlings. *Armillaria mellea* and *Fomes annosus*, which also cause extremely important tree root diseases, exhibit very restricted growth in soil apart from host roots and are classed as root-inhabiting pathogens.

B. Distribution

Terrestrial fungi are primarily located in the upper 20 cm of soil horizons (Pirozynski, 1968). Soils may contain approximately one million fungal spores per gram of dry soil. In general, soil-inhabiting pathogens and nonpathogens tend to be quite cosmopolitan in their distribution. Local variations are presumed primarily due to competition for food, biological interactions between antagonistic organisms, surface vegetation, physiochemical properties, and soil microclimate (Pirozynski, 1968). Root-inhabiting pathogens and nonpathogens may have relatively wide distributions or may be extremely restricted. Those capable of infecting or utilizing a large number of plants may have extensive geographical ranges. *Armillaria mellea*, because of its broad host range, is ubiquitous. *Fomes annosus*, on the other hand, is restricted to temperate climates because it parasitizes hosts which grow only in these regions (Pirozynski, 1968).

Air is not truly a fungal habitat. Fungal fragments and spores may be isolated from the air but they all have terrestrial origins. Many asexual and sexual spores are specially adapted for aerial distribution, however. Many air-borne spores play exceedingly important roles in the life cycles of plant pathogens.

C. Entrance into Host Plant

Fungi enter plants primarily in one of three ways: natural openings, wounds, and direct penetration.

As in the case of bacteria, stomata, lenticels, hydathodes, and other natural openings provide very suitable ingress routes for pathogenic fungi.

Fungi exploit wounds of all types in order to enter plant hosts. Wounds significant in tree disease phenomena vary considerably from conspicuous fire or branch scars to inconspicuous leaf scars and insect wounds.

An important distinction between bacterial and fungal plant pathogens is that many of the latter are capable of directly penetrating unbroken plant surfaces. Present evidence indicates that this penetration is basically a mechanical process and that chemical factors do not play primary roles. Active fungal ingress frequently involves a specialized hyphal structure, termed the appressorium. This is a flattened hyphal filament that serves as a pressing organ for the infection peg. These structures are illustrated in Fig. 29 which shows the germ tube of a rust urediospore (Chapter 17) entering a stomate. Similar structures are involved in direct penetration through intact plant surfaces.

D. Growth in Host Plant

Once inside host plants, fungal parasites exhibit considerable variation with respect to extent and location of development (Wheeler, 1968). Many ascomycetous leaf pathogens are restricted to epidermal cells. Phycomycetous seedling root pathogens, for example, Pythium spp. and Phytophthora spp., are characteristically confined to the roots and fail to colonize tissues above the root collar. Several fungi which cause wilt symptoms in plants, for example, Verticillium spp. and Ceratocystis spp., develop principally in vascular tissues. In contrast to these fungi, some varieties, especially those which parasitize perennial hosts, become more generally distributed. Numerous examples of the latter type can be found in the smut and rust fungal groups.

With respect to the relation between fungal hyphae and individual host cells, some fungi are intercellular, some intracellular and some exhibit development both in and between cells.

E. Survival and Growth Outside Host Plant

The mycelium of many fungal plant parasites is incapable of persisting for extended periods in the soil apart from a host food base due to poor compet-

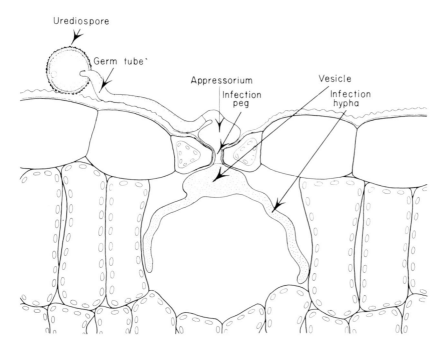

Fig. 29. Stomatal penetration, showing the infection structures produced from a urediospore germ tube. [From Maheshwari *et al.* (1967). Reproduced by permission of American Phytopathological Society.]

itive saprophytic ability and antagonism. Since colonization of soil organic matter is very competitive; fungi that lack rapid growth and efficient enzyme production, that fail to produce materials toxic to other organisms, and those that are susceptible to antibiotics released by other microbes tend to be excluded from nonliving soil substrates. Many parasitic fungi, therefore, produce spores or other specialized structures which enable them to persist under conditions mycelia could not tolerate. These structures frequently require specific dormancy periods or external stimuli, for example leaf or root exudates, to induce germination.

Other plant parasites circumvent soil competition by remaining as mycelia in plant tissues. *Fomes annosus*, for example, is an extremely poor soil competitor but is able to persist for many years in the root systems of dead host trees.

Wheeler (1968) suggests that fungi derive two primary benefits by parasitizing plants. First, they reduce competitive influences from strictly saprophytic fungi. Second, they ameliorate the effects of changes in environmental conditions which may be deleterious to their growth. Levels of parasitism of fungal pathogens vary considerably, however, from an unspecialized primitive nature to a more specialized advanced type. A summary of some characters of these two groups is presented in Table XX.

TABLE XX

CHARACTERS ASSOCIATED WITH PRIMITIVE AND SPECIALIZED FUNGAL PARASITES[a]

Character	Primitive	Specialized
Entry into the plant	Through wounds	Through stomata, and by direct penetration of intact surfaces
Type of tissue invaded	Confined to immature or senescent tissues	Not so confined
Mycelium	Inter- and intracellular	Intracellular, intercellular, or intercellular with haustoria
Effect on host cells	Necrosis	No necrosis
Existence outside the plant	Saprobic	"Resting" stage only
Host range	Wide	Limited

[a]From Wheeler (1968). Reproduced by permission of Academic Press, Inc.

REFERENCES

Ainsworth, G. C., and Sussman, A. S., eds. (1968). "The Fungi," Vol. 3. Academic Press, New York.

Brock, T. D. (1966). "Principles of Microbial Ecology." Prentice-Hall, Englewood Cliffs, New Jersey.

Garrett, S. D. (1956). "Biology of Root-infecting Fungi." Cambridge Univ. Press, London and New York.

Gawetz, E., Melnick, J. L., and Adelberg, E. A. (1966). "Review of Medical Microbiology." Lange Med. Publ., Los Altos, California.

Ingold, C. T. (1967). "The Biology of Fungi." Hutchinson, London.

Ludwig, R. A. (1960). Toxins. In "Plant Pathology" (J. G. Horsfall and A. E. Dimond, eds.), Vol. 2, pp. 315–357. Academic Press, New York.

Maheshwari, R., Allen, P. J., and Hildebrandt, A. C. (1967). Physical and chemical factors controlling the development of infection structures from urediospore germ tubes of rust fungi. *Phytopathology* **57**, 855–862.

Park, D. (1968). The ecology of terrestrial fungi. In "The Fungi" (G. C. Ainsworth and A. S. Sussman, eds.), Vol. 3, pp. 5–39. Academic Press, New York.

Pirozynski, K. A. (1968). Geographical distribution of fungi. In "The Fungi" (G. C. Ainsworth and A. S. Sussman, eds.), Vol. 3, pp. 487–504. Academic Press, New York.

Robinson, R. K. (1967). "Ecology of Fungi." English Univ. Press, London.

Wheeler, B. E. J. (1968). Fungal parasites of plants. *In* "The Fungi" (G. C. Ainsworth and A. S. Sussman, eds.), Vol. 3, pp. 179–210. Academic Press, New York.

GENERAL REFERENCES

Alexopoulos, C. J. (1962). "Introductory Mycology." Wiley, New York.

Bollard, E. G., and Matthews, R. E. F. (1966). The physiology of parasitic diseases. *In* "Plant Physiology" (F. C. Steward, ed.), pp. 417–550. Academic Press, New York.

Buxton, E. W. (1960). Heterokaryosis, saltation, and adaptation. *In* "Plant Pathology" (J. G. Horsfall and A. E. Dimond, eds.), Vol. 2, pp. 359–405. Academic Press, New York.

Cochrane, V. W. (1958). "Physiology of Fungi." Wiley, New York.

Fincham, J. R. S., and Day, P. R. (1963). "Fungal Genetics." Blackwell, Oxford.

Foster, C. T. (1953). "Dispersal in Fungi." Oxford Univ. Press, London and New York.

Griffin, D. M. (1969). Soil water in the ecology of fungi. *Ann. Rev. Phytopathol.* **7**, 289–310.

Ilag, L., and Curtis, R. W. (1968). Production of ethylene by fungi. *Science* **159**, 1357–1358.

Ksser, K., and Raper, J. R. (1965). "Incompatibility in Fungi." Springer, Berlin.

Lilly, V. G., and Barnett, H. L. (1951). "Physiology of the Fungi." McGraw-Hill, New York.

Parmeter, J. R., Jr., Snyder, C. W., and Reichle, R. E. (1963). Heterokaryosis and variability in plant-pathogenic fungi. *Ann. Rev. Phytopathol.* **1**, 51–76.

Raper, J. R. (1966). "Genetics of Sexuality in Higher Fungi." Ronald Press, New York.

Society of General Microbiology. (1957). "Microbial Ecology," 7th Symp. Cambridge Univ. Press, London and New York.

Tinline, R. D. and MacNeill, B. H. (1969). Parasexuality in plant pathogenic fungi. *Ann. Rev. Phytopathol.* **7**, 147–170.

West Virginia Agricultural Experiment Station. (1963). The physiology of fungi and fungus diseases. *West Va. Univ., Agr. Expt. Sta., Bull.* **488T**, 1–106.

Wright, D. E. (1968). Toxins produced by fungi. *Ann. Rev. Microbiol.* **22**, 269–282.

16

FUNGI THAT CAUSE DECAY
AND DISCOLORATION

The phenomenon of wood decay by fungi is both an asset and a liability. Because of their relatively unique capacity to degrade lignified tissues, these fungi play a critical role in the carbon cycle. As the fungi decay wood, forest debris is diminished, organic materials are added to the soil and carbon is returned to the atmosphere in the form of carbon dioxide (Fig. 30).

In commercially important trees, however, wood decay fungi are a liability since these organisms destroy valuable raw material. Certain fungi also attack wood in service, an additional significant loss (Cowling, 1961). Basham and Morawski (1964) documented the cost of wood decay fungi to the forest industries in Ontario, Canada. These investigators found that approximately 22 million cubic feet of timber, which is roughly 6.3% of the annual harvest, is culled annually in Ontario because of heart rot or stain.

I. WOOD ANATOMY

In order to appreciate the wood decay process, it is important to realize the general nature of the wood substrate.

In living trees, microbial decay is primarily restricted to the heartwood. Heartwood is the interior core of tissue in stems and branches of mature trees and consists of xylem devoid of living parenchyma or less living parenchyma than that contained in the outermost (or younger) portions of stems or branches. The primary function of heartwood is presumed to be mechanical support. Since decay fungi persist on essentially nonliving material, they are actually operating saprophytically. Sapwood decay occurs only infrequently

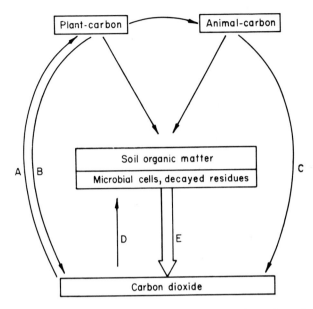

Fig. 30. The carbon cycle. (A) Photosynthesis; (B) respiration, plant; (C) respiration, animal; (D) autotrophic microorganisms; (E) respiration, microbial. [From Alexander (1961). Reproduced by permission of John Wiley and Sons, Inc.]

and, when it does, it is usually associated with large wounds. Sapwood exists as a vital cylinder around the heartwood and consists of xylem containing living parenchyma. Principal sapwood functions are thought to be sap conduction and the storage of reserve materials. It is interesting to note that shortly after a tree dies, the sapwood characteristically becomes considerably more susceptible to decay than the heartwood.

An awareness of wood microstructure is also important in understanding decay phenomena. Individual wood cells are joined by an intercellular substance termed the middle lamella. The actual cell walls consist of primary and secondary layers. The primary layer (the outermost cell layer), when combined with the middle lamella is commonly referred to as the compound middle lamella. The compound middle lamella is, to a considerable extent, lignin. Lignin is a complex aromatic compound whose chemistry is not fully understood. The secondary cell wall layer may be additionally divided into three layers termed the S1, S2, and S3 regions. The S1 and S3 layers are relatively thin, while the S2 is quite thick and represents the bulk of the secondary wall (Fig. 31). The secondary wall layers are made up of microfibrils consisting primarily of cellulose molecules (Table XXI).

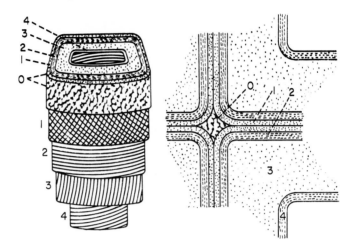

Fig. 31. Cell walls and intercellular layer. Left, side view, with walls cut away to show the various layers of the cell wall. Right, transverse section. (0) Intercellular layer or middle lamella; (1) primary wall, secondary wall consisting of: (2) outer layer; (3) middle layer; and (4) inner layer. [From Hägglund (1951). Reproduced by permission of Academic Press, Inc.]

II. WOOD AS A MICROBIAL SUBSTRATE

Fungi which decay wood possess some unique characteristics enabling them to use wood as a source of required nutrients. Two factors relating to the nutritional aspects of wood make it relatively unsuitable for general microbial decomposition. Since most microorganisms cannot use cellulose,

TABLE XXI

CONSTITUENTS OF PRIMARY AND SECONDARY LAYERS OF WOOD CELL WALLS

Constituent	Approximate percentage
Cellulose, linear glucose polymers	51
Hemicellulose, short polymers of various sugars (glucose, mannose, galactose, xylose, arabinose)	23
Lignin	22
Extraneous organics (waxes, fats, oils, tannins, resins)	4
Miscellaneous inorganics	Trace

hemicelluloses, or lignin as a source of carbon, they are restricted from colonizing wood. In addition, and perhaps more importantly, wood is deficient in nitrogen. The amount of nitrogen in wood is rarely greater than 0.3% by weight and more commonly may be only 0.03-0.10%. The carbon/nitrogen ratio of common artificial laboratory media is approximately 10/1-20/1. The carbon/nitrogen ratio of wood, however, may vary from approximately 350/1 to 1250/1 (Merrill and Cowling, 1966).

The widespread and important occurrence of fungal wood decay attests to the relative efficiency with which certain microbes have overcome these obstacles. Wood decay fungi, which are primarily members of the series Hymenomycetes, are capable of synthesizing enzymes that enable the utilization of the polymeric organic wood materials. These enzymes, termed lignases and carbohydrases, have the capacity to depolymerize or cleave the large carbon-containing molecules into smaller, readily assimilated units. These enzymes are released from hyphal filaments growing inside the wood. They readily move through the wood by diffusion and catalyze the breakdown of cell walls. There is evidence to suggest that this enzymatic action occurs considerably in advance of the growing hyphae.

The process which enables wood decay fungi to grow on such a nitrogen deficient substrate is still unclear. Cowling and Merrill (1966), however, have proposed three hypotheses. The first suggests that fungi may preferentially allocate nitrogen obtained from wood to materials and metabolic pathways highly efficient in the use of wood constituents. The second suggests that fungi may recycle nitrogen obtained from wood by a dynamic and continuous process of autolysis and reuse. Levi et al. (1968) recently found that, in the presence of glucose, representative wood decay fungi were able to utilize fractions of their own mycelium as the sole source of nitrogen. The third proposes that certain fungi have the capacity to utilize nitrogen sources outside the wood itself, for example, via the fixation of atmospheric nitrogen.

III. TYPES OF WOOD DECAY

Three principal types of wood decay are recognized; soft rot, white rot and brown rot.

a. Soft rot.   The significance of soft rot has been recognized only relatively recently. This type of rot is most important in wood in service. It is very prevalent, for example, in wood exposed to excessive moisture, such as in cooling tower slats, pilings, and boats. It is also present in fence posts, telephone poles, ponded logs, and unpainted building siding. Soft rot may be present in standing trees but it is presumed to be of little economic or biological significance.

The fungi which cause soft rot are primarily members of the Ascomycetes and Deuteromycetes classes. The organisms mainly attack the polysaccharide constituents of the secondary cell walls, while the lignin is left relatively unaffected. The fungi characteristically move through the secondary walls of the wood elements.

b. White rot and brown rot. White and brown rots are commercially and ecologically extremely important as they are the types found in standing trees.

Although a few Ascomycetes, principally those in the family Xylariaceae, cause these types of rots, most are the result of Basidiomycetes. Table XXII lists a representative group of Basidiomycetes and the rots they cause.

In contrast to the soft-rot fungi, organisms which cause white and brown rots generally move through and between, as well as within, wood cell walls.

White and brown rot decay types are characterized by numerous dissimilarities. Fungi causing brown rots generally result in decayed wood brown in color. This coloration is presumed to be due to the lignin residue resulting from the preferential utilization of wood carbohydrates. Fungi which cause white rots, however, generally result in wood with a white or bleached appearance. This lack of color is generally attributed to the utilization or modification of some unknown wood constituent. It is not presumed to result from a selective utilization of lignin. White rotting fungi frequently cause dark lines, termed zone lines, in the wood they decay. These lines are probably strings of tightly woven hyphae.

Brown rotted wood generally exhibits abnormal longitudinal swelling and shrinkage which frequently gives rise to a characteristic cubical checking pattern. White rotted wood, in contrast, typically has normal shrinkage properties and is quite similar to uninfected wood in terms of dimensional stability. In terms of strength properties, brown rotted wood shows considerable strength reduction, while white rotted wood exhibits only slight strength reduction.

Pulp yields of brown rotted woods are considerably lower than white rotted woods. The latter may, on a weight basis, have yields not greatly different from those obtained from sound wood.

White and brown rotted woods can generally be distinguished both chemically and microscopically. The former has a solubility in 1% aqueous sodium hydroxide only slightly greater than uninfected wood. The latter, however, is very soluble in the same solution. White rot fungi act primarily on the internal surfaces of cell walls and microscopic examination will show degradation in this area. Brown rot fungi have a tendency not to degrade entire cell walls but to leave a lattice of lignin.

The fungi which cause white rots are generally assumed capable of me-

TABLE XXII

REPRESENTATIVE BASIDIOMYCETES THAT CAUSE WHITE AND BROWN DECAYS OF WOOD

Family	Species	Disease common name	Host	Decay type
Agaricaceae	Collybia velutipes	—	Hardwoods	White
	Lentinus lepideus	Brown cubical rot	Conifers	Brown
	Pholiota adiposa	Brown mottled rot	Hardwoods	Brown
	Pleurotus ulmarius	Elm brown rot	Elm	Brown
	Schizophyllum commune	—	Hardwoods	White
Hydnaceae	Echinodotium tinctorium	Brown stringy rot	Western conifers	Brown
	Hydnum abietis	Fir hydnum	Western firs	White
Polyporaceae	Daedalea quercina	Brown cubical rot	Oaks	Brown
	Fistulina hepatica	Brown cubical rot	Oaks	Brown
	Fomes pini	Red ring rot	Conifers	White
	Ganoderma lucidum	Red ring rot	Eastern hemlock	White
	Lenzites tigrinus	White butt rot	Southern hardwoods	White
	Merulius lacrymans	Dry rot	—	Brown
	Polyporus sulphureus	Brown cubical rot	Hardwoods	Brown
	Poria weirii	Yellow ring rot	Conifers	Brown
	Trametes suaveolens	—	Willows, poplars	White
Thelephoraceae	Coniophora cerebella	Brown cubical rot	Conifers	Brown
	Hymenochaete rubiginosa	White pocket rot	Chestnut	White
	Peniophora gigantea	—	Conifers, hardwoods	White
	Stereum gausapatum	White pocket rot	Eastern oaks	White

tabolizing both wood carbohydrates and lignin. This ability to degrade lignin may be due to the possession of laccase-type enzymes. Brown rot fungi are restricted to carbohydrate utilization.

In general, fungi causing brown rots tend to infect gymnosperms, while those causing white rots are typically associated with angiosperms.

IV. ECOLOGY OF WOOD DECAY FUNGI

Natural distribution of most wood decay fungi is accomplished by spores. These spores may be airborne or soilborne. In a study conducted in an Adirondack mixed hardwood–conifer forest, DeGroot (1968) found that airborne basidiospore release exhibited diurnal cycles with nocturnal peaks.

Wood decay fungi have a very restricted competitive capacity and a limited ability to grow through living tissue. As a result, only those spores which come in contact with exposed heartwood, either above or below ground, are generally successful in initiating infection. Direct contact with heartwood is typically provided by wounds of various kinds. Above ground wounds of significance include: dead or broken branches, fire, logging and pruning scars, bird and insect damage, and wind breakage. In the south-central United States it has been estimated that approximately 95% of the decay probably results from entrance of fungi through fire scars. Subterrainian wounds include areas of mechanical abrasion, nematode punctures, and insect feeding sites.

If a spore from a wood decay fungus comes in contact with the exposed heartwood of a susceptible host, and if the moisture, temperature, and nutritional conditions are appropriate, it may germinate and introduce a filament into the heartwood. Manion and French (1969) have observed that the germination of basidiospores of Fomes igniarius var. populinus is enhanced by contact with outer sapwood of freshly cut host stems. This may be due to glucose present in the cut tissues. In addition to external nutrients, Brown (1968) suggested that high carbon dioxide concentration and proximity to certain other fungi may enhance the germination of Fomes applanatus basidiospores (Fig. 32). Levi and Cowling (1968) have observed that decreased nitrogen content in oak sapwood during foliation was correlated with a reduction in the susceptibility of the oak wood to decay by white and brown rot fungi.

Once in the heartwood, wood decay fungi exhibit variable rates of growth, from 0.01 to 11–15 feet per year. Following artificial inoculation of white pine with Fomes pini (Fig. 33), Silverborg and Larsen (1967) found that the fungus showed a yearly vertical extension of 0.84 feet. After varying periods of growth in the heartwood, generally several years, decay fungi typically produce fruiting bodies (sporophores, brackets, conks) on the branches or main stem of the host tree. The fruiting bodies function to release spores

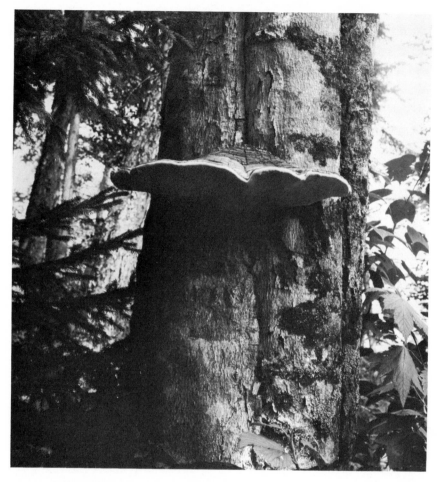

Fig. 32.   Fruiting body of *Fomes applanatus* on an American beech. The decay column in this tree caused by this white rotting organism may approximate 15 feet in length. (Photograph courtesy U.S. Forest Service.)

which, in turn, may initiate new decay cycles. For many decay fungi, estimates are available for the amount of decay which probably exists above and below a fruiting body. Silverborg (1954), for example, states that a single fruiting body of *Fomes igniarius* on beech or hard maple indicates a decay column approximately 6–7 feet both above and below the fungus structure. Excellent photographs of the extent of decay in diseased trees have been provided by Shigo and Larson (1969).

Wood decay fungi are frequently classified as either top-rotting organisms

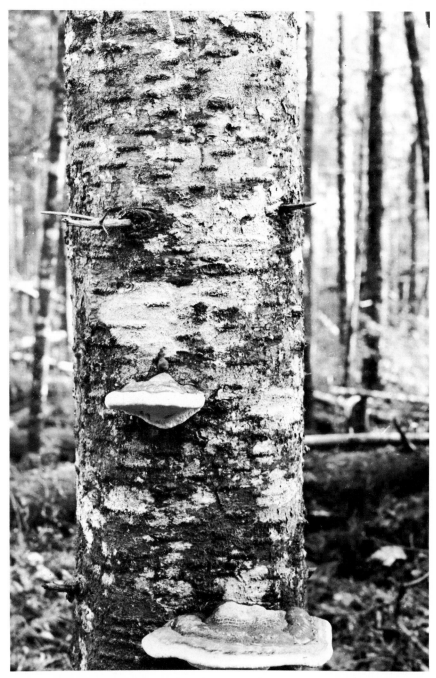

Fig. 33. Fruiting bodies of *Fomes pini* on a balsam fir. This fungus is one of the most important wood decay organisms of North American conifers. It has an extremely wide geographical and host distribution. (Photograph courtesy U.S. Forest Service.)

or butt- or root-rotting organisms, depending on where they generally reside in the host tree. Under certain conditions, wood decay fungi already well advanced in the heartwood may be capable of advancing into the sapwood.

For years it was felt that wood decay was caused by fungi, primarily Hymenomycetes, acting independently of other organisms. Evidence is being accumulated, however, that a succession of microorganisms may be involved in the decay process. Shigo (1965) made in excess of 70,000 isolations from northern hardwood trees with decay and discoloration symptoms and obtained bacteria and non-Hymenomycetes as well as Hymenomycetes fungi. The principal bacteria cultured were gram negative, motile, short rods that were characterized by abundant slime production. Many were apparently members of the *Pseudomonas* genus. Non-Hymenomycetes were variable and included many Ascomycetes and Deuteromycetes.

Certain Hymenomycetes fungi may be dependent on other organisms present in wood for growth factor supplies. Other wood decay fungi appear inhibited by bacteria and non-Hymenomycetes. The interaction between organisms in the decay process is of fundamental importance in the understanding of this stress factor. Shigo (1967) reviews this phenomenon.

V. MANAGERIAL AND SILVICULTURAL ASPECTS OF WOOD DECAY

In forests managed for the commercial production of timber, rotation lengths (number of years trees are grown until harvest) are determined by a complex of biologic and economic factors. Rotation lengths determined exclusively by pathological considerations are probably nonexistent. Wood decay considerations, however, underscore the importance of including disease phenomena in the establishment of rotation lengths. In general, there is a positive correlation between the amount of wood decay and the age of the tree crop. French et al. (1967) cite the example of Fomes pini which causes a top rot of numerous conifers including Douglas fir. In general, this fungus causes insignificant damage in Douglas fir until the trees reach approximately 50 years of age. As the trees age the amount of decay caused by F. pini increases accordingly. An appropriate management objective would be to insure that the cutting cycle comes before the steep increase in decay volume. In the case of Douglas fir, this would be shortly before or after 160 years. In a recent investigation of decay in upland oak stands of Kentucky, Berry (1969) found that the decay percentage increased progressively with age for most oak species (Table XXIII). In general, however, losses due to decay can be minimized if the trees are harvested prior to 90 years of age. Rotation lengths not to exceed 90 years, therefore, were suggested for natural upland oak stands.

Hardwood silviculture presents some interesting problems with respect to

TABLE XXIII

COMPARISON OF AGE AND DECAY IN UPLAND OAK
STANDS (ALL SPECIES) OF KENTUCKY[a]

Age class (yrs)	Decay (%)[b]
30	0.43
40	0.35
50	1.32
60	1.11
70	1.18
80	1.06
90	5.56
100	5.97
110	5.68

[a]From Berry (1969). Reproduced by permission of U.S. Forest Service.
[b]Decay indicated as percentage of gross merchantable volume.

decay incidence. Many hardwood stands are reproduced by sprouts by procedures described as coppice silviculture. In sprout stands, as much as 86%
of the decay which develops in stems originates from the connection between sprout heartwood and parent stump heartwood (French et al., 1967).
In recognition of this fact, certain guidelines have been suggested for mini-
mizing decay in sprout stems. First, since the sprouts that form highest on the
stump are most subject to decay, the lower sprouts should be favored. This
selection must be accomplished before the sprouts are 15–20 years of age as
beyond this time it is difficult to ascertain which are of low or high origin.
Second, smaller stumps are to be favored over larger stumps as the former
generally have experienced less decay development. Finally, when sprouts
are thinned, those with a V-shaped intersection should not be cut while
those with a U-shaped intersection may be cut (Fig. 34).

VI. STAINS

Stain or discoloration phenomena are frequently considered along with
decay but are actually important independent processes in themselves.
Decay is typically associated with some degree of stain. Stain, however, may
exist in the absence of any decay.

Stains may be divided into those which occur in trees under natural conditions in the forest and those which develop in the wood of harvested trees.
The former may be of considerable significance in the preconditioning of
wood for decay organisms and in direct tree mortality (Ohman and Spike,
1966). These stains are presumably caused by numerous bacteria and fungi.

Siegle (1967) has suggested that microbial phenol oxidases may convert heartwood phenols to colored materials and thereby induce stain formation.

Four types of stains are recognized in harvested wood (French *et al.*, 1967). Fungal stains occur in freshly cut logs during storage and in green lumber. The causal fungi generally develop mainly in the sapwood, cause little strength reduction, and are of principal importance in warm and humid regions. The fungi may be surface molds, for example, *Penicillium* spp., or interior sap stain fungi, such as *Ceratocystis* spp. or *Cladosporium* spp. The

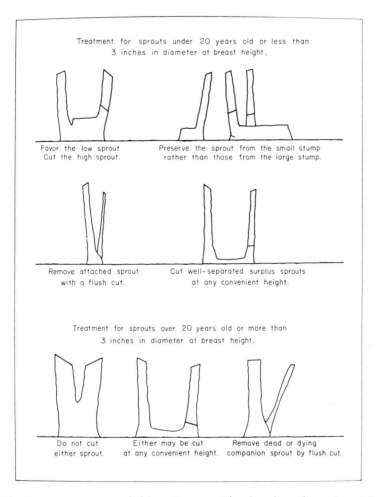

Fig. 34. Procedures recommended in cutting sprout stands to keep decay at a minimum. [From Hepting and Fowler (1962). Reproduced by permission of U.S. Forest Service.]

common blue stain is caused by organisms of the latter type. The three remaining stains result from abiotic factors including; exposure to air (again resulting in oxidation of wood phenols), manufacturing discoloration (for example, by heat used in drying), and weathering (for example, that caused by ultraviolet sunlight or ozone).

REFERENCES

Alexander, M. (1961). "Introduction to Soil Microbiology." Wiley, New York.

Basham, J. T., and Morawski, Z. J. R. (1964). Cull studies, the defects and associated basidiomycete fungi in the heartwood of living trees in the forests of Ontario. *Dept. Forestry (Canada), Publ.* **1072**, 1-68.

Berry, F. H. (1969). Decay in the upland oak stands of Kentucky. *Res. Paper, Northeast. Forest Exptl. Sta.* **NE-126**, 1-16.

Brown, T. S., Jr. (1968). Germination of *Fomes applanatus* basidiospores. *Phytopathology* **58**, 1044 (abstr.).

Cowling, E. B. (1961). Comparative biochemistry of the decay of sweetgum sapwood by white-rot and brown-rot fungi. *U.S. Dept. Agr., Tech. Bull.* **1258**, 1-79.

Cowling, E. B., and Merrill, W. (1966). Nitrogen in wood and its role in wood deterioration. *Can. J. Botany* **44**, 1539-1554.

DeGroot, R. C. (1968). Diurnal cycles of airborne spores produced by forest fungi. *Phytopathology* **58**, 1223-1229.

French, D. W., Kelman, A., and Cowling, E. B. (1967). "An Introduction to Forest Pathology." D. W. French, University of Minnesota, St. Paul, Minn.

Hägglund, E. (1951). "Chemistry of Wood." Academic Press, New York.

Hepting, G. H., and Fowler, M. E. (1962). Tree diseases of eastern forests and farm woodlands. *U.S. Dept. Agr., Agr. Inform. Bull.* **254**, 1-48.

Levi, M. P., and Cowling, E. B. (1968). Role of nitrogen in wood deterioration. V. Changes in decay susceptibility of oak sapwood with season of cutting. *Phytopathology* **58**, 246-249.

Levi, M. P., Merrill, W., and Cowling, E. B. (1968). Role of nitrogen in wood deterioration. VI. Mycelial fractions and model nitrogen compounds as substrates for growth of *Polyporus versicolor* and other wood-destroying and wood-inhabiting fungi. *Phytopathology* **58**, 626-634.

Manion, P. D., and French, D. W. (1969). The role of glucose in stimulating germination of basidiospores of *Fomes igniarius* var. *populinus*. *Phytopathology* **59**, 293-296.

Merrill, W., and Cowling, E. B. (1966). Role of nitrogen in wood deterioration: Amount and distribution of nitrogen in fungi. *Phytopathology* **56**, 1083-1090.

Ohman, J. H., and Spike, A. B. (1966). Effect of staining caused by sapstreak disease on sugar maple log and lumber values. *Res. Note, North Central Forest Exptl. Sta.,* **NC-12** , 1-4.

Shigo, A. L. (1965). Organism interactions in decay and discoloration in beech, birch, and maple. *Res. Paper, Northeast Forest Exptl. Sta.,* **NE-43**, 1-23.

Shigo, A. L. (1967). Successions of organisms in discoloration and decay of wood. *In* "International Review of Forestry Research" (J. A. Romberger and P. Mikola, eds.), Vol. 2, pp. 237-299, Academic Press, New York.

Shigo, A. L., and Larson, E. vH. (1969). A photo guide to the patterns of discoloration and decay in living northern hardwood trees. *Res. Paper, Northeast. Forest Exptl. Sta.* **NE-127**, 1-100.

Siegle, H. (1967). Microbiological and biochemical aspects of heartwood stain in *Betula papyrifera* Marsh. *Can. J. Botany* **45**, 147-154.

Silverborg, S. B. (1954). Northern hardwoods cull manual. *Bull., N.Y. State Coll. Forestry* **31**, 1-45.

Silverborg, S. B., and Larsen, M. N. (1967). Rate of decay in *Pinus strobus* following artificial inoculation with *Fomes pini. Plant Disease Reptr.* **51**, 829-831.

GENERAL REFERENCES

Amburgey, T. L. (1967). Decay capacities of monokaryotic and dikaryotic isolates of *Lenzites travea. Phytopathology* **57**, 486-491.

Anderson, A. B. (1964). On the chemistry of wood durability and decay. Structure of fungicidal components in some cedars. *In* "Symposium on Phytochemistry" (H. R. Arthur, ed.), pp. 101-116. Hong Kong Univ. Press, Hong Kong.

Basham, H. G. (1968). Pathogenicity of some blue-stain fungi in the genus *Ceratocystis. Phytopathology* **58**, 1042 (abstr.).

Boyce, J. S. (1961). "Forest Pathology." McGraw-Hill, New York.

Byler, J. W., and True, R. P. (1966). Root and butt rot in young yellow-poplar stump sprouts. *Phytopathology* **56**, 1091-1097.

Cartwright, K. St. G., and Findlay, W. P. K. (1958). "Decay of Timber and its Prevention." Her Majesty's Stationery Office, London.

Darbyshire, B., Wade, G. C., and Marshall, K. C. (1969). *In vitro* studies of the role of nitrogen and sugars on the susceptibility of apple wood to decay by *Trametes versicolor. Phytopathology* **59**, 98-102.

Findlay, W. P. K. (1967). "Timber Pests and Diseases." Pergamon Press, Oxford.

Jensen, K. F. (1969). Effect of constant and fluctuating temperature on growth of four wood-decaying fungi. *Phytopathology* **59**, 645–647.

Kistler, B. R., and Merrill, W. (1968). Effects of *Strumella coryneoidea* on oak sapwood. *Phytopathology* **58**, 1429–1430.

Levi, M. P., and Cowling, E. B. (1969). Role of nitrogen in wood deterioration. VII. Physiological adaptation of wood-destroying and other fungi to substrates deficient in nitrogen. *Phytopathology* **59**, 460–468.

Manion, P. D., and French, D. W. (1968). Inoculation of living aspen trees with basidiospores of *Fomes igniarus* var. *populinus. Phytopathology* **58**, 1302–1304.

Merrill, W., and Cowling, E. B. (1966). Role of nitrogen in wood deterioration: Amounts and distribution of nitrogen in tree stems. *Can. J. Botany* **44**, 1555–1580.

Norkrans, B. (1963). Degradation of cellulose. *Ann. Rev. Phytopathol.* **1**, 325–350.

Ohman, J. H. (1968). Decay and discoloration of sugar maple. *Forest Pest Leaflet, U.S. Forest Serv.* **110**, 1–6.

Peace, T. R. (1962). "Pathology of Trees and Shrubs." Oxford Univ. Press, London and New York.

Schubert, W. J. (1965). "Lignin Biochemistry." Academic Press, New York.

Shigo, A. L. (1965). Decay and discoloration in sprout red maple. *Phytopathology* **55**, 957–962.

Shigo, A. L. (1966). Decay and discoloration following logging wounds on northern hardwoods. *Res. Paper, Northeast. Forest Exptl. Sta.,* **NE-47**, 1–43.

Shigo, A. L. (1969). The death and decay of trees. *Nat. His.* **78**, 43–47.

Shigo, A. L., and Sharon, E. M. (1968). Discoloration and decay in hardwoods following inoculations with Hymenomycetes. *Phytopathology* **58**, 1493–1498.

True, R. D., and Tryon, E. H. (1966). Butt decay in yellow-poplar sprouts in West Virginia. *West Vir. Agr. Exp. Sta., Bull.* **541T**, 1–67.

Whitney, R. D., and Denyer, W. B. G. (1968). Rates of decay by *Coniophora puteana* and *Polyporus tomentosus* in living and dying white spruce. *Forest Sci.* **14**, 122–126.

Wilcox, W. W. (1968). Changes in wood microstructure through progressive stages of decay. *Res. Paper, U.S. Forest Serv.* **FPL-70**, 1–46.

Zabel, R. A., Silverborg, S. B., and Fowler, M. E. (1958). A survey of forest tree diseases. *Sta. Paper, Northeast. Forest Expt. Sta.* **110**, 1–30.

17

FUNGI THAT CAUSE VARIOUS SYMPTOMS (RUST FUNGI)

Diseases caused by fungi belonging to the Uredinales order are among the most ecologically and economically important of all plant maladies. Geographically, the rust fungi are located on all major land masses, with the exception of Antarctica. The greatest number of species, however, are found in the temperate regions. Almost all major groups of green plants are parasitized by rust fungi. Rusts are known to infect primitive ferns as well as phylogenetically advanced orchids, mints, and composites.

The various species of the Uredinales order exhibit considerable diversity, but all have three major characteristics in common. First, without exception, the rust fungi as they occur in nature are obligate plant parasites. Shaw (1967), in a comprehensive treatment of the relationships between plant hosts and obligate fungal parasites, suggests two criteria which distinguish obligate parasites. (1) These organisms in nature can complete their life cycle only on the living tissues of their hosts. These organisms cannot, at present, be grown in axenic (or pure) culture. (2) The second major characteristic of rust organisms is that many species of these microbes require two unrelated (often widely unrelated) host plants in order to consumate their life cycles. This is a condition unique among fungi. Species which exhibit this two-host phenomenon are termed heteroecious. The final distinguishing feature is that most rust fungi produce several different types of spores in regular and almost unchanging succession. This phenomenon is termed pleomorphism. Numerous fungi produce two kinds of spores, but several rust fungi produce as many as five spore types.

Diseases caused by rust fungi have been historically and, are presently, especially significant. Stem diseases caused by rust fungi on cereal plants are a notable example. Several civilizations have been significantly dependent on one or more cereal crops; rice, Orient; corn, Middle and South America; barley, Mediterranean; and wheat, North America. All of these cereals are infected by one or more rust fungi and these organisms have often acutely reduced yields. In addition to cereals, numerous other plants of economic importance are seriously effected by rust fungi, including many forest tree species.

I. SPORE TYPES OF RUST FUNGI

Life cycles of the Uredinales are quite complex. An appreciation of the various spore types produced is basic to an understanding of the life patterns of rust fungi. Many rust fungi, but not all, produce five spore types (Table XXIV).

Since all rust fungi do not produce all five spore types, three general life cycles are recognized; macrocyclic, demicyclic, and microcyclic. Macrocyclic fungi produce all five spore types if they complete their life cycle. These fungi may be autoecious (one host) or heteroecious (two hosts). An example of an autoecious, macrocyclic fungus is *Puccinia helianthi,* which causes a disease of sunflower. *Cronartium ribicola,* the causal agent of white pine blister rust, is a heteroecious, macrocyclic organism. The fungi which exhibit the demicyclic life cycle produce all spore types with the exception of urediospores. As in the case of macrocyclic fungi, demicyclic species may be autoecious or heteroecious. *Gymnoconia peckiana* is an autoecious, demicyclic organism which causes a rust disease of *Rubus* spp., while *Gymnosporangium juniperi-virginianae* is a heteroecious, demicyclic fungus which is the causal agent of cedar-apple rust (Fig. 35). Many demicyclic species have a perennial mycelium in one or more of their host plants. The life cycles of microcyclic rust fungi involves only pycniospores, teliospores, and basidiospores. In some cases, only the latter two spore types are evident. All microcyclic rust fungi are autoecious, and only a few have been documented to infect forest trees. *Coleosporium pinicola* is a microcyclic species which causes a needle rust of Virginia pine.

II. GENERALIZED LIFE CYCLE OF A MACROCYCLIC RUST FUNGUS

This life cycle description will involve a heteroecious species which alternates between host X and Y.

In early spring, the fungus produces pycniospores on host X. These spores are noninfective and have a sexual function. They act as gametes (that is, + or −, male or female) and function to bring nuclei of the two mating strains together. After plasmogamy, but not karyogamy, has occurred, and while

TABLE XXIV

SPORE TYPES AND CHARACTERISTICS OF RUST FUNGI

Designation of life stage	Spore type	Spore bearing structure	Alternate host
0	Pycniospore	Pycnium	X
I	Aeciospore	Aecium	X
II	Urediospore	Uredium	Y
III	Teliospore	Telium	Y
IV	Basidiospore	Probasidium	Y

the fungus is still on host X, aecia are produced, bearing aeciospores. Each aeciospore contains two nuclei, one from each of the two pycniospores which fused to form the aecium. The aeciospores are typically produced in some quantity and are windborne. These spores function to initiate infection of host Y.

Following aeciospore infection of host Y, a mycelium is produced in this host which eventually gives rise to uredia and dicaryotic urediospores. Urediospores function to spread the fungus to uninfected Y individuals during the summer. After urediospores germinate and enter host Y, a mycelium is produced which eventually produces additional uredia and urediospores. Because several successions of urediospores may be rapidly produced during the summer, this spore-type is commonly referred to as the repeating spore-type.

After a number of crops of urediospores have been produced on Y hosts, the mycelium which gave rise to them initiates the production of telia, which bear teliospores. Teliospores may either germinate at once or lie dormant over the winter and germinate in the early spring. Teliospores germinate in place and following germination these spores form a probasidium into which the paired nuclei migrate, undergo fusion (or karyogamy), and finally divide meiotically to form four haploid basidiospores.

Basidiospores, which are generally relatively short-lived, are carried by the wind back to host X. Following germination and successful penetration of X, a sparse mycelium develops. Eventually this mycelium produces pycnia which bear +and − pycniospores.

III. RUST DISEASES OF FOREST TREES

Rust fungi infect various tree organs, and diseases caused by these organisms are characterized by a wide variety of symptoms. Rust diseases are commonly associated with tree leaves, cones (fruit), and stems. Those fungi which cause stem galls or cankers are generally the most devastating.

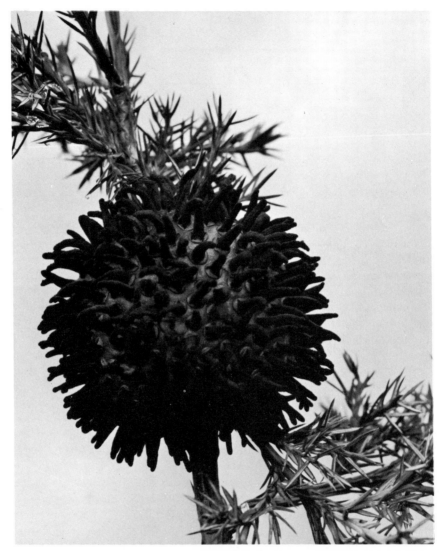

Fig. 35. Gall on eastern red cedar resulting from infection by *Gymnosporangium juniperi-virginianae*. "Hornlike" protrusions from the gall are the dry telia of the fungus. (Photograph courtesy U.S. Forest Service.)

A. Angiosperms

The influence of diseases caused by rust fungi on angiosperms is less significant than on gymnosperms. The leaves of several hardwoods, however, are infected by heteroecious rust fungi which usually have coniferous alternate hosts. Poplars have several leaf rust diseases caused by members of the

Melampsora genus. Ash rust caused by *Puccinia sparganoides* results in the swelling of twigs and petioles and distortion of leaves in various ashes. The alternate host for this fungus is *Spartina*, a common marsh grass.

B. Gymnosperms

1. Needle rusts.   Many rust fungi infect the needles of conifers. The majority of these fungi are heteroecious and have pycnia and aecia on coniferous leaves and uredia and telia on leaves of ferns or on various other higher plants. Boyce (1961) lists the following approximate numbers of needle rust fungi which infect various conifers; pine 18, balsam fir 24, Douglas fir 2, hemlock 6, spruce 10, larch 2, and cedar and juniper 15.

2. Cone rusts.   Longleaf, slash and Chihuahua pine; Sitka, black, blue, Engelmann, Norway, red and white spruce; and eastern hemlock all have cone rust diseases. Infection may result in reduced seed production, but rarely in complete crop failure.

3. Stem rusts.   By far the most serious rust diseases of all trees are the stem rusts of conifers. In these rusts, the mycelium of the causal fungus is typically perennial in the bark or wood of the host tree. This resident mycelium causes various host malformations including, for example, galls, other tumefactions, cankers, and fasciculations (witches' brooms or dense proliferations of twigs or branches about a common point). In the case of seedling and sapling size trees, infection by stem rust fungi frequently results in mortality. Infection of older individuals commonly results in disfigurement and reduced vigor.

Nearly all of the fungi which cause stem rust diseases are heteroecious with their alternate stages on annual and perennial herbaceous plants or on broad-leaved trees and shrubs.

C. Cronartium spp. — Stem Rust Fungi

Blister rusts are extremely important coniferous stem rust diseases caused by fungi belonging to the genus *Cronartium*. Members of this genus are widely distributed throughout North America, Europe, and Asia, where they primarily infect hard pines. Until approximately 1900, the most important *Cronartium* stem rust diseases in the United States were: eastern gall rust on Virginia and shortleaf pine caused by *C. cerebrum* and southern fusiform rust on southern hard pines caused by *C. fusiforme* and western gall rust on western hard pines caused by *C. coleosporiodes*.

At the turn of the twentieth century, another *Cronartium, C. ribicola*, was spreading westward from its native Siberia into Europe. This migration was widespread in northern and western Europe. An interesting aspect of *C. ribicola* was that it did not infect hard pines but rather members of the soft pine group (5 needles per fasicle).

Unfortunately, also during this period United States foresters were shipping native soft-pine seed to Europe for germination and initial seedling development. Seedlings were then returned to the United States for planting. As a result of this practice, C. ribicola was introduced into this country on returning seedlings. In 1906, stem rust disease caused by C. ribicola was observed on 3-year-old seedlings from Germany in Geneva, New York. In 1921, this fungus was also introduced into Vancouver, British Columbia, on a shipment of white pines from France.

From these two points of initial introduction, C. ribicola has spread almost entirely throughout the ranges of our native white pines and has caused destruction of hosts resulting in economic loss and great ecological impact.

Evolution over extended time periods results in equilibration of organisms with their environment, including a balance between host populations and their parasites and pathogens. When foreign disease agents are introduced into suitable host populations where natural selection has not operated to produce equilibrium, catastrophic losses may ensue. Diseases which result from introduced, nonnative pathogens are typically the most damaging of all disease types. Disease caused by C. ribicola represents the first of several of this type which we will consider.

1. *Life Cycle of Cronartium ribicola.* Basidiospores (sporidia) of the fungus land on the needles of susceptible pine species and enter a stomate by producing a germ tube. Following stomatal penetration, hyphae are produced which penetrate the vascular elements of the leaf, eventually grow into the phloem of the twig, and ultimately extend into the stem. Germ tube penetration of the stomates is within 8–24 hours of deposition on the needle. Spots on infected needles may become visible within 4–10 weeks of fungal entrance. The base of infected needle bundles often turns yellow-orange and exhibits swelling.

In 2–4 years following basidiospore infection, pycnidia are formed on a branch or on the main stem. Pycnidia are typically formed just below the bark and erupt through its surface. Pycniospores are released in a honey-colored liquid and are disseminated by insects, birds, and rain. If a + and – pycniospore successfully fuse, then, in approximately 12 months, aecia will be formed at the approximate site of the pycnidia (Fig. 36). This pycnidial-aecial sequence is repeated each growing season as the perennial mycelium of C. ribicola advances through the bark. Continued growth of the fungus up and down the branch and/or trunk eventually results in the production of a spindle-shaped canker. In young trees this canker may soon girdle the trees and cause their death.

Aeciospores which are produced in aecia are viable for 9–12 months and are windborne. These spores may be transmitted over several hundred miles. If aeciospores happen to land on a suitable *Ribes* spp. (gooseberry, currant), the alternate host for C. ribicola, they infect it by penetrating a sto-

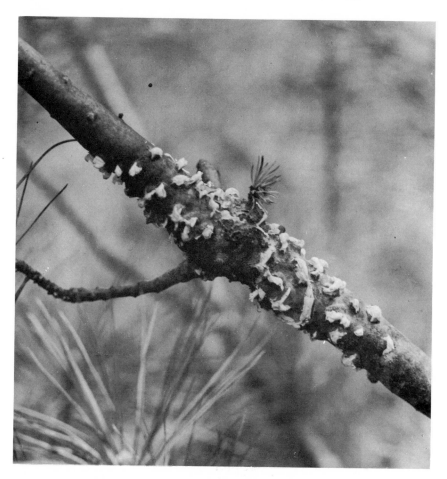

Fig. 36. Small eastern white pine branch infected by *Cronartium ribicola*. Note branch swelling and the mature aecia of the fungus. Upon rupture, these aecia will release large orange aeciospores. (Photograph courtesy U.S. Forest Service.)

mate with a germ tube. *Ribes* spp. vary in their susceptibility to *C. ribicola* infection. There are approximately 80 native *Ribes* in the United States.

One to three weeks after aecial infection, uredia are formed on the underside of infected *Ribes* leaves. These uredia produce urediospores which have the capacity to infect additional *Ribes* plants only. Urediospores, which are viable for 9-12 months, are commonly carried by wind for distances averaging 300-500 yards. These spores germinate on the underside of *Ribes* leaves, enter the plant, and, shortly, more uredia are formed. There may be several generations of urediospores per growing season.

Eventually, in late summer and early fall, telia are formed on old uredial pustules on *Ribes* leaves. Teliospores are borne on the telia in the form of telial columns. The teliospores are viable for 90 days. These spores germinate *in situ* and produce a probasidium. In 8–24 hours four basidiospores are produced on each probasidium. Basidiospore release represents a weak point in the life cycle of the fungus. Basidiospores are viable for only 30 hours and must reach a susceptible pine host within that time in order to initiate infection. Since these spores are typically carried only 900–1000 feet from their source in 30 hours, isolation of pine stands by barriers of approximately 1000 feet devoid of *Ribes* has proved an effective protective scheme. This life cycle is summarized in Fig. 37.

As in the case of all rust diseases, microclimate plays an extremely critical role in pathogen and disease development. The significance of weather will be discussed more completely in Chapter 22.

2. Mechanism of disease development.   The hyphae of most rust fungi grow intercellularly in their host tissues and penetrate individual cells with absorbing organs termed haustoria.

The toxin relationships in obligate parasitism are presumed to be more subtle than those in facultative parasitism. Since obligate parasites are restricted to development in living host tissues, outright death of host cells would also result in death of the fungus. In certain investigations of rust disease phenomena, a suggestion of the "stimulation" of host metabolism by infecting rust fungi has been observed. So called "green islands" have been observed in tissues surrounding older rust infections. It has been proposed that growth-regulating substances (IAA or kinetin?) may induce metabolically dependent accumulation of amino acids and other substances in infected areas. A working hypothesis is that the interaction of host and rust fungus results in the release of a diffusable substance during incipient infection which "stimulates" the metabolic activity of the host tissue in the area of infection (Ludwig, 1960).

Krebill (1968) studied six canker rusts in pines and concluded that the bark swelling was due to the space requirements of the intercellular hyphae of the causal fungi. It was also suggested that a slight increase in number and size of host parenchyma cells may also contribute to swelling. This investigator further suggested that desiccation of host cells following the rupture of periderm by aecial structures or other wounding may be responsible for bark necrosis.

IV. CONTROL OF RUST DISEASES

Because of the very great economic significance of rust diseases, a considerable effort has been directed to achieve suitable controls. The significance of *Tuberculina maxima* (Deuteromycete), a hyperparasite of *C. ribicola*, has

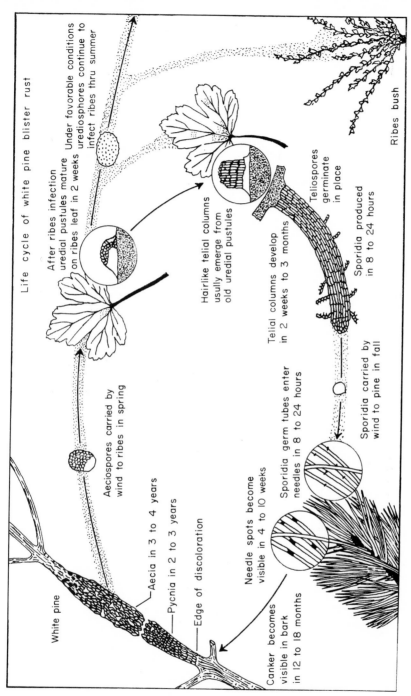

Life cycle of white pine blister rust

Under favorable conditions urediosphores continue to infect ribes thru summer

After ribes infection uredial pustules mature on ribes leaf in 2 weeks

Aeciospores carried by wind to ribes in spring

Hairlike telial columns usully emerge from old uredial pustules

Teliospores germinate in place

Telial columns develop in 2 weeks to 3 months

Sporidia produced in 8 to 24 hours

Sporidia carried by wind to pine in fall

Ribes bush

Aecia in 3 to 4 years

Pycnia in 2 to 3 years

Edge of discoloration

Needle spots become visible in 4 to 10 weeks

Sporidia germ tubes enter needles in 8 to 24 hours

White pine

Canker becomes visible in bark in 12 to 18 months

Fig. 37. Life cycle of *Cronartium ribicola*. [From Miller *et al.* (1959). Reproduced by permission of U.S. Forest Service.]

been explored. Under certain conditions, the former fungus appears to "inactivate" cankers caused by the latter. Systemic antibiotics, for example, cycloheximide derivatives and phytoactin, have also been evaluated in blister rust control programs. These efforts will receive greater attention in the chapters on control.

REFERENCES

Boyce, J. S. (1961). "Forest Pathology." McGraw-Hill, New York.

Krebill, R. G. (1968). Histology of canker rusts in pines. *Phytopathology* **58**, 155-164.

Ludwig, R. A. (1960). Toxins. *In* "Plant Pathology" (J. G. Horsfall and A. E. Dimond, eds.), Vol. 2, pp. 315-357. Academic Press, New York.

Miller, D. R., Kimmey, J. W., and Fowler, M. E. (1959). White pine blister rust. *Forest Pest Leaflet, U.S. Forest Serv.* **36**, 1-8.

Shaw, M. (1967). Cell biological aspects of host-parasite relations of obligate fungal parasites. *Can. J. Botany* **45**, 1205-1220.

GENERAL REFERENCES

Allen, P. J. (1959). Metabolic considerations of obligate parasitism. *In* "Plant Pathology, Problems and Progress 1908-1958" (C. S. Holton *et al.*, eds.), pp. 119-129. Univ. of Wisconsin Press, Madison, Wisconsin.

Anderson, N. A., and French, D. W. (1964). Sweet-fern rust on jack pine. *J. Forestry* **62**, 467-471.

Cordell, C. E., and Wolfe, R. D. (1969). Comandra blister rust, a threat to southern hard pines. *Phytopathology* **59**, 1022 (abstr.).

Eleuterius, L. N. (1968). Morphology of *Cronartium fusiforme* in *Quercus nigra*. *Phytopathology* **58**, 1487-1492.

Jewell, F. F., and Walker, N. M. (1967). Histology of *Cronartium quercuum* galls in shortleaf pine. *Phytopathology* **57**, 545-550.

Koenigs, J. W. (1968). Culturing the white pine blister rust fungus in callus of western white pine. *Phytopathology* **58**, 46-48.

Krebill, R. G. (1968). *Cronartium comandrae* in the Rocky Mountain States. *Res. Paper, Intermount. Forest and Range Expt. Sta.* **INT-50**, 1-28.

Mielke, J. L., Krebill, R. G., and Powers, H. R., Jr. (1968). Comandra blister rust of hard pines. *Forest Pest Leaflet, U.S. Forest Serv.* **62**, 1-8.

Nicholls, T. H., Patton, R. F., and Van Arsdel, E. P. (1968). Life cycle and seasonal development of *Coleosporium* pine needle rust in Wisconsin. *Phytopathology* **58**, 822-829.

Peterson, R. S. (1968). Limb rust of pine: The causal fungi. *Phytopathology* **58**, 309-315.

Peterson, R. S., and Jewell, F. F. (1968). Status of American stem rusts of pine. *Ann. Rev. Phytopathol.* **6**, 23-40.

Shaw, M. (1963). The physiology and host-parasite relations of the rusts. *Ann. Rev. Phytopathol.* **1**, 259-294.

Van Arsdel, E. P. (1968). Stem and needle inoculations of eastern white pine with the blister rust fungus. *Phytopathology* **58**, 512-514.

White, B. L., and Merrill, W. (1969). Pathological anatomy of *Abies balsamea* infected with *Melampsorella caryophyllacearum*. *Phytopathology* **59**, 1238-1242.

Wicker, E. F., and Woo, J. Y. (1969). Differential response of invading *Tuberculina maxima* to white pine tissues. *Phytopathology* **59**, 16 (abstr.).

18

FUNGI THAT CAUSE CANKER AND FOLIAR SYMPTOMS

I. CANKER DISEASES

Cankers may be defined as localized regions of necrosis in the bark of stems or branches of trees. There are many fungi which cause diseases of trees that are manifested in canker symptoms. Diseases of this type occur in both the gymnosperm and angiosperm groups. There are more canker-type diseases and their significance is greater, however, in the angiosperm class.

In 1958, the estimated mortality and growth losses from hardwood canker diseases on the growing stock of commercial forest land in the United States and coastal Alaska was 152 million cubic feet of wood annually (Hepting and Jemison, 1958). Cankers are very frequently located ρn the lower bole, potentially the highest quality portion of the tree. Secondary significances of cankered regions include; predisposition of cankered stems to wind, ice, and snow damage; and provision of entrance courts for wood staining and decaying microorganisms.

Most fungi which cause diseases expressed in canker symptoms belong to the Ascomycetes class. Several fungi belonging to the Deuteromycetes class are also capable of inducing canker diseases. Only a few Basidiomycetes have been implicated in canker formation.

Diseases expressed in canker symptoms may be conveniently grouped into three classes depending on whether the cankers formed are diffuse, perennial, or annual. In diffuse cankers, the causal pathogen generally has the capacity to grow rapidly through host bark. Cankers of this type may completely girdle the stem and result in host mortality. Fungi which induce perennial cankers, on the other hand, appear to grow much more slowly in

186

host tissue. In this instance, the fungus and host tree seem to be in a delicate balance such that the canker enlarges slowly and coincidently with tree development. Annual cankers are formed by fungi which are normally saprophytic but which become temporarily pathogenic. These fungi are most significant on hosts that are exposed to unusual environmental stresses. The association of these fungi with the host tree is short-lived in the absence of continued, additional stress factors.

In an effort to illustrate more clearly the characteristics of the three canker types, examples of each class will be discussed.

A. Diffuse Canker Types

1. Hypoxylon canker of poplar.   This canker disease is responsible in the Lake States for annual losses exceeding $1 million. It is the most important disease recognized on quaking aspen, bigtooth aspen, and balsam poplar (Anderson, 1956). The causal fungus is *Hypoxylon pruinatum,* an Ascomycete (Berbee and Rogers, 1964).

The life cycle of *H. pruinatum* is quite simple and representative of ascomyceteous canker-inducing pathogens. Ascospores are presumed to be the major inoculum for natural infections. Ascospores are discharged throughout the year during periods of rain or snow precipitation. Ascospore discharge has been documented even when the temperature was below 0°C. Dissemination of the ascospores is thought to be either by wind or insects. Following ascospore germination, which may be stimulated by some host bark substance, the resulting germ tube must encounter a wound or natural opening in order to successfully enter the host plant. Bark boring insects may provide extremely favorable infection sites. Fungal hyphae, once inside the epidermis, penetrate the cell walls of the bark cortex, phloem, and outer wood but appear to be excluded from the cork cambium (periderm). After appreciable hyphal development in the host, perithecia are formed on ruptured bark surfaces (Berbee and Rogers, 1964). These ruptured bark surfaces constitute the diffuse canker and may coalesce to girdle and ultimately kill the host tree.

Anderson (1964) has enumerated several peculiar characteristics which appear to be associated with this disease. These include: (*1*) No direct relationships are obvious which relate various sites to disease severity. (*2*) Periods of high disease intensity seem to be correlated with low rainfall. (*3*) No uniform relation appears to exist between disease and stand density. (*4*) Thinning operations have produced both more and less disease, depending on the individual stand being evaluated. All of these observations suggest we need additional information on this important disease.

2. Chestnut blight.   Perhaps the most infamous of all diffuse-canker diseases is chestnut blight, caused by *Endothia parasitica.* At the turn of the present century, American chestnut (*Castanea dentata*) was the most important hardwood tree species in the eastern United States. It was a dominant component of the eastern hardwood forests whose range extended from Vermont southward along the southern Appalachians to northern Georgia. Mature trees were commonly 3–5 feet in diameter and 60–90 feet in height (Fig. 38). Trees had considerable commercial value for; tannin (greater than 55,000 tons in 1923), lumber (more than 600 million board feet in 1909), pulpwood, poles (telephone and others), railway ties, and edible nut production.

In 1904 in the New York Zoological Park, mature chestnuts suddenly began to die. The fungus *Endothia parasitica* (Ascomycete) was consistently isolated from diseased individuals. This organism, which is a native of Japan, China, and Korea, was presumed to have been introduced into the United States on nursery stock imported from the Orient. Spreading at the rate of approximately 24 miles per year, the pathogen rapidly became distributed throughout the natural range of chestnut. Despite all manner of control efforts, in less than 50 years *E. parasitica* destroyed practically every mature chestnut within its natural range. The impact of *E. parasitica*, as in the case of *Cronartium ribicola*, can be attributed to the fact that natural selection had not produced any chestnut variants resistant to infection by the fungus due to the absence of the microbe throughout the natural range of the tree. *Castenea dentata* persists today because its root collar region resists infection by the fungus and fosters sprouts which occasionally reach 20–30 feet in height before they are killed by *E. parasitica*. The nuts which are occasionally produced on these sprouts are typically not viable.

The life cycle of *E. parasitica* is basically identical with that of *Hypoxylon pruinatum*, previously discussed. Three significant differences do, however, exist. (1) *Endothia parasitica* has a greater capacity to grow more deeply into the host stem. Outer rings of the sapwood are commonly colonized. In this region, toxins produced by the fungus are presumed to induce the formation of tyloses. Tyloses are balloon-like enlargements of the membranes of pits in the wall between xylem cells and a vessel or tracheid which act to restrict the normal flow of water through these conducting elements. (2) *Endothia parasitica* has the ability to grow relatively rapidly in the phloem, cambium, and outer xylem which frequently results in complete girdling in a single year. When a stem is completely girdled, water conduction is inhibited and the tree rapidly wilts and dies. This rapid necrosis accounts for the term chestnut "blight." (3) *Endothia parasitica* grows relatively efficiently saprophytically on the bark of at least twelve oak species and on the bark of several plants in a dozen other genera. These three characteristics, coupled with the absence of any inherent resistance in the chestnut, have resulted in the near extinction of *C. dentata*.

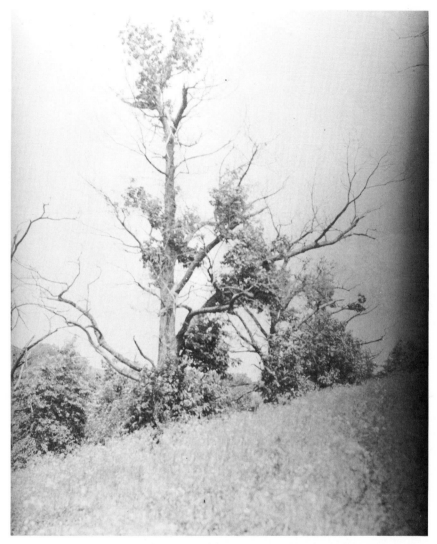

Fig. 38.   American chestnut in final stages of deterioration resulting from infection by *Endothia parasitica*. This picture was taken in Ohio in 1934. Today, even photographs of chestnuts this size, living or dead, are becoming scarce. (Photograph courtesy U.S. Forest Service.)

Castanea spp. which naturally exist in Asia are resistant to infection by *E. parasitica*. Considerable effort has been directed at attempting to hybridize Asian species with American and European species (also susceptible) to achieve a resistant, desirable chestnut. These efforts have enjoyed only limited success and will be discussed more fully in the chapters on control.

3. *Scleroderris canker.* This disease is one of the most important canker diseases on coniferous hosts. The malady is caused by *Scleroderris lagerbergii*, an Ascomycete. Red and jack pines appear to be the most seriously damaged, especially in the Lake States. The pathogen is present and causing mortality on every ranger district in the national forests in upper Michigan and northern Wisconsin. In this area the fungus has been found in 66% of the red pine plantations and in 86% of the jack pine plantations sampled. Mortality in these red and jack pine stands is averaging 40 and 39%, respectively. In Ontario, *S. lagerbergii* has recently caused the destruction of approximately 900,000 red pine seedlings (Punter, 1967).

Airborne ascospores of *S. lagerbergii* are the primary agent of dissemination. These spores are released from May to October with maximum release levels in July and August. Most ascospores are released within 48 hours after a rain period. Free moisture is required for release and germination of ascospores. Temperature is also critical for ascospore release, and the maximum release appears to be at approximately 17°C.

B. Perennial Canker Types

These cankers characteristically develop more slowly than diffuse cankers as the causal fungi grow more slowly in their hosts. Perennial canker diseases are nevertheless very important.

1. *Nectria cankers.* These cankers are the most important canker diseases of hardwoods in the northeast. The pathogens responsible are members of the *Nectria* genus. The most widespread and damaging species is *Nectria galligena* (Ascomycete). Actually, no North American hardwood species can be considered immune to infection by *N. galligena*. The forest tree species most frequently attacked include; red and sugar maple, black walnut, black, yellow, and white birch, beech, and largetooth aspen. Ornamental shrubs, shade trees, and fruit trees, as well as forest trees, are commonly infected. It is interesting to note that hickory, ash, and elm species are rarely infected (Brandt, 1964).

The degree and seriousness of *Nectria* canker damage is very closely correlated with general host vigor. Trees weakened by one or more stresses are most severely damaged. Infection by *Nectria* fungi very infrequently results in outright host mortality. Death occurs only after cankers have completely girdled the stem. Birch species and black walnut are most susceptible to death as the result of girdling. Predisposition to breakage at cankered points by several abiotic stress factors is the most significant aspect of *Nectria* infection. In northeastern areas, where snow and ice are important factors, 60–70% of the trees in a young hardwood stand may have *Nectria* cankers. Cankers also frequently result in culling the basal portion of the stem which is the most valuable portion of the tree from a lumber standpoint. The ability of *Nectria* cankers to serve as infection courts for wood decay fungi is not fully appreciated.

Well-developed *Nectria* cankers are very distinctive and easily recognized because of their "target-like" appearance (Fig. 39). Incipient stages, however, are somewhat more difficult to detect. The first visible symptom is usually a dark red or blackened water-soaked appearance of the bark adjacent to the opening through which the pathogen gained ingress. Subsequent symptoms include further discoloring, depression, and fissuring of the bark at the margins of the initial discoloration.

The characteristic "target" appearance of older cankers results from the continued alteration between necrosis of bark tissue caused by the fungus in the autumn and winter months and growth of host callus in spring and early summer. Cankers are usually open, but dead bark tissue may remain in place and produce a covered canker.

Nectria spores, both sexual and asexual, gain entrance to host trees through openings (natural or wounds) in the outer bark which expose the inner bark or cambium. If a viable spore lands on exposed cambium and if moisture and temperature conditions are appropriate, germination occurs and the fungus may become established in the tree in 3-4 hours. As the hyphae develop through the host they are presumed to release a metabolic product (toxin) which kills the cambial and phloem cells in advance of the mycelium. The fungi apparently lack the ability to grow through living cells.

Evidence of necrosis may become evident within days of infection or may fail to be expressed for 2 or 3 years depending upon the pathogenicity of the particular *Nectria* strain and inherent susceptibility of the host.

Each year while the tree is dormant or semidormant, the mycelium grows outward as much as ¼-1½ inches. As tree growth resumes in the spring the advance of the fungus is delayed or stopped by the production of callus tissue.

In the autumn, usually with the advent of more rain, the causal fungi produce spores. Asexual conidia are borne on hyphae which protrude through cracks or lenticels in the bark along the outer ridges of the canker. Conidia are disseminated by wind, rain, insects, and birds. Ascospores are formed in red perithecia which occur singly or in groups generally on the dead callus tissue. Ascospores are efficiently transported by air currents.

2. Beech bark disease. This canker disease of American beech is the apparent result of an interaction of several organisms (Shigo, 1964). The primary causal agents are thought to be several bark scale insects and species of *Nectria* fungi.

The fungi invade the stylet punctures of the scale insects and rapidly form

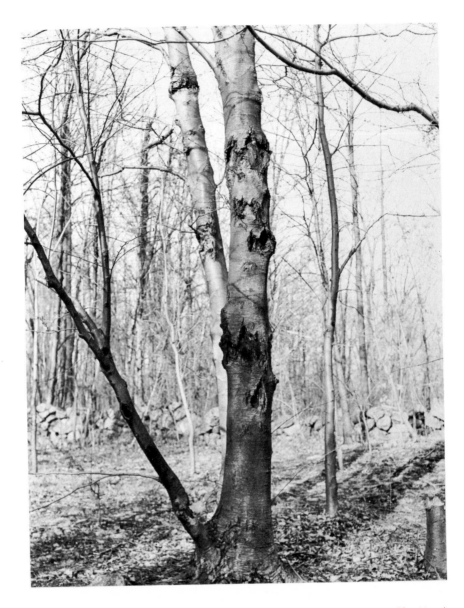

Fig. 39.   Black birch with extensive canker symptoms. These cankers were caused by *Nectria galligena*, the most important canker inducing fungus on deciduous species in the east (Photograph courtesy U.S. Forest Service.)

large cankers which may quite quickly girdle and kill host trees. Beetles associated with the diseased bark may play important roles as long range *Nectria* vectors.

Another example of an important perennial canker is *Eutypella* canker of maple (Fig. 40).

C. Annual Canker Types

Canker diseases of this type have generally been considered relatively unimportant. There is, however, additional research required in this area.

Fusarium solani (Deuteromycete) is the causal agent of a significant annual canker on sugar and red maples (Wood and Skelly, 1964). Trees under insect or temperature-extreme stress appear to be predisposed to infection by *F. solani.* Pawuk (1968) has suggested that extracts from sugar maple bark regions stimulate spore germination of the causal fungus. Weidensaul (1968), however, concluded that airborne spores are probably not a major source of inoculum for natural infections. Dochinger (1967) considered *F. solani* an important canker-inducing agent of eastern cottonwood and hybrid poplars in Iowa.

Annual cankers have frequently been associated with various dieback diseases as a possible contributing factor. Silverborg and Ross (1968), for example, have hypothesized that ash dieback is induced by periods of low rainfall followed by severe stem and branch cankering by fungi such as *Cytophoma pruinosa* and *Fusicoccum* spp.

II. FOLIAGE DISEASES

There are numerous fungi which belong to the Ascomycetes and Deuteromycetes classes which cause foliage diseases on both angiosperms and gymnosperms. Foliage diseases are only of minor importance in angiosperms. The diseases are usually expressed only in a partial defoliation, if any. Even complete defoliation, which is very rare, would only have great significance if it occurred early in the growing season and in several consecutive years. Defoliation does, however, result in reduced growth and reduced resistance to other stress factors.

Defoliation, complete or partial, is substantially more important in the case of gymnosperms. In this case the growth of the trees is dependent on the photosynthetic activity of several years of leaf (needle) growth. Three-, four-, and five-year-old needles may be functioning. Any appreciable loss of needles is not followed by a complete replenishment the following year as occurs in angiosperms. Complete coniferous defoliation is typically fatal. Foliage diseases generally are ecologically and economically more important in gymnosperms.

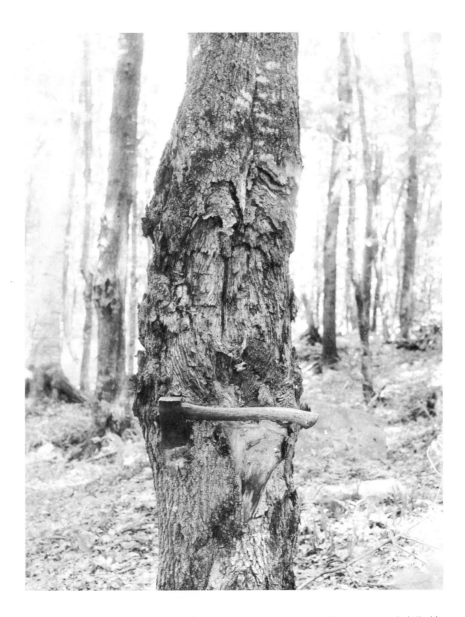

Fig. 40. Sugar maple canker caused by *Eutypella parasitica*. Trees this size are rarely killed by the fungus and the cankers may persist for many years and may reach approximately 5 feet in length. (Photograph courtesy U.S. Forest Service.)

Examples of relatively important foliar diseases will be used to illustrate the significance of these disease types in the two classes.

A. Angiosperms

1. Tar spot.   This malady, caused by *Rhytisma acerinum* (Ascomycete), is common on red and silver maples. During the summer black, thick-walled sclerotia (Fig. 41) develop on host leaves. These sclerotia release conidia which serve to infect additional maple leaves. In the autumn, ascospores are formed in asci on the fallen leaves. Ascospores overwinter on these leaves and serve to initiate infection of new foliage in the spring.

2. Anthracnose.   Anthracnose leaf disease caused by *Gnomonia veneta* (Ascomycete) is prevalent on sycamores and oaks. In the east, sycamores are occasionally severely infected and, if defoliated for several consecutive years, they may exhibit some dieback symptoms.

Ascospores which have overwintered in leaf litter infect young leaves in the spring by entering through stomates. Toxins released by the fungus may result in rapid leaf necrosis. Infection is frequently confused with spring frost injury. Within approximately 5 weeks of a heavy initial infection, a new leaf crop may be produced by host trees. As these leaves become infected, large irregular necrotic areas may develop along the veins. Acervuli (hyphal mats which give rise to dense asexual spore bearing structures) are formed on these necrotic areas and masses of conidia are produced. The causal fungus may occasionally grow through the petiole and produce twig cankers. Ascospores are ultimately formed in the autumn on infected, fallen leaves.

B. Gymnosperms

1. Rhabdocline needle cast.   This very important needle disease of Douglas fir is caused by *Rhabdocline pseudotsugae* (Ascomycete) (Brandt, 1960). In regions of severe infection, annual loss of needles occurs until the tree dies.

Infection normally takes place in early summer. The young needles are infected by ascospores produced on needles of the previous year. In late summer, the needles yellow, eventually turning brown in winter as the fungus grows intracellularly through the chlorenchyma tissue. The following spring, orange-brown apothecia erupt through the epidermis of infected needles and release ascospores.

2. Brown-spot needle blight. *Scirrhia acicola* (Ascomycete) infects longleaf pine and causes the most serious disease of this tree in its seedling stage. The life cycle of this fungus is similar to those of the other ascomycetous foliar pathogens discussed. *Scirrhia acicola*, by delaying growth and

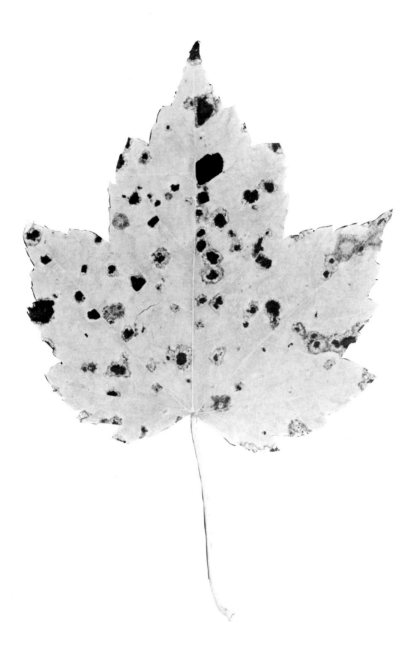

Fig. 41. Tar spot disease of red maple. The dark blotches are the result of infection by *Rhytisma acerinum* and are actually sclerotia of the fungus. (Photograph courtesy U.S. Forest Service.)

killing seedlings, causes a total annual growth loss estimated to equal 16 million cubic feet of timber (Lightle, 1960).

III. SUMMARY

Most important diseases which are expressed in canker or foliar symptoms are caused by fungi belonging to the Ascomycetes class. Canker diseases of angiosperms are considerably more prevalent and significant than similar diseases of gymnosperms. Only diffuse cankers generally result in outright mortality. Perennial and annual canker diseases are most important because they reduce host vigor or reduce merchantability.

Fungi which cause leaf necrosis are considerably more important on gymnosperms than on angiosperms. Those microbes having the capacity to significantly reduce the number of functioning needles commonly cause mortality. The life cycles of these fungi are quite simple, with conidia acting to spread the pathogen during the summer, and ascospores formed in abscissed foliage, permitting survival over the dormant season.

REFERENCES

Anderson, R. L. (1956). Hypoxylon canker of Aspen. *Forest Pest Leaflet, U.S. Forest Serv.* **6**, 1-3.

Anderson, R. L. (1964). Hypoxylon canker impact on Aspen. *Phytopathology* **54**, 253-257.

Berbee, J. G., and Rogers, J. D. (1964). Life cycle and host range of *Hypoxylon pruinatum* and its pathogenesis on poplars. *Phytopathology* **54**, 257-261.

Brandt, R. W. (1960). The rhabdocline needle-cast of Douglas fir. *Tech. Publ., N.Y. State Coll. Forestry* **84**, 1-66.

Brandt, R. W. (1964). Nectria canker of hardwoods. *Forest Pest Leaflet, U.S. Forest Serv.* **84**, 1-7.

Dochinger, L. S. (1967). Occurrence of poplar cankers caused by *Fusarium solani* in Iowa. *Plant Disease Reptr.* **51**, 900-903.

Hepting, G. H., and Jemison, G. M. (1958). Forest protection. *In* "Timber Resources for America's Future," *Forest Res. Rept., U.S. Forest Serv.* **14**, 185-220.

Lightle, P. C. (1960). Brown-spot needle blight of longleaf pine. *Forest Pest Leaflet, U.S. Forest Serv.* **44**, 1-7.

Pawuk, W. H. (1968). The effect of sugar maple stem tissue extracts on spore germination of *Fusarium solani*. *Phytopathology* **58**, 402 (abstr.).

Punter, D. (1967). *Scleroderris lagerbergii* in and near Ontario forest nurseries. *Plant Disease Reptr.* **51**, 357.

Shigo, A. L. (1964). Organism interactions in the beech bark disease. *Phytopathology* **54**, 263-269.

Silverborg, S. B., and Ross, E. W. (1968). Ash dieback disease development in New York State. *Plant Disease Reptr.* **52**, 105-107.

Weidensaul, T. C. (1968). The occurrence of *Fusarium* in the air in northern hardwood forests. *Phytopathology* **58**, 1071 (abstr.).

Wood, F. A., and Skelly, J. M. (1964). The etiology of an annual canker on maple. *Phytopathology* **54**, 269-272.

GENERAL REFERENCES

Anderson, R. L., and Anderson, G. W. (1969). Hypoxylon canker of Aspen. *Forest Pest Leaflet, U.S. Forest Serv.* **6**, 1-6.

Batson, W. E., Jr., and Witcher, W. (1968). Live oak cankers caused by *Endothia parasitica*. *Phytopathology* **58**, 1473-1475.

Berry, C. R., and Hepting, G. H. (1959). Pitch canker of southern pines. *Forest Pest Leaflet, U.S. Forest Serv.* **35**, 1-4.

Bier, J. E. (1964). The relation of some bark factors to canker susceptibility. *Phytopathology* **54**, 250-253.

Bramble, W. C. (1938). The effect of *Endothia parasitica* on conduction. *Am. J. Botany* **25**, 61-65.

Bynum, H. H., and Miller, D. R. (1969). A new needle disease of hard pines in Oregon and California. *Plant Disease Reptr.* **53**, 232-234.

Childs, T. W. (1968). Elytroderma disease of ponderosa pine in the Pacific Northwest. *Res. Paper, Pac. Northwest For. and Range Exp. Sta.* **PNW-69**, 45 pp.

Cobb, F. W., Jr., and Libby, W. J. (1968). Susceptibility of Monterey, Guadalupe Island, Cedros Island and Bishop Pines to *Scirrhia (Dothistroma) pini*, the cause of red band needle blight. *Phytopathology* **58**, 88-90.

Cobb, F. W., Jr., and Miller, D. R. (1968). Hosts and geographic distribution of *Scirrhia pini*—the cause of red band needle blight in California. *J. Forestry* **66**, 930-933.

Cobb, F. W., Jr., Uhrenholdt, B., and Krohn, R. F. (1969). Epidemiology of *Dothistroma* pine needle blight on *Pinus radiata*. *Phytopathology* **59**, 1021-1022.

Cordell, C. E., Skilling, D. D., and Benzie, J. W. (1968). Susceptibility of three pine species to *Scleroderris lagerbergii* in Upper Michigan. *Plant Disease Rptr.* **52**, 37-39.

DeVay, J. E., Lukezic, F. L., English, H., Trujillo, E. E., and Moller, W. J. (1968). Ceratocystis canker of deciduous fruit trees. *Phytopathology* **58**, 949-954.

Diller, J. D. (1965). Chestnut blight. *Forest Pest Leaflet, U.S. Forest Serv.* **94**, 1-7.

Filer, T. H., Jr. (1967). Pathogenicity of Cytospora, Phomopsis, and Hypomyces on *Populus deltoides. Phytopathology* **57**, 978-980.

French, W. J. (1969). Eutypella canker on *Acer* in New York. *Tech. Publ., N.Y. State Coll. Forestry* **94**, 1-56.

Froyd, J. D., and French, D. W. (1967). Ejection and dissemination of ascospores of *Hypoxylon pruinatum. Can. J. Botany* **45**, 1507-1517.

Gross, H. L. (1967). *Cytospora* canker of black cherry. *Plant Disease Reptr.* **51**, 261-263.

Houston, D. R. (1969). Basal canker of white pine. *Forest Sci.* **15**, 66-83.

Lightle, P. C. (1960). Brown-spot needle blight of longleaf pine. *Forest Pest Leaflet, U.S. Forest Serv.* **44**, 1-7.

Lortie, M. (1964). Pathogenesis in cankers caused by *Nectria galligena. Phytopathology* **54**, 261-263.

Manion, P. D., and French, D. W. (1967). *Nectria galligena* and *Ceratocystis fimbriata* cankers of aspen in Minnesota. *Forest Sci.* **13**, 23-28.

Moller, W. J., DeVay, J. E., and Backman, D. A. (1969). Effect of some ecological factors on *Ceratocystis* canker in stone fruits. *Phytopathology* **59**, 938-942.

Neely, D., and Himelick, E. B. (1967). Characteristics and nomenclature of the oak anthracnose fungus. *Phytopathology* **57**, 1230-1236.

Peacher, P. H. (1969). Live oaks in Mississippi infected by *Endothia parasitica. Plant Disease Reptr.* **53**, 304.

Peterson, G. W. (1967). *Dothistroma* needle blight of Austrian and ponderosa pines: Epidemiology and control. *Phytopathology* **57**, 437-441.

Ross, E. W. (1964). Cankers associated with ash die-back. *Phytopathology* **54**, 272-275.

Schreiber, L. R., and Dochinger, L. S. (1967). Fusarium canker on paper mulberry (*Broussonetia papyrifera*). *Plant Disease Reptr.* **51**, 531-532.

Shigo, A. L. (1969). How *Poria obliqua* and *Polyporus glomeratus* incite cankers. *Phytopathology* **59**, 1164-1165.

Skilling, D. D. (1969). Spore dispersal by *Scleroderris lagerbergii* under nursery and plantation conditions. *Plant Disease Reptr.* **53**, 291-295.

Skilling, D. D., and Cordell, C. E. (1966). *Scleroderris* canker on National Forests in Upper Michigan and Northern Wisconsin. *Res. Paper, North Central Forest Expt. Sta.* **NC-3**, 1-10.

Tree Nut Section (A.R.S.). (1959). Chestnut blight and resistant chestnuts. *U.S. Dept. Agr., Farmers' Bull.* **2068**, 1-21.

Wood, F. A., and Skelly, J. M. (1969). Relation of the time of year to canker initiation by *Fusarium solani* in sugar maple. *Plant Disease Reptr.* **53**, 753-755.

19

FUNGI THAT CAUSE VASCULAR
DISCOLORATION AND WILTING

Diseases that are expressed in wilting symptoms are among the most dramatic and important diseases. Many of the most significant wilt diseases are found in the larger woody perennials.

Several generalizations can be made concerning wilt diseases and the fungi which cause them. Since the casual microbes generally proliferate in the vascular elements, discoloration of these elements and loss of turgor due to impeded water transport are the two most characteristic symptoms. Infection frequently results in a relatively rapid killing of host trees or in the necrosis of large portions of these trees. Fungi which cause diseases of the wilt type are typically either Ascomycetes or Deuteromycetes. These fungi are usually distributed from tree to tree by one of three mechanisms; direct infection of roots from the soil, root grafting between infected and uninfected hosts, and insect vector transmission. Even though many wilt-inducing fungi are confined to single-cell types, for example, vessels or tracheids, and can generally only very poorly move through cell walls, most are capable of becoming systemically distributed through the tree in the vascular system.

Wilt diseases are of primary importance on angiosperms. Until recently, they were considered essentially nonexistent on gymnosperms. In a recent study of a root disease of several western conifers caused by *Verticicladiella wagenerii* (Deuteromycete), Smith (1967) suggested that this pathogen and the disease it causes have numerous similarities to pathogens and vascular diseases of angiosperms. During disease development, for example, the fungus appears to be restricted to the xylem. In addition, the microbe grows only in nonliving mature tracheids and migrates through bordered pits. *Ver-*

ticicladiella wagenerii causes a discoloration of the xylem as it becomes systemic in its host. Tylose formation is also observed in infected xylem.

I. EXAMPLES OF IMPORTANT ANGIOSPERM WILT DISEASES

A. Maple Wilt

Infection of Norway, sugar, red, silver, Japanese, bigleaf, and sycamore maples and boxelder by *Verticillium albo-atrum* (Deuteromycete) causes this important disease.

The most common symptom is necrosis of one or more limbs with subsequent dieback. In certain instances, infected trees will wilt very rapidly, but, more typically, disease progression is quite slow. Diseased individuals commonly develop a greenish discoloration in the outer rings of the infected sapwood. The discoloration may be in petioles, twigs, and the main trunk. It is not uncommon for trees with trunk diameters of 1-2 inches to be killed within 1 year of infection. Other individuals may live many years following infection, but typically, they gradually deteriorate.

Verticillium albo-atrum is a root-inhabiting soil fungus and it is presumed that the majority of host entries are made below the ground. Some aboveground infection does occur, probably from airborne spores reaching wounds or direct introduction, for example, via contaminated pruning tools. Once inside the host, the fungus develops in the vascular system. It is not clear where sporulation occurs.

The significance of the disease has been occasionally great, especially in nurseries and ornamental trees.

B. Oak Wilt

This disease is one of the most important afflictions of members of the *Quercus* genus. The malady has been observed in 50 species and varieties of *Quercus,* 3 of *Castanea,* 1 of *Castanopsis* and 1 of *Lithocarpus.* In the United States, no native oak species can safely be considered immune. Trees of any age, size or vigor appear susceptible to infection by *Ceratocystis fagacearum* (Ascomycete), the causal agent (Fowler, 1958; True et al., 1960).

The major damage resulting from this disease has been in forest stands in Wisconsin, Minnesota, and Iowa. In a study conducted in southeastern Minnesota and central Wisconsin, Anderson and Anderson (1963) observed that the average rate of increase in the radii of individual infection centers was 3.2 feet per year and that the annual rate of new infection centers established was 1.7 for each 100 acres sampled. In 1965, oak wilt disease had been detected in twenty states (Rexrode and Lincoln, 1965).

Symptoms of oak wilt disease vary considerably, depending on whether the host tree is a member of the red oak (Erythrobalanus) or white oak

(Leucobalanus) group. The initial symptoms in the red oak group include wilting and bronzing of the foliage in the upper crown. These symptoms first appear at the ends of branches and rapidly spread through the crown, downward from the top, and inward along the lateral branches. The entire crown may exhibit symptoms in a few weeks following onset of symptom expression. Large trees may be killed within 1 or 2 months following infection. In contrast, infected members of the white oak group develop wilt symptoms much more slowly. Typically, only a single branch or two will die each year. Disease progression is continual, however, and infected trees may be killed in 3–7 years. Vascular discoloration may be associated with infection by *C. fagacearum* in members of the white oak group.

Ceratocystis fagacearum develops in the vascular system of host oaks. Its movement in this system is accomplished by mycelial growth and asexual spore production. Local spread of the fungus is accomplished when the roots of an infected tree graft with the roots of an uninfected individual. The fungus is capable of persisting for approximately 4 years in the roots of dead host trees (Skelly and Merrill, 1968).

Since *C. fagacearum* is capable of more rapid spread than could be accounted for via root grafting, alternative distribution mechanisms must exist. Therefore, the role of insects as vectors of this pathogen has been extensively investigated. In most trees following death, the fungus forms "mycelial mats" just below the bark surface. These mats exert pressure against the bark and usually crack or split it. Volatile materials released from the fungus mats attract numerous insects. Among the most commonly attracted insects are sap-feeding beetles of the family Nitidulidae. Large numbers of *C. fagacearum* spores adhere to the bodies of these beetles and it has been suggested that these insects may transmit the fungus to healthy trees during their feeding efforts. Wood and Skelly (1968) found that, under controlled conditions, nitidulid beetles transferred *C. fagacearum* from wounds on infected trees to wounds on healthy trees in seven of 162 attempts. *Ceratocystis fagacearum* is a bipolar species and requires the fusion of A and B mating type nuclei for ascospore production. Insects may also function to transfer these nuclei from mycelia of opposite mating types. The significance of insects under natural conditions, however, is still unresolved (Rexrode, 1968).

C. Dutch Elm Disease

This disease is caused by *Ceratocystis ulmi* (Ascomycete) in all native American and European elms. Dutch elm disease occurs from the east coast to the Rocky Mountains and from Tennessee to Ontario and Quebec. Even though an important forest malady, Dutch elm disease has had its greatest impact on shade and ornamental elms (Fig. 42).

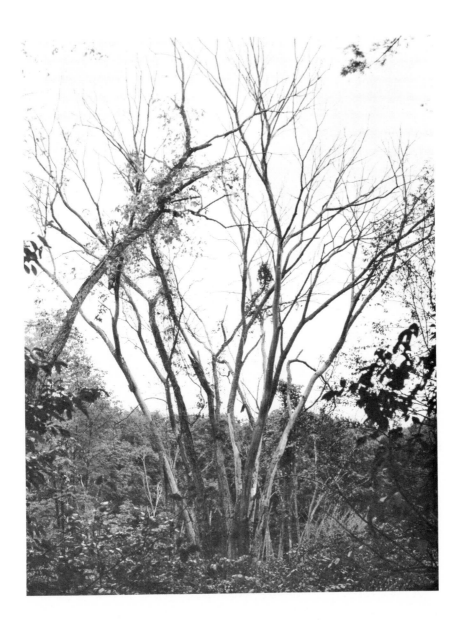

Fig. 42.   American elms recently killed as a result of infection by *Ceratocystis ulmi*. Trees this size may die within 1 or 2 months of the appearance of initial foliar symptoms.

The causal pathogen, like those which cause white pine blister rust and chestnut blight, is not a native of North America, nor for that matter, Holland. *Ceratocystis ulmi* originated, as did *Cronartium ribicola* and *Endothia parasitica*, in Asia. The fungus spread to Europe, from where it was introduced into the United States on elm burls for veneer manufacture in the early 1930's.

Symptoms of Dutch elm disease include wilting, curling, and yellowing of leaves on one or more branches. In some instances, only a few branches are involved and in others the entire tree may die within a few weeks. Internal brown spots or streaks may develop in the sapwood of infected branches.

In some rare instances, diseased trees may recover in the absence of repeated annual reinfection. This phenomenon may be due to the inability of the fungus to grow outward from one annual ring to the next.

Ceratocystis ulmi gains ingress into a host tree when it is brought into contact with xylem tissue exposed by injury. Once inside the functional vessels, asexual spores (conidia), which reproduce by yeast-like budding, are passively distributed by water movement. The fungus is also capable of active penetration of vessel walls and, consequently, of movement between adjacent vessels. Once an infected branch or tree is dead, *Ceratocystis ulmi* is capable of leaving the vessels and colonizing other cells of the xylem. Eventually sexual and asexual fructifications are produced in damp, sheltered locations, such as bark cracks and galleries, or larval tunnels of elm bark beetles. Sexual ascospores from perithecia, and asexual conidia from coremia (clusters of upright hyphae), are borne in mucilaginous drops. These spores adhere to bark beetles. Inter-tree spore transmission is accomplished by the European small elm bark beetle (*Scolytus multistriatus*, principal vector in United States) and the native elm bark beetle (*Hylurgopinus rufipes*). These beetles also cause the injuries resulting in xylem exposure which permit initial fungal invasion. Inter-tree transmission of the fungus can also be achieved via root grafts.

II. MECHANISM OF VASCULAR DISEASE

The mechanisms through which fungi, and bacteria, cause diseases expressed in wilt symptoms has received considerable research attention (Beckman, 1964; Sadasivan, 1961). In general, two conclusions have evolved from these efforts: (1) Wilting is induced by abnormal host–water relations and (2) this abnormal physiology is initiated by the release of toxins by the causal pathogen. It still remains unclear as to what microbial metabolites are involved and exactly how and where these materials act.

Histological changes typically associated with wilt diseases in the vascular system are: formation of gums and gels, tyloses, and discoloration.

In the instance of gum and gel formation in plants infected by wilt-in-ducing bacteria, much of this viscous material is assumed to arise from the bacterial cells themselves. In the case of fungal pathogens, however, gum and gel materials are presumed to be of host origin. Pectic enzymes may be involved in the formation of these blocking materials. These enzymes may release small residues from the large molecules of the compound middle lamellae. These residues may be moved in the transpiration stream until they accumulate on vessel end walls in sufficient numbers to impede water transport. Struckmeyer *et al.* (1954) observed extensive gum plugging of northern pin oak vessels infected with *C. fagacearum* prior to wilting.

The association of tyloses with wilt diseases is well documented. Nair *et al.* (1967) have observed that 3–5 days before foliage wilting in red oaks infected with *C. fagacearum* tyloses form in the xylem vessels. These structures, which are balloon-like enlargements of the pit membranes between xylem parenchyma cells and vessels or tracheids, can effectively restrict water transport. Tyloses may be induced by numerous biotic and abiotic agents. During infection by wilt inducing microbes, the pathogens may stimulate the host to produce growth regulators which cause tylose formation.

The full significance of the vascular discoloration associated with wilt diseases is not realized. Phenolic materials of host plants are thought to be released from complex compounds by enzymes from invading pathogens. These free phenolics may be oxidized by polyphenoloxidase enzymes of the host. Ultimately, these oxidized compounds may polymerize to form pigments.

Presumably, abnormal water balance resulting in wilting could be caused either by insufficient water supply or by excessive water loss. Extensive evidence is not available to support the latter contention, and the wilting caused by infective agents is thought to involve insufficient water resulting from blockage of the transpiration stream.

A good recent review of the mechanisms of abnormal water transport resulting from vascular diseases has been provided by Talboys (1968).

REFERENCES

Anderson, G. W., and Anderson, R. L. (1963). The rate of spread of oak wilt in the Lake States. *J. Forestry* **61**, 823–825.

Beckman, C. H. (1964). Host responses to vascular infection. *Ann. Rev. Phytopathol.* **2**, 231–252.

Fowler, M. E. (1958). Oak wilt. *Forest Pest Leaflet, U.S. Forest Serv.* **29**, 1–7.

Nair, V. M. G., Kuntz, J. E., and Sachs, I. B. (1967). Tyloses induced by *Ceratocystis fagacearum* in oak wilt development. *Phytopathology* **57**, 823 (abstr.).

Rexrode, C. O. (1968). Tree-wounding insects as vectors of the oak wilt fungus. *Forest Sci.* **14**, 181–189.

Rexrode, C. O., and Lincoln, A. C. (1965). Distribution of oak wilt. *Plant Disease Reptr.* **49**, 1007–1010.

Sadasivan, T. S. (1961). Physiology of wilt disease. *Ann. Rev. Plant Physiol.* **12**, 449–468.

Skelly, J. M., and Merrill, W. (1968). Susceptibility of red oaks to infection by *Ceratocystis fagacearum* during the dormant season in Pennsylvania. *Phytopathology* **58**, 1425–1426.

Smith, R. S., Jr. (1967). *Verticicladiella* root disease of pines. *Phytopathology* **57**, 935–938.

Struckmeyer, B. E., Beckman, C. H., Kuntz, J. E., and Riker, A. J. (1954). Plugging of vessels by tyloses and gums in wilting oaks. *Phytopathology* **44**, 148–153.

Talboys, P. W. (1968). Water deficits in vascular disease. *In* "Water Deficits and Plant Growth" (T. T. Kozlowski, ed.), Vol. 2, pp. 255–311. Academic Press, New York.

True, R. P., Barnett, H. L., Dorsey, C. K., and Leach, J. G. (1960). Oak wilt in West Virginia. *West Va. Univ., Agr. Expt. Sta., Bull.* **448T**, 1–119.

Wood, F. A., and Skelly, J. M. (1968). Nitidulid transmission of *Ceratocystis fagacearum* from wounds on infected red oaks. *Phytopathology* **58**, 1247–1249.

GENERAL REFERENCES

Amos, R. E., and True, R. P. (1967). Longevity of *Ceratocystis fagacearum* in roots of deep-girdled oak-wilt trees in West Virginia. *Phytopathology* **57**, 1012–1015.

Banfield, W. M. (1968). Dutch elm disease recurrence and recovery in American elm. *Phytopathol. Z.* **62**, 21–60.

Benedict, W. G. (1969). Anatomy of young branches of American elms naturally infected with *Ceratocystis ulmi. Phytopathology* **59**, 1200–1202.

Boyce, J. S. (1961). "Forest Pathology." McGraw-Hill, New York.

Brener, W. D., and Beckman, C. H. (1968). A mechanism of enhanced resistance to *Ceratocystis ulmi* in American elms treated with sodium trichlorophenylacetate. *Phytopathology* **58**, 555–561.

Cobb, F. W., Jr., and Platt, W. D. (1967). Pathogenicity of *Verticicladiella wagenerii* to Douglas Fir. *Phytopathology* **59**, 998–999.

Dimond, A. E. (1967). Physiology of wilt disease. *In* "The Dynamic Role of Molecular Constituents in Plant-Parasite Interaction" (C. J. Mirocha and I. Uritana, eds.), pp. 100–120. Bruce Publ. Co., St. Paul, Minnesota.

Filer, T. H., Jr., McCracker, F. I., and Toole, E. R. (1968). *Cephalosporium wilt of elm in lower Mississippi Valley. Plant Disease Reptr.* **52**, 170-171.

French, D. W., Kelman, A., and Cowling, E. B. (1967). "An Introduction to Forest Pathology." D. W. French, University of Minnesota, St. Paul, Minn.

Holmes, F. W. (1967). Resistance of certain elm clones to *Ceratocystis ulmi* and *Verticillium albo-atrum. Phytopathology* **57**, 1247-1249.

Landis, W. R., and Hart, J. H. (1968). Respiratory changes in *Ceratocystis ulmi*-infected *Ulmus americana. Phytopathology* **58**, 1057 (abstr.).

May, C. (1961). Diseases of shade and ornamental maples. *U.S. Dept. Agr., Agr. Handbook* **211**, 1-22.

Neely, D. (1968). Twig inoculations on American elm with *Ceratocystis ulmi. Phytopathology* **58**, 1566-1570.

Rexrode, C. O. (1967). Preliminary study on the time and frequency of oak bark beetle attacks on oak wilt trees. *Plant Disease Reptr.* **51**, 755-756.

Roberts, B. R. (1966). Transpiration of elm seedlings as influenced by inoculation with *Ceratocystis ulmi. Forest Sci.* **12**, 44-47.

Singh, D., and Smalley, E. B. (1969). Changes in amino acid and sugar constituents of the xylem sap of American elm following inoculation with *Ceratocystis ulmi. Phytopathology* **59**, 891-896.

Smith, R. S., Jr. (1969). The inability of *Verticicladiella wagnenerii* to break down cellulose. *Phytopathology* **59**, 1050 (abstr.).

Wysang, D. S., and Willis, W. A. (1968). Recorded distribution of Dutch elm disease west of the Mississippi River as of 1967. *Plant Disease Reptr.* **52**, 652-653.

20

FUNGI THAT CAUSE ROOT DISCOLORATION, NECROSIS, ROTTING, AND OTHER ROOT SYMPTOMS

The above-ground portion of the environment of a tree is actually approximately one-half the environment in which the tree persists. The roots, which exist in the below-ground environment, comprise a substantial portion of the mass of the tree. For many trees the root length is measured in miles, and the root area may exceed that of the above-ground portion. Numerous microorganisms cause disease of plant root systems. The most important agents of tree root disease are fungi.

I. ROOT ENVIRONMENT

The above- and below-ground environments differ greatly in several characteristics:

	Physical characteristics	Chemical characteristics	Macrobial population	Microbial population
Above ground	More variable	Less complex	Less variable	Less variable
Below ground	Less variable	More complex	More variable	More variable

The above-ground environment exhibits greater variation in several physical parameters, for example, temperature extremes, insolation, and air movements, than the below-ground area. However, the below-ground environment is characterized by a more complex and diverse chemical constitution and flora and fauna. This latter complexity and the inaccessibility of roots has restricted research efforts directed toward a greater appreciation of root disease phenomena.

One of the most interesting aspects of the root environment is the rhizosphere. This term was introduced by L. Hiltner in 1904 to describe the zone of soil in which the microflora was influenced by plant roots. This zone of soil is the most important soil region with respect to microorganisms which are capable of inducing root disease. The rhizosphere which surrounds plant roots is discontinuous and has a tendency to be most pronounced in the zone of cell elongation and root hair induction. Perhaps the most outstanding characteristics of the rhizosphere region are the greater number of microorganisms and greater microbial activity in rhizosphere soil compared to nonrhizosphere soil (soil devoid of roots). These phenomena constitute the "rhizosphere effect."

A. Character of the Rhizosphere Populations

In quantitative terms, rhizosphere populations are commonly expressed in R/S ratios:

$$R/S = \frac{\text{Number of organisms in rhizosphere soil per unit weight}}{\text{Number of organisms in nonrhizosphere soil per unit weight}}$$

R/S ratios are generally greatest for bacterial species with values from 10 to 20 relatively common. Lower, yet significant, R/S values have been reported for actinomycetes and fungi. Certain rhizospheres may also support higher nematode populations than nonrhizosphere soil. Absolute numbers of soil microorganisms must, however, be interpreted with caution, as one nematode or fungus hypha may be pathologically and metabolically as significant as several thousand bacterial cells.

With respect to the qualitative nature of rhizosphere populations, plants do not appear to support specific populations with the exception of those possessing specific rhizobial and mycorrhizal associations. Certain generalizations, nevertheless, may be made with respect to rhizosphere microbes. Rhizosphere bacteria are typically gram negative, nonsporulating, and rod shaped. These bacteria are frequently characterized by greater physiological activity and greater dependence on exogenous amino acid supplies than nonrhizosphere bacteria. Representative genera include *Pseudomonas, Arthrobacter, Norcardia,* and *Agrobacterium.* More research is required on the actinomycetes of soil adjacent to roots but several investigators have reported a greater number of actinomycetes with antibacterial and antifungal properties in the rhizosphere compared with nonrhizosphere areas. In the instance of fungi of the rhizosphere most studies have been taxonomic in character. Typical components of rhizosphere mycofloras include members of the following genera: *Fusarium, Cylindrocarpon, Mucor, Rhizopus, Penicillium,* and *Rhizoctonia.*

B. Cause of the Rhizosphere Effect

The increased numbers of microbes surrounding plant roots can probably be attributed to one or more of the following factors: (1) sloughed-off root material and decomposition of moribund root hairs, epidermal cells, and cortex; differences in (2) oxygen or carbon dioxide concentration, (3) pH, (4) moisture availability, (5) mineral nutrients, and (6) exudation of organic materials. One of the most interesting and perhaps the most important factor is the last. This exudation occurs through intact, unsuberized roots by a mechanism as yet not fully appreciated. The character of the root exudate is generally quite diverse and may include: carbohydrates, amino acids, organic acids, nucleotides, enzymes, flavonones, growth factors, and other miscellaneous materials. The nature of the root exudates from several forest tree seedlings has recently been described by Smith (1969a).

C. Significance of Root Exudates

The importance of root exudates to plant growth is probably profound. These materials may be significant to nutrient availability, effect beneficial rhizosphere microbes and root symbionts, play a role in the competition among higher plants, that is, phytosociology, and influence root pathogens.

The significance of the release of organic materials into the rhizosphere is extremely great for many microbes that infect plant roots. Root exudates have been shown to play an important chemotaxic role. Motile spores or zoospores present in certain members of the parasitic Phycomycetes class have been shown to be attracted by proteins, amino acids, and sugars, certain of which are contained in root exudates. Zentmyer (1961) showed that zoospores of *Phytophtora cinnamomi* were rapidly attracted to the region of elongation of avocado roots. Root exudates have the capacity to induce the germination of spores of pathogenic fungi.

Many of the most important root diseases are caused by root-inhabiting fungi that have poor competitive saprophytic ability and do not grow freely in the soil. When apart from the host's roots, they exist in some dormant form, for example, a resistant spore or sclerotium. The dormancy of these structures has been shown in several instances to be broken by root exudate materials. Smith and Peterson (1966) presented evidence that clover root-exudate carbohydrates were capable of inducing the germination of chlamydospores of *Fusarium roseum, F. solani,* and *F. oxysporum,* all important clover root pathogens. Recently, the germination of sclerotia of *Macrophomina phaseoli,* which is an important root pathogen of many forest tree species, was shown to be enhanced by sugar pine root exudate (Smith, 1969b).

Root exudates may also act to support vegetative growth of root-infecting fungi prior to their entrance into the root. Unless a parasitic fungus is located on the root surface, it must grow vegetatively through the rhizosphere to reach the root. This growth may be mediated to a considerable extent by the availability of utilizable substrates released in the root exudate. Ullah and Preece (1966) found that wheat root exudate caused the germ tubes of *Helminthosporium sativum* to branch profusely. Agnihortri and Vaartaja (1967) observed that certain components of red pine seedling root exudate stimulated the germ tube growth of *Pythium ultimum*.

Root exudates may further play a role in infection structure formation. Once in contact with a host root, many pathogens require the development of a specialized structure, for example, a fungus pad or appressorium, to provide the basis for actual physical penetration of the host root. Husain and McKeen (1963) found that amino acids in strawberry root exudate enhanced the formation of fungus pads in *Rhizoctonia fragariae*.

Root exudate compounds may also have direct or indirect inimical effects on root pathogens. Evidence has been presented indicating that certain root exudate materials contain components toxic to bacteria. Krasilnikov (1934) has reported that the exudates of wheat, corn, and flax suppressed the growth of *Azotobacter* and other bacteria. With respect to fungal pathogens, no conclusive evidence has been presented that indicates whether a toxic root exudate plays a direct role in contributing to disease resistance. Vrany et al. (1962), however, applied the antibiotic chloramphenicol as an aerial spray to wheat plants and detected this compound in the root exudate. Root exudate stimulation of antagonistic microbes may play an important role in nature by indirectly inhibiting root pathogens. Timonin (1966) found that the incidence of spore-forming bacteria antagonistic to *Fusarium culmorum* and *Rhizoctonia solani* was nearly six times greater in the rhizosphere of healthy lodgepole pine seedlings than in that of diseased seedlings. Physiochemical alterations, for example, changes in pH, moisture, and oxygen tension, occasioned in the rhizosphere by release of root exudates may also exert a deleterious effect on root-infecting microorganisms.

II. SPECIFIC ROOT DISEASES OF FOREST TREES

For discussion purposes, tree root diseases will be divided into seedling and nonseedling categories.

A. Seedling Root Disease

Because germinating seeds and young seedlings are succulent and in other ways generally susceptible to microbial attack, many are rapidly rotted by various Phycomycetes and Deuteromycetes fungi. This rotting which may involve the seed itself, radicle, hypocotyl, or older seedling root is referred to as dampingoff. Dampingoff diseases, which represent the most important diseases of the nursery, effect the seedlings of almost all tree species. Coniferous species, whose roots and stems have a tendency to remain unlignified and unsuberized for longer periods, are particularly susceptible.

Generally, four types of dampingoff may be distinguished; preemergence, normal, late, and top (French et al., 1967). In preemergence dampingoff, the seedling is infected prior to eruption above the soil line. Since the only obvious indication of preemergence dampingoff is failure of the seedling to appear, this phenomenon is apt to be confused with poor seed viability or animal ingestion. Tree species most susceptible to preemergence dampingoff probably have seeds which exude considerable amounts of carbohydrates and amino acids into the soil during germination. Normal dampingoff refers to the infection of the roots or stems of young seedlings. Stem infection, which is characteristically located at the ground line, generally causes diseased seedlings to topple over. Root infection, on the other hand, may be expressed in a gradual browning of the standing seedling. If infection of new succulent portions of roots occurs after lignification of stems and roots is initiated, late dampingoff occurs. This type of disease may be less common than normal dampingoff but is extremely important for certain species, such as sugar pine. This tree is importantly infected by Macrophomina phaseoli (Deuteromycete) during its first several months of growth. Top dampingoff, which is much less common than the other types mentioned, may occur when fungi infect cotyledons that are kept for abnormally extended periods inside the seed coat following emergence.

The fungi which cause dampingoff are generally soil inhabitors. Typical Phycomycetes include Pythium spp. and Phytophthora spp.; Deuteromycetes include Fusarium spp. and Rhizoctonia solani. These fungi directly penetrate the cell walls of root and stem epidermis and grow intracellularly. While cell wall material may be decomposed to a limited extent, these fungi persist primarily by metabolizing cell contents.

B. Nonseedling Root Disease

The majority of the most damaging root diseases of mature trees are caused by root-inhabiting Basidiomycetes. A representative and extremely important member of this group of pathogens is Fomes annosus.

Root diseases caused by F. annosus are currently the most important diseases on several European conifers. In North America the fungus also causes considerable damage. Hosts include several species in the following genera; Abies, Acer, Fraxinus, Juniperus, Larix, Liquidambar, Picea, Pinus, Pseudotsuga, Quercus, Rhus, Tsuga, and Ulmus. Infection of Juniperus and Pinus is most significant as F. annosus is capable of causing relatively rapid root decay in these groups. Geographically the fungus is widely distributed throughout the temperate regions.

The life cycle of *F. annosus* is comparatively simple. It is generally accepted that spores produced by *F. annosus* are the primary inoculum for initial infection. Of the two spore types produced, basidiospores and conidia, the former are thought to be of much greater significance. Conidial production is infrequently observed in nature. Basidiospores, on the other hand, are frequently abundantly produced in woody, perennial fruiting bodies, formed on the trunks of infected trees usually at the ground line (Fig. 43). These spores are very light and apparently quite effectively transported from their position of origin by air movements. Basidiospores are not long-lived but in the presence of favorable humidity they may remain viable for several weeks. Several investigations have attempted to correlate basidiospore release with season of the year, time of day, and various other environmental parameters. Much of the evidence which has been presented is somewhat conflicting or inconclusive, but it appears that basidiospores are produced in all seasons and released in largest numbers, in many areas, primarily in the spring and fall.

Since *F. annosus* is not a vigorous microbial competitor, the basidiospores are most efficient in initiating infection when they directly intercept interior root tissue or the heartwood of the lower bole of susceptible hosts. In coniferous plantations, where this pathogen is particularly damaging, stump surfaces of recently cut individuals are excellent infection courts. Because these stump surfaces are also colonized by other microbes, several of which are more vigorous competitors than *F. annosus,* the length of susceptibility of these areas is quite short. In the case of most species, susceptibility estimates have been less than 1 month. Cobb and Schmidt (1964) have suggested that the susceptibility of white pine stump surfaces may be only 1-3 days after cutting. While other wounds, for example, those resulting from pruning, animal feeding, or logging, may be important infection courts, their significance is generally thought to be less important than that of stump surfaces.

Following basidiospore germination on the stump, the mycelium of the fungus grows through the heartwood into the root system at a variable rate which may approximate 20-40 centimeters per week. *Fomes annosus* is classified as a white rot fungus; movement through the stump and in the roots involves decay of both lignin and cellulose. The specific tissues decayed, however, depend on the particular host infected. Before the death of infected trees, for example, *F. annosus* primarily decays the sapwood of ponderosa pine and the heartwood of eastern white pine (Cobb and Wilcox, 1967). The mechanism of decay by *F. annosus* is thought to be via the production of typical extracellular enzymes of the white rot group. Studies of *F. annosus in vitro* by Bassett *et al.* (1967), however, have revealed the presence of fomannosin. This compound is a sesquiterpene which when applied artificially to host roots will produce symptoms similar to those in natural

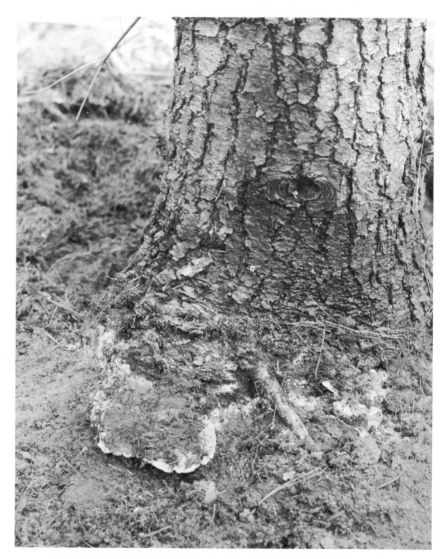

Fig. 43.   Base of red pine infected with *Fomes annosus*. Duff has been removed to expose the fruiting body of the fungus. Conks are extremely variable in morphology and range from small pustules to the bracket-like structures shown here. (Photograph courtesy U.S. Forest Service.)

infections. Demonstration of this material in diseased tissue would support the suggestion that it is a fungal toxin.

Once *F. annosus* is established in the root system of a stump or intact tree, spread to surrounding trees is accomplished by growth through root grafts or points of contact between adjacent roots. Relatively long-term survival of the fungus is possible during the decomposition of woody material in the soil (Kuhlman, 1968). As the fungus spreads in a stand of trees, semicircular infection centers are developed. Annual rates of spread from established infection centers in northeastern red pine stands may approximate 1-3 meters per year.

C. Role of Mycorrhizae in Root Diseases

Mycorrhizae are specialized roots which are formed when certain fungi infect the roots of higher plants (Hacskaylo, 1967; Meyer, 1966). These infections result in a symbiotic relationship in which both members presumably benefit. If the fungus component of the mycorrhizal symbiosis is located primarily outside the root, the relationship is termed ectotrophic; if inside, endotrophic. Fungi involved in ectotrophic mycorrhizal formation are mostly Basidiomycetes belonging to such genera as: *Amanita, Boletus, Hebeloma, Cortinarius, Lactarius,* and *Russula.*

While it is generally recognized that mycorrhizae facilitate tree development and may be necessary for persistence on certain sites, the specific benefits for the tree are not clear. The contribution of mycorrhizal roots is frequently ascribed to improved nutrition of these roots relative to nonmycorrhizal roots.

The suggestion has recently been made that mycorrhizal roots may be more resistant to infection by pathogenic microbes than nonmycorrhizal roots (Marx, 1966; Marx and Davey, 1967; Zak, 1964). Zak (1964) has proposed four ways in which ectrotrophic mycorrhizae may protect tree roots. Mycorrhizal fungi may; (1) reduce root exudation of compounds capable of stimulating pathogens, (2) serve as a physical barrier to penetration, (3) secrete antibiotics and (4) favor protective rhizosphere populations. *Cenococcum graniforme,* a common mycorrhizal fungus of eastern white pine, red pine, and Norway spruce, is known to produce an antibiotic material *in vitro* (Grand, 1966). Katznelson *et al.* (1962) found higher bacterial and actinomycete numbers in the rhizospheres of mycorrhizal than in nonmycorrhizal roots of yellow birch seedlings.

REFERENCES

Agnihortri, V. P., and Vaartaja, O. (1967). Root exudates from red pine seedlings and their effects on *Pythium ultimum. Can. J. Botany* **45**, 1031-1040.

Bassett, C., Sherwood, R. T., Kepler, J. A., and Hamilton, P. B. (1967). Production and biological activity of fomannosin, a toxic sesquiterpene metabolite of *Fomes annosus. Phytopathology* **57**, 1046-1052.

Cobb, F. W., Jr., and Schmidt, R. A. (1964). Duration of susceptibility of eastern white pine stumps to *Fomes annosus. Phytopathology* **54**, 1216-1218.

Cobb, F. W., Jr., and Wilcox, W. W. (1967). Comparison of susceptibility of *Abies concolor* and *Pinus ponderosa* wood to decay by *Fomes annosus*. *Phytopathology* **57**, 1312–1314.

French, D. W., Kelman, A., and Cowling, E. B. (1967). "An Introduction to Forest Pathology." D. W. French, University of Minnesota, St. Paul, Minn.

Grand, L. F. (1966). An antibiotic associated with the mycorrhizal fungus *Cenococcum graniforme*. *Phytopathology* **56**, 147 (abstr.).

Hacskaylo, E. (1967). Mycorrhizae: Indispensable invasions by fungi. *Agr. Sci. Rev.* **5**, 13–20.

Husain, S. S., and McKeen, W. E. (1963). Interactions between strawberry roots and *Rhizoctonia fragariae*. *Phytopathology* **53**, 541–545.

Katznelson, H., Rouatt, J. W., and Peterson, E. A. (1962). The rhizosphere effect of mycorrhizal and non-mycorrhizal roots of yellow birch seedlings. *Can. J. Botany* **40**, 377–382.

Krasilnikov, N. A. (1934). The influence of root secretion on the development of *Azotobacter* and of other soil microbes. *Mikrobiologiya* **3**, 343–359.

Kuhlman, E. G. (1968). Survival of *Fomes annosus* in the presence of competing fungi in loblolly pine roots. *Phytopathology* **58**, 729 (abstr.).

Marx, D. H. (1966). The role of ectotrophic mycorrhizal fungi in the resistance of pine roots to infection by *Phytophthora cinnamomi* Rands. Ph.D. Dissertation, North Carolina State University.

Marx, D. H., and Davey, C. B. (1967). Ectrotrophic mycorrhizae as deterrents to pathogenic root infections. *Nature* **213**, 1139.

Meyer, F. H. (1966). Mycorrhiza and other plant symbioses. *In* "Symbiosis" (S. M. Henry, ed.), pp. 171–257, Academic Press, New York.

Smith, W. H. (1969a). Release of organic materials from the roots of tree seedlings. *Forest Sci.* **15**, 138–143.

Smith, W. H. (1969b). Germination of *Macrophomina phaseoli* sclerotia as effected by *Pinus lambertiana* root exudate. *Can. J. Microbiol.* **15**, 1387–1391.

Smith, W. H., and Peterson, J. L. (1966). The influence of the carbohydrate fraction of the root exudate of red clover, *Trifolium pratense* L., on *Fusarium* spp. isolated from the clover root and rhizosphere. *Plant Soil* **25**, 413–424.

Timonin, M. I. (1966). Rhizosphere effect of healthy and diseased lodgepole pine seedlings. *Can. J. Microbiol.* **12**, 531–537.

Ullah, A. K. M. O., and Preece, T. F. (1966). Wheat root exudate and early stages of infection by *Helminthosporium sativum* Panm., King and Bakke. *Nature* **210**, 1369–1370.

Vrany, J., Vancurra, V., and Macura, J. (1962). The effects of foliar application of some readily metabolized substances, growth regulators and antibiotics on rhizosphere microflora. *Folia Microbiol. (Prague)* **7**, 61-70.

Zak, B. (1964). Role of mycorrhizae in root disease. *Ann. Rev. Phytopathol.* **2**, 377-392.

Zentmyer, G. A. (1961). Chemotaxis of zoospores for root exudates. *Science* **133**, 1595-1596.

GENERAL REFERENCES

Cobb, F. W., Jr., and Barber, H. W., Jr. (1968). Susceptibility of freshly cut stumps of redwood, Douglas fir, and ponderosa pine to *Fomes annosus*. *Phytopathology* **58**, 1551-1557.

Driver, C. H., and Ginns, J. H., Jr. (1968). Practical control of *Fomes annosus* in intensive forest management. *Contrib., Inst. Forest Prod., Wash.* **5**, 1-8.

Driver, C. H., and Ginns, J. H., Jr. (1969). Ecology of slash pine stumps: Fungal colonization and infection by *Fomes annosus*. *Forest Sci.* **15**, 2-10.

Hendrix, F. F., Jr., and Campbell, W. A. (1968). Pythiaceous fungi isolated from southern forest nursery soils and their pathogenicity to pine seedlings. *Forest Sci.* **14**, 292-297.

Hodges, C. S. (1962). Diseases of southeastern forest nurseries and their control. *Sta. Paper, Southeast Forest Expt. Sta.* **142**, 1-16.

Hodges, C. S. (1969). Modes of infection and spread of *Fomes annosus*. *Ann. Rev. Phytopathol.* **7**, 247-266.

Koenigs, J. W. (1969). Root rot and chlorosis of released and thinned western redcedar. *J. Forestry* **67**, 312-315.

Kuhlman, E. G. (1969). Survival of *Fomes annosus* spores in soil. *Phytopathology* **59**, 198-201.

Kuhlman, E. G. (1969). Number of conida necessary for stump root infection by *Fomes annosus*. *Phytopathology* **59**, 1168-1169.

Leaphart, C. D. (1963). Armillaria root rot. *Forest Pest Leaflet, U.S. Forest Serv.* **78**, 1-8.

Mook, P. V., and Eno, H. G. (1961). *Fomes annosus*. What it is and how to recognize it. *Sta. Paper, Northeast Forest Expt. Sta.* **146**, 1-33.

Nelson, E. E. (1968). Survival of *Poria weirii* in conifer, alder, and mixed conifer-alder stands. *Res. Note, Pacific Northwest Forest Range Expt. Sta.* **PNW-83**, 1-5.

Nelson, E. E. (1969). Occurrence of fungi antagonistic to *Poria weirii* in a Douglas-fir forest soil in Western Oregon. *Forest Sci.* **15**, 49-54.

Punter, D., and Cafley, J. D. (1968). Two new hardwood hosts of *Fomes annosus*. *Plant Disease Reptr.* **52**, 692.

Smith, R. S., Jr. (1967). Verticicladiella root disease of pine. *Phytopathology* **57**, 935–938.

van Vloten, H. (1962). Present and potential significance of root rots in intensive forest management. *Proc. 5th World Forestry Congr.,* Vol. 2, pp. 887–890, Aug. 29–Sept. 10, 1960, Seattle, Washington.

Witcher, W., Lane, C. L., and Baxter, L. W., Jr. (1968). Delayed symptoms expression of *Fomes annosus* root rot of pine. *Phytopathology* **58**, 732 (abstr.).

21

DELETERIOUS HIGHER PLANTS

Microorganisms are not the only biotic plant disease agents. Numerous and frequently important diseases, especially of trees, are caused by certain macroscopic spermatophytes. These higher plant disease agents may act parasitically or nonparasitically to induce abnormal physiology. The former group, which obtains nutrients from their hosts, include among others mistletoes and dodder. The latter group, which does not act parasitically but causes mechanical damage, includes several vine species.

I. PARASITIC ANGIOSPERMS

A. True Mistletoes

The mistletoes are dicotyledonous seed plants of the family Loranthaceae. All typical higher plant parts are present, including leaves, flowers, fruits, seeds, and an absorbing system, although somewhat modified and/or reduced in size. These perennial evergreens are parasitic on numerous plants. Three genera, *Loranthus, Phoradendron*, and *Viscum*, are important parasites of stems and branches of several shrub and tree species.

1. Anatomy. The leaves of true mistletoes, which characteristically have a low chlorophyll content, vary in size from scalelike structures to organs several centimeters in width. Flowers may be monoecious or dioecious and possess or lack a corolla. Nectar seeking birds may play a greater role in pollen dispersal than insects.

Fruits enclosing true mistletoe seeds are characterized by a fleshy coat surrounding a mucilaginous outer seed layer. This outer layer, termed viscin, functions to attach the fruits to host organs by virtue of its adhesive property and facilitates seed germination by providing favorable moisture conditions.

The seed itself is technically a naked embryo embedded in endosperm tissue. In certain species in the genus *Viscum*, seeds are explosively discharged a distance of 1 or 2 feet. Most mistletoes, however, lack this mechanism and have their seed distributed primarily by animal vectors.

The "root system" of mistletoes is more appropriately termed the "haustorial system" and consists of cortical strands and sinkers (Fig. 44). The radicle of a germinating seed gives rise to the primary haustorium. The cortical strand, which contains xylem elements, represents lateral protrusion of this primary haustorium. Sinkers are wedge-shaped structures that develop from the primary haustorium or from the cortical strand. Generally, sinkers are located within the rays of host xylem tissue, where they appear to grow coincidentally with the host. Sinkers may displace host cells but they do not penetrate them. Since these structures do develop vascular elements in direct contact with those of the host, they presumably function to extract water and nutrient materials. In several instances, haustorial systems have been shown capable of persistence for extended periods in the absence of aerial parts.

2. *Life cycle.*   In the typical true mistletoe life cycle, birds eliminate the seed after digesting the outer pulp. If this seed happens to contact the foliage, branch, or trunk of a tree, the gelatinous viscin may cause it to be held secure. During exposure to alternate wettings and dryings, the viscin loses much of its hygroscopic quality and begins to function as a firm cement. Fol-

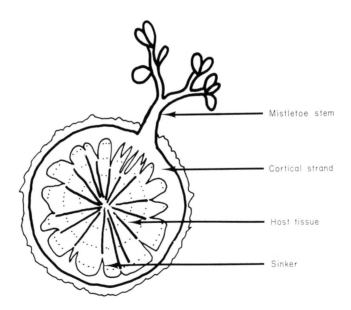

Fig. 44.   Diagrammatic cross section of a host branch parasitized by a mistletoe.

lowing this rather rigid attachment, the seed germinates, and the hypocotyl or radicle grows along the host surface. If a suitable location for penetration is encountered, typically an obstacle (for example, a needle if development is along a twig), a holdfast is formed. The holdfast is a domelike structure which becomes attached to the host along its rim. This attachment is accomplished by the release of a viscous substance which produces an air-tight seal. Projections, termed papillae, originate on the inner, upper surface of the holdfast and attach themselves to host bark. Growth of the holdfast causes the periderm to lift until a crack forms that is of sufficient size to permit the primary haustorium of the mistletoe to enter the host. Further penetration of the host may be accomplished by both mechanical and enzymatic means. The tip of the haustorium has been shown to produce enzymes capable of degrading pectic materials of host middle lamellae. The development of mistletoe leaves, stems, and fruits reflects the expansion of the haustorial system within the host.

3. *True mistletoes as disease agents.*   These parasites are disease agents of economic importance throughout the world. In Europe, important trees infected are apple, almond, and cherry. Serious infection in citrus and tea is caused in Africa. In southeast Asia, tea, mango, and teak, and in Malaysia, rubber may be severely damaged. Commercial timber, for example, eucalyptus, frequently sustains appreciable losses due to mistletoe infection in Australia. In South America, rubber, cacao, cashew, avocado, and coffee may be importantly damaged. In North America, however, the economic impact of true mistletoe infection is insignificant with the exception of very minor importance in the southwest. Actually, members of the genus *Phoradendron* collected from low-value hosts in the south and southwest have an economic value as Christmas decorations.

B. Dwarf Mistletoes

These plants are also members of the Loranthaceae, but all are classified in the genus *Arceuthobium*. The members of this genus are the most destructive of all the mistletoes. They are restricted to coniferous hosts and are most prevalent in the western portions of North America. *Arceuthobium* spp. are able to infect almost all conifers of commercial importance. The economic importance of dwarf mistletoe infection is greatest in the Pacific Northwest. Dwarf mistletoes have been considered the agents of the most important tree disease problem in California (Scharpf and Parmeter, 1967).

The stem and endophytic systems of dwarf mistletoes are anatomically very similar to those discussed for the true mistletoes. In dwarf mistletoes, however, leaves are reduced to scalelike structures.

1. *Life cycle.*   Generally, the life cycle patterns of dwarf mistletoes are comparable to those of true mistletoes. In the former group, three primary

mechanisms for seed dispersal are presumed important. The first, forcible ejection, occurs following imbition of water and abscission-layer formation. Dissemination by this method may be relatively slow but it is relatively effective in local intensification. If older infected trees remain in areas of reproduction, disease intensification due to ejected seeds may be considerable (Fig. 45). The second means of spread is by animal vectors. Unlike true mistletoes, there is little evidence that birds pass dwarf mistletoe seeds through their digestive systems. The adhesive character of the seed, however, is presumed to cause the seeds to become attached to birds and other animals and to be passively distributed. The third possible mechanism of transport is wind. In consideration of the size of the seeds, only winds of relatively high velocity are probably important.

Once the seeds are liberated, they have been found more likely to adhere to needles than to branches. The needles yield under the impact and reduce the tendency of the seed to bounce away. Generally, the seeds remain on the intercepting needle until rain washes them down the needle toward the sheath. Most infection apparently results when the seeds come in contact with the axils of the needles. Natural openings generally occur at these axils and presumably allow relatively unobstructed entrance of the radicle. The probability that any particular seed will actually initiate infection is not very high. Even after deposition on the needles of suitable hosts, seeds may be removed or destroyed by snow, rain, wind, insects, fungi, birds, or high temperature (Wicker, 1967).

2. *Expression of host symptoms.* The first obvious symptom of dwarf mistletoe infection is an increase in the thickness and succulence of the inner bark. As the infection progresses, the basal portions of invaded branches frequently become three to five times as large as uninfected branches in the same whorl. This symptom may not be obvious until approximately two years following initial infection. Another two years may be required for the production of aerial dwarf mistletoe parts and still another two years (six years after initial infection) for seed production. Cankers may also develop on infected branches. Ultimately, dwarf mistletoe infection results in the development of fasciculations (witches' brooms). These fasciculations, characterized by dense foliage, tend to be long-lived and may become quite heavy. Branches with these malformations are extremely susceptible to wind and snow breakage.

3. *Significance of dwarf mistletoe infection.* Most importantly, infection by *Arceuthobium* spp. results in reduced growth rate and, to a lesser extent,

Fig. 45. Intensification of dwarf mistletoe infection in an area of southwestern ponderosa pine during 90 years. [From Hawksworth and Hinds (1965). Reproduced by permission of American Museum of Natural History.]

SPREAD OF INFECTION IN PONDEROSA PINE

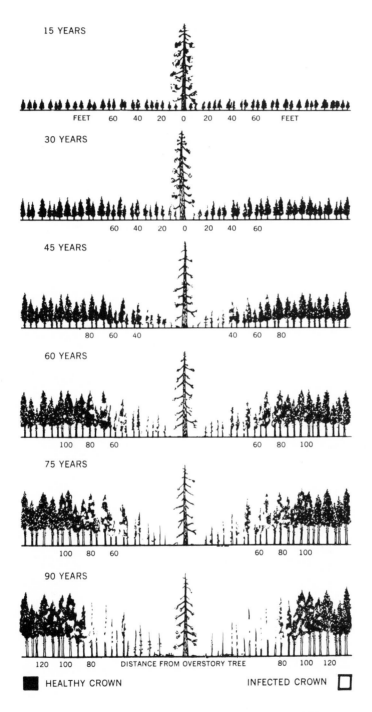

15 YEARS

FEET 60 40 20 0 20 40 60 FEET

30 YEARS

60 40 20 0 20 40 60

45 YEARS

80 60 40 40 60 80

60 YEARS

100 80 60 60 80 100

75 YEARS

100 80 60 60 80 100

90 YEARS

120 100 80 DISTANCE FROM OVERSTORY TREE 80 100 120

HEALTHY CROWN   INFECTED CROWN

increased chance of mortality. In Colorado, lodgepole pine infected by *A. americanum* showed a reduction of height and diameter growth which averaged approximately 0.7% per year (Hawksworth and Hinds, 1964). In a recent study, Childs and Edgren (1967) concluded that infection by dwarf mistletoe results in a greater depression of height growth than diameter growth in ponderosa pine. In some instances, production and germination of seed of infected trees may be impaired. Wood quality may be importantly effected in individuals with extensive cankering or fasciculation. In certain cases, outright mortality may be occasioned by the mistletoe itself. More commonly, however, dwarf mistletoe infection causes significant predisposition to damage by other biotic and abiotic stress factors.

4. Hyperparasities of dwarf mistletoes.   Mistletoes are, of course, subject to infection by various microorganisms. The question of the ecological significance of certain fungal parasites has recently been raised. *Colletotrichum gloeosporioides* (Deuteromycete) is an important disease agent of *A. americanum* in western Canada (Muir, 1967). Peterson (1966) has reported the simultaneous occurrence of *A. americanum* and *Cronartium comandrae* (rust fungus) on lodgepole pine. The evidence presented by the author in this case, however, did not permit the suggestion that the fungus was actually parasitizing the mistletoe.

C. Dodders

These plants are members of the genus *Cuscuta* and are related to the familiar *Ipomoea* spp. (morning glories). Of the 100 recognized species of *Cuscuta*, 32 are native to the United States and 18 others have been introduced (Gill, 1953).

Unlike the mistletoes, seed of the dodder plant germinates, and the plant initially develops, in contact with the ground. The young plant, which consists of a yellow, leafless stalk, "gropes" in the air. If contact is made with another plant, coils are formed by the dodder around the host stem. Ultimately, haustoria are formed by the dodder inside host tissues. Soon after haustorial formation is initiated, the basal portion of the parasite, that is, that attached to the ground, aborts, and the growth of the dodder is henceforth entirely on the host plant (Fig. 46).

The reports of dodder occurrence are scattered, and the significance of the plant as a direct agent of tree disease is probably slight. The greatest damage caused by dodder occurs in nurseries. Hocking (1966) recently described an important outbreak of *Cuscuta cassytoides* on hardwood seedlings in an African nursery. Dodders may have an indirect disease importance as vectors of virus diseases.

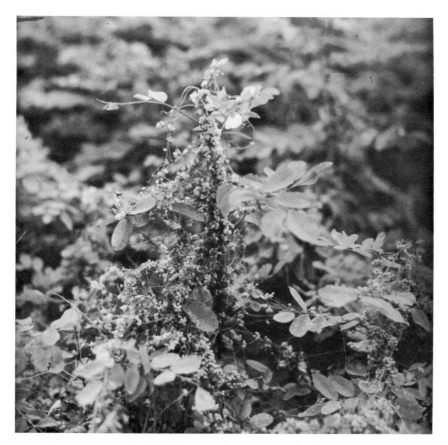

Fig. 46. Dodder growing on a black locust seedling. (Photograph courtesy U.S. Forest Service.)

D. Other Parasitic Higher Plants.

Numerous other flowering plants are parasitic on trees. Many of these parasitize roots, for example, *Castilleja* spp. (Indian paintbrush), *Orobanche* spp. (broomrapes), and *Lathraea* spp. (toothwort). The significance of these and other parasitic genera is considered to be slight.

II. NONPARASITIC ANGIOSPERMS

Numerous vines and climbers act to cause poor tree health by mechanically constricting stems, shading leaves, or otherwise interfering with normal development. These plants do not, however, obtain any nutrients directly from the trees on which they grow.

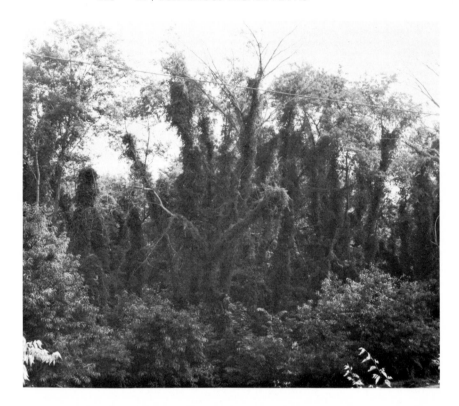

Fig. 47. Deteriorating stand of American elm with extensive growth of Virginia creeper. Shading caused by the vines may have played some role in the decline of these trees.

A. Plants Causing Stem or Branch Constriction

1. Bittersweet (Celastrus scandens). This climber is relatively abundant in the forests of the eastern United States. Since it is a relatively intolerant species, it is generally confined to situations with ample light, for example, young stands, understocked stands, areas of windfall, or near forest borders.

The injury resulting from bittersweet is caused by the vines twining tightly around the stems and branches of supporting trees. This constriction particularly impairs the downward translocation of organic materials (Lutz, 1943). The accumulation of food materials above the restriction frequently results in the appearance of sarcody (swelling) symptoms. Trees are not generally killed by bittersweet, since the constricting action is slow and new conductive tissues are formed which enable continued, albeit impaired, translocation. The upward movement of organic compounds supplied via root grafts may also play an important role in supplying severely constricted trees.

2. *Grape (Vitis spp.).* The tendrils of grape cause deformation of tree parts similar to those resulting from bittersweet. In general, however, since the tendrils are small, the constrictions have a tendency to be smaller than those caused by bittersweet. Breakage of stems and branches at points of constriction by wind, snow, and ice is not uncommon. The large leaves of grape vines frequently result in considerable shading of the leaves of the supporting tree.

B. Plants not Causing Stem or Branch Constriction

The damage caused by these plants is not due to constriction but rather to shading and deforming the crown of supporting trees. Vines causing this kind of injury are numerous and widely distributed. Important examples in the eastern United States include; *Parthenocissus quinquefolia* (Virginia creeper) (Fig. 47), *Rhus radicans* (poison ivy), *Lonicera japonica* (Japanese honeysuckle) and *Smilax* spp. (greenbriers). In general, vine damage is more severe with older angiosperms than with older gymnosperms. The shade beneath most coniferous stands is typically sufficient to inhibit the development of most intolerant vines. Young stands of any tree species, however, may be significantly damaged by uncontrolled vine growth.

REFERENCES

Childs, T. W., and Edgren, J. W. (1967). Dwarfmistletoe effects on ponderosa pine growth and trunk form. *Forest Sci.* **13**, 167-174.

Gill, L. S. (1953). Broomrapes, dodders, and mistletoes. *In* "Plant Diseases -Yearbook of Agriculture, 1953" (A. Stefferud, ed.), pp. 73-78, U.S. Government Printing Office, Washington, D.C.

Hawksworth, F. G., and Hinds, T. E. (1964). Effects of dwarfmistletoe on immature lodgepole pine stands in Colorado. *J. Forestry* **62**, 27-32.

Hawksworth, F. G., and Hinds, T. E. (1965). Spread of a parasite. *Nat. Hist., N.Y.* **74**, 52-57.

Hocking, D. (1966). *Cuscuta* parasitic on hardwood seedlings. *Plant Disease Reptr.* **50**, 593-594.

Lutz, H. J. (1943). Injuries to trees caused by *Celastrus* and *Vitis*. *Bull. Torrey Botan. Club* **70**, 436-439.

Muir, J. A. (1967) Occurrence of *Colletotrichum gloeosporioides* on dwarfmistletoe (*Arceuthobium americanum*) in western Canada. *Plant Disease Reptr.* **51**, 798-799.

Peterson, R. S. (1966). *Cronartium* mycelium parasitizing gymnosperm and angiosperm tissue simultaneously. *Mycologia* **58**, 474-477.

Scharpf, R. F., and Parmeter, J. R., Jr. (1967). The biology and pathology of dwarfmistletoe, *Arceuthobium campylopodum* f. *abietinum*, parasitizing true firs (*Abies spp.*) in California. *Tech. Bull., U.S. Forest Serv.* **1362**, 1-42.

Wicker, E. F. (1967). Seed destiny as a klendusic factor of infection and its impact upon propagation of *Arceuthobium* spp. *Phytopathology* **57**, 1164-1168.

GENERAL REFERENCES

Boyce, J. S. (1961). "Forest Pathology." McGraw-Hill, New York.

Childs, T. W., and Wilson, E. R. (1966). Dwarfmistletoe effects in mature ponderosa pine forest in south-central Oregon. *J. Forestry* **64**, 246-250.

Gill, L. S. (1935). *Arceuthobium* in the United States. *Trans. Conn. Acad. Arts Sci.* **32**, 111-245.

Gill, L. S., and Hawksworth, F. G. (1961). The mistletoes: A literature review. *Tech. Bull., U.S. Dept. Agr.* **1242**, 1-87.

Hawksworth, F. G. (1959). Distribution of dwarfmistletoes in relation to topography on the Mescalero Apache Reservation, New Mexico. *J. Forestry* **57**, 919-922.

Hawksworth, F. G. (1969). Rapid intensification and upward spread of dwarf mistletoe in inoculated digger pines. *Plant Disease Reptr.* **53**, 615-617.

Hawksworth, F. G., and Gill, L. S. (1960). Rate of spread of dwarfmistletoe in ponderosa pine in the Southwest. *Res. Note, Rocky Mt. Forest Range Expt. Sta.* **42**, 1-2.

Heidmann, L. J. (1968). Silvicultural control of dwarf mistletoe in heavily infected stands of ponderosa pine in the Southwest. *Res. Paper, Rocky Mt. Forest Range Expt. Sta.* **RM-36**, 1-11.

Kuijt, J. (1955). Dwarfmistletoes. *Botan. Rev.* **21**, 569-627.

Lant, J. G. (1967). Eastern dwarf mistletoe on jack pine in Manitoba. *Plant Disease Reptr.* **51**, 899-900.

Leaphart, C. D. (1963). Dwarfmistletoes: A silvicultural challenge. *J. Forestry* **61**, 40-46.

Leben, C. (1965). Epiphytic microorganisms in relation to plant disease. *Ann. Rev. Phytopathol.* **3**, 209-230.

McCartney, W. O. (1968). European mistletoe, *Viscum album,* an unusual phanerogamic parasite in California. *Plant Disease Reptr.* **52**, 198-201.

Ozenda, P. (1965). Recherches sur les phanerogames parasites. I. Revue des travaux récents. *Phytomorphology* **15**, 311-338.

Parmeter, J. R., Jr., and Platt, W. D. (1968). Dwarf mistletoe infection at girdle and segment regions of fir branches. *Plant Disease Reptr.* **52**, 452-455.

Peace, J. R. (1962) "Pathology of Trees and Shrubs." Oxford Univ. Press, London and New York.

Roth, L. F. (1967). Resistance of ponderosa pine to dwarf mistletoe. *Phytopathology* **57**, 1008 (abstr.).

Scharpf, R. F. (1969). *Cytospora abietis* associated with dwarf mistletoe on true firs in California. *Phytopathology* **59**, 1048 (abstr.).

Scharpf, R. F. (1969). Dwarf mistletoe on red fir—infection and control in understory stands. *Res. Paper, Southwest. Forest Range Expt. Sta.* **PSW-50**, 1-8.

Scharpf, R. F., and Hawksworth, F. G. (1968). Dwarf mistletoe on sugar pine. *Forest Pest Leaflet, U.S. Forest Serv.* **113**, 1-4.

Tainer, F. H., and French, D. W. (1968). Further observations of dwarf mistletoe on eastern larch in Minnesota. *Phytopathology* **58**, 880-881.

Wicker, E. F. (1969). Susceptibility of coastal form and central Montana Douglas-fir to *Arceuthobium douglasii. Plant Disease Reptr.* **53**, 311-314.

Wicker, E. F., and Shaw, C. G. (1967). Target area as a klendusic factor in dwarf mistletoe infections. *Phytopathology* **57**, 1161-1163.

PART III

Special Topics

22

CLIMATE AND TREE DISEASE

After several chapters in which specific pathogens and tree hosts have been discussed, it might be concluded that the simple joining of a pathogenic microorganism and a susceptible host will result in disease. Actually, the condition of the physical environment plays an extremely important role in microbial and higher plant development and as such is an integral component of any disease cycle. Environmental conditions, or climate, are especially important in determining pathogenicity by regulating spore production and mycelial growth of pathogens, and in influencing host susceptibility by weakening or predisposing them to infection and by providing infection courts.

The significance of these three interacting factors can be recognized as equivalent components of any disease phenomenon:

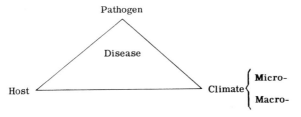

Trees are long-lived individuals and, as a result, climate has significance not only in a "micro" sense, that is, the climate in the immediate vicinity of particular tree organs at particular points in time, but also in a "macro" sense, referring to weather changes throughout large areas over extended time periods.

I. MICROCLIMATE AND TREE DISEASE

Microclimatic conditions are the conditions of the physical environment in the immediate vicinity of a particular plant part. In the interest of standardization, meterologists commonly measure physical parameters in specific ways and at specific sites. Temperature and humidity are commonly measured in a Stevenson screen, approximately 4 feet above the ground. Wind velocity is frequently taken at approximately 30 feet, and light intensity and other variables are generally measured in exposed situations.

The microclimatic conditions of importance in plant disease development are not those measured by the meteorologist by standard procedures. The condition of the environment within a few millimeters or centimeters of a particular plant or pathogen is the condition which is relevant. The nature of the environment close to a plant surface is very much different from that measured even a short distance from the plant. In the proximity of plants, air circulation is greatly retarded and evaporation potential is lowered. In addition, plants transpire water and may thus increase the relative humidity of their environment over that of ambient air. Plants also absorb and reflect light and many are exposed to light which has been previously filtered by other vegetative components, as in a forest. Temperature values are very critical in disease development and are very much conditioned by the plants themselves. Plants have, for example, a depressing influence on soil temperatures. Temperature conditions of aerial plant parts are frequently appreciably different than those at some distance from the plant. Leaf temperatures, for example, are commonly several degrees warmer in bright sunlight and several degrees cooler at night than the surrounding air. The specific estimation of these temperature differences, however, is not a simple task, since the actual value is the result of a complex of factors including insolation, ventilation, and relative humidity (Waggoner, 1965).

The majority of microclimatological data concerning plant pathogens has been in reference to spore dispersal and infection. It is important to realize, however, that the microclimate exerts influences on the pathogen throughout its life cycle and also directly on the host plant itself. Yarwood (1959) has summarized the significance of several microclimatic parmeters to the infection process.

A. Temperature

Tree leaves and bark areas exposed to direct insolation have higher temperatures than the ambient air. Up to approximately 30°–40°C, these higher values favor pathogen development. Spore germination, germ-tube development, and mycelial growth are facilitated. Temperature values in excess of approximately 40°C exert deleterious effects on several pathogens. Certain microbes which infect grape plants, for example, are unable to enter grape leaves on vines on the ground as these leaves have surface temperatures which may approach 45°C (Yarwood, 1959). Pine stump temperatures in North Carolina have been recorded in excess of 40°C. Temperatures this high are probably capable of restricting colonization of the cut surfaces by fungi such as *Fomes annosus*. Under controlled conditions, Houston et al. (1965) found that seedlings grown at 32°C were restricted from developing oak wilt symptoms. The investigators suggested that the extended periods of high temperatures which occur in some southern areas may delay or prevent the development of oak wilt. Smith (1966), in an interesting study, presented evidence indicating that the importance of *Macrophomina phaseoli* as a tree seedling root pathogen was controlled not only by the absolute temperature value, but by the magnitude of the temperature fluctuation. In controlled tests, greater sugar pine mortality resulted when the soil temperature had mean values of 77° and 86°F and fluctuated 16°F than with the same means and fluctuations of 8°F and 0°F.

B. Moisture

Moisture availability is an absolute requirement for the growth of microorganisms. Most plant pathogens are favored by free water or high relative humidity.

Moisture sources are many in natural environments and include precipitation, fog, and water of condensation and guttation (water exuded from leaf margins). The obvious importance of rain, snow, and fog in supplying moisture to microorganisms commonly leads to an underestimation of the significance of condensed water or dew (Yarwood, 1959). Conditions necessary for dew formation include plant surface temperature below the dew point of surrounding air and condensation nuclei. The former is frequently realized through the loss of infrared radiation from plant parts at night, which depresses their surface temperatures below that of the ambient air. Clear skies and restricted air turbulence facilitate this temperature decrease. Condensation nuclei are abundantly present on tree leaf, twig, and bark surfaces.

Nighswander and Patton (1965) found moisture conditions extremely important in the epidemiology of the jack pine–oak gall rust caused by *Cronartium quercuum*. Initial infection of the oak host by the aeciospores of the fungus resulted only following at least 10 hours of saturated air plus free water when the temperature was between 8° and 28°C. The spread of the pathogen via urediospores was limited by dry weather, in addition to other factors. The production and germination of basidiospores followed periods of measurable rainfall and required periods of at least 13 hours of 100% relative humidity.

The lack of available soil moisture is of paramount importance in predisposing trees to infection by biotic disease agents. Several perplexing hardwood maladies currently important in the northeast, including, birch and ash dieback and oak mortality, are presumed to have drought as an important contributing factor.

C. Light

Microorganisms are sensitive to the light conditions of their environment. Bacteria are characteristically more sensitive than fungi. Numerous microbes can respond to light values approximately 10^{-9} the intensity of full sunlight (Yarwood, 1959). Full sunlight for extended periods is probably lethal for most plant pathogens.

The deleterious effect of sunlight exposure has led to the suggestion that many pathogens are distributed and enter their host primarily at night. Van Arsdel (1967) has recently presented evidence indicating that *Cronartium ribicola* pycniospores and basidiospores are released primarily at night. This nocturnal release may be a significant selective advantage to the pathogen as these spores are sensitive to ultraviolet light.

Plants importantly alter the quality and intensity of light received by potential pathogens by absorbing and reflecting radiation. In general, it might be suggested that these alterations typically favor the development of the pathogens.

D. Wind

The relationships between spore distribution and air movements have received a great deal of research attention. Perhaps the most useful principle to glean from these researches is that most spores behave in the atmosphere like smoke particles and that their movement and deposition is similar to all small aerosols as described by established aerodynamic laws (Waggoner, 1965).

In addition to its significance in spore movements, wind is extremely important for other reasons. Air movements over plant surfaces in large measure determine the temperature of these surfaces and the relative humidity of the air immediately adjacent to these surfaces.

E. Development of White Pine Blister Rust as Influenced by Microclimate

One of the most informative applications of microclimatological detail to forest tree disease development was a study conducted by Van Arsdel et al. (1961) on white pine blister rust in Wisconsin. Observations on the occurrence of white pine blister rust in Europe, New England, and Wisconsin indicated that the disease was not uniformly distributed throughout areas of *Cronartium ribicola* occurrence. In Wisconsin, for example, white pines located in certain southern regions were typically free of *C. ribicola* infection despite the fact that diseased *Ribes* were prevalent. In the northern portion of the State, parts of which were cooler and more moist than southern areas, blister rust appeared more common. The Van Arsdel investigation was conceived to interpret the influence of temperature and moisture conditions on the spread of *C. ribicola*.

The conclusion of the study was that infection of white pine occurred only under specific environmental conditions. Fertile teliospores were formed on *Ribes* only after 2 weeks of cool weather. It was necessary for the second week of this fortnight to have less than three consecutive days with temperatures over 82°F. When the temperatures of the fortnight were under 68°F, the germination of teliospores was enhanced over higher temperature 2-week periods. In general, the lower the temperatures when telia were being formed on currant leaves, the greater the number of basidiospores which were formed. With greater numbers of basidiospores, the probability of pine infection is increased. It was further ascertained that pine infection required at least 48 hours with saturated air at less than 68°F.

With this knowledge at hand, the investigators embarked on an ambitious study to correlate local temperature and moisture conditions with topography and vegetative cover. These studies permitted several generalizations. Bottoms of narrow valleys were under 68°F for longer periods than level ground. Shoulders of valleys remained warmer longer than either the valleys or level ground. Slope bases were cool, like the valleys, but the temperature depression was less pronounced. Kettle holes, or small depressions of glacial origin, were generally cooler than flat land sites.

The research further revealed that openings in the forest with diameters less than the height of surrounding trees were at temperatures under 68°F longer than sites in the open or under the forest canopy. Humidities were found to be generally higher near the ground, in the bottoms of narrow valleys, in kettle holes, and in small forest openings.

In an effort to render their findings practically useful, the investigators quantified their observations. By assigning numerical values to the various topographic and vegetative features, they developed a means to estimate the likelihood of blister rust occurrence on a given site (Table XXV).

If all of the values pertaining to a particular site were added together and a sum of nine resulted, then blister rust was in all probability located on the pines present on the site. If the sum of the values was as high as eighteen, then serious damage was probably occurring or would occur if *C. ribicola* were introduced. The application of the estimator to 112 Wisconsin plots resulted in correct prediction on 99 plots, for an 89% accuracy.

Subsequent to the Van Arsdel study, several other investigators have correlated environmental parameters with the development of rust fungi that infect trees. Weather conditions have been found critical in the infection process of slash pines by *Cronartium fusiforme* (Davis and Snow, 1968;

TABLE XXV

TOPOGRAPHIC AND VEGETATIVE FACTORS AND VALUES
ASSIGNED FOR BLISTER RUST HAZARD FOR SOUTHERN
WISCONSIN BELOW 1000 FT ELEVATION[a]

Topographic factors	Tentative value assigned
Special conditions	
kettle holes	6
sheltered valley	6
Position classes	
base of slope	6
on the slope	2
shoulder of the slope	−2
flat	0
Slope-percent classes	
0–3%	0
3–20%	5
20–50%	3
50–100%	0
over 100%	−2
Vegetative cover classes	
covered with a complete crown canopy	0
small opening (D/H = 1.0 or less)	9
large opening or in the open	
(D/H greater than 1.0)	0
brush (nondescript broken vegetation)	3

[a]From Van Arsdel et al. (1961). Reproduced by permission of U.S. Forest Service.

Snow 1968a,b; Snow and Froelich, 1968; Snow et al., 1968). Aeciospore release is also critically controlled by environmental conditions. Pady et al. (1968) found aeciospore liberation by Gymnosporangium juniperi-virginianae to be dependent on the relative humidity of the air.

II. MACROCLIMATE AND TREE DISEASE

Macroclimate as used here refers to weather conditions over extended time periods as well as over large areas. Macroclimate is significant to tree health because trees are long-lived and weather over time is subject to considerable change.

A. Changing Climate

The climate of the world is not stable. In geological terms, the climate of the earth is most typically characterized by extended "moderate periods" with equable weather the year round, lack of icecaps, and generally warm seas. Man evolved after the last "moderate period" and his development has been in a period of climatic revolution (Hepting, 1963).

This period of revolutionary climatic alteration has been characterized by a complex of "cycles within cycles." Over the past 3000 years, for example, the general evidence suggests that the northeast has become cooler and more moist. This observation led Raup (1937) to suggest that northern hardwoods, including sugar maple, red oak, beech, white ash, and the birches, may be selectively favored over species characteristic of more moderate climates, for example, white, black, and chestnut oaks, hickories, and tulip trees. Over the past several hundred years, however, and particularly during the first half of the present century, there is evidence for a moderating trend. The average annual world temperature has increased 1°F from 1885 to 1945. Mean annual temperature increases in excess of 5°F have been recorded in Iceland, Greenland, and Spitzbergen. Most United States regions have witnessed warmer summers and winters. Additional support for the warming theory is given by the receding glaciers in Alaska and the northward migration of the tree line in Finland (Hepting, 1963).

1. *Causes of climatic change.* Numerous hypotheses have been proposed to explain the forces behind climatic change. The most plausible of these include: (1) an alteration in the angle between the axis of the earth and the ecliptic plane, (2) sunspot activity, (3) variation in the energy emitted by the sun, (4) variation in the amount of the energy of the sun received by the earth, and (5) the development and spread of urban areas. This last hypothesis is an intriguing possibility recently proposed by Lowry (1967).

A hypothesis which has received considerable attention with respect to the recent warming trend relates to the amount of energy from the sun intercepted and held by the earth. The carbon dioxide theory has frequently been associated with the amount of heat energy retained by the earth (Plass, 1959). Since approximately 1850, we have placed into the atmosphere enormous quantities of carbon dioxide, mainly through the combustion of fossil fuels. By the year 2000, emissions will have increased by approximately 18-fold from 1890. In 1965–85, an emission rate increase of roughly 4% per year, compounded, is expected. It is presumed that the advent of expanded nuclear power generation will lower this rate of increase after 1985 (Kigoshi, 1967). It has been suggested that carbon dioxide acts to enforce the warming trend by absorbing reradiation from the earth. The trapped radiation acts to warm the atmosphere.

In contrast to the warming hypothesis, McCormick and Ludwig (1967) have suggested that a cooling tendency has been in evidence during the two decades between 1940 and 1960. These authors theorize that emission of long-lived aerosol pollutants have had a tendency to increase the earth's reflectance and have resulted in this cooling.

2. *Climatic change and tree health.* The influence of climatic alteration on tree health may be expressed directly or indirectly. The significance of

climatic change is indirect if the primary effect of the alteration is on tree pathogens. Many plant pathogens are relatively insensitive to weather changes, but most operate within fairly well-defined tolerance limits. Any prolonged climatic change, like the current warming trend, may act to enhance the pathogenicity of members of this latter group.

Phytophthora cinnamomi, which caused significant losses of American chestnut in the southeast prior to the chestnut blight, is considered essentially a tropical organism whose influence was moving northward in response to subtle warming (Woods, 1953). It has also been suggested that an advance in oak budbreak, aecial fruiting, and pine shoot growth has resulted in greater fusiform rust occurrence in the south.

Climatic variation may also operate directly to influence tree welfare. It has been suggested, for example, that dieback and decline diseases of maple, birch, ash, and others may be in response to subtle climatic change (Weaver, 1965). This hypothesis involves the "climax" concept of ecologists. This concept suggests that any forest left undisturbed for extended periods of time will become stable in character by virtue of attaining equilibrium with its environment. Since climate is not static, however, and is presumably continually changing, vegetation may be constantly adjusting to reflect its new environment. Holloway (1954) has suggested, for example, that this adjustment may show a lag period during which the response to a particular change may still be in progress when the next change occurs. Dieback and decline diseases may therefore reflect the adjustment of species not ideally suited to the climate extant at the present time.

With respect to tree health, climatic change may not always be deleterious. A further and sustained increase in temperature would presumably reduce the importance of white pine blister rust and oak wilt.

REFERENCES

Davis, R. T., and Snow, G. A. (1968). Weather systems related to fusiform rust infection. *Plant Disease Reptr.* **52**, 419–422.

Hepting, G. H. (1963). Climate and forest diseases. *Ann. Rev. Phytopathol.* **1**, 31–50.

Holloway, J. T. (1954). Forests and climate in the South Island of New Zealand. *Trans. Roy. Soc. New Zealand* **82**, Part 2, 329–410.

Houston, D. R., Drake, C. R., and Kuntz, J. E. (1965). Effects of environment on oak wilt development. *Phytopathology* **55**, 1114–1121.

Kigoshi, K. (1967). Industrial emissions of carbon dioxide in the United States: A projection. *Science* **156**, 931–934.

Lowry, W. P. (1967). The climate of cities. *Sci. Am.* **217**, 15–23.

McCormick, R. A., and Ludwig, J. H. (1967). Climate modification by atmospheric aerosols. *Science* **156**, 1358–1359.

Nighswander, J. E., and Patton, R. F. (1965). The epidemiology of the jack pine-oak gall rust (*Cronartium quercuum*) in Wisconsin. *Can. J. Botany* **43**, 1561-1581.

Pady, S. M., Kramer, C. L., and Clary, R. (1968). Periodicity in aeciospore release in *Gymnosporangium juniperi-virginianae. Phytopathology* **58**, 329-331.

Plass, G. N. (1959). Carbon dioxide and climate. *Sci. Am.* **201**, 41-47.

Raup, H. M. (1937). Recent changes of climate and vegetation in southern New England and adjacent New York. *J. Arnold Arboretum* **18**, 79-117.

Smith, R. S., Jr. (1966). Effect of diurnal temperature fluctuations on the charcoal root disease of *Pinus lambertiana. Phytopathology* **56**, 61-64.

Snow, G. A. (1968a). Time required for infection of pine by *Cronartium fusiforme* and effect of field and laboratory exposure after inoculation. *Phytopathology* **58**, 1547-1550.

Snow, G. A. (1968b). Basidiospore production by *Cronartium fusiforme* as affected by suboptimal temperatures and preconditioning of teliospores. *Phytopathology* **58**, 1541-1546.

Snow, G. A., and Froelich, R. C. (1968). Daily and seasonal dispersal of basidiospores of *Cronartium fusiforme. Phytopathology* **58**, 1532-1536.

Snow, G. A., Froelich, R. C., and Popham, T. W. (1968). Weather conditions determining infection of slash pines by *Cronartium fusiforme. Phytopathology* **58**, 1537-1540.

Van Arsdel, E. P. (1967). The nocturnal diffusion and transport of spores. *Phytopathology* **57**, 1221-1229.

Van Arsdel, E. P., Riker, A. J., Kouba, T. F., Suomi, V. E., and Bryson, R. A. (1961). The climatic distribution of blister rust on white pine in Wisconsin. *Sta. Paper, Lake States Forest Expt. Sta.* **87**, 1-34.

Waggoner, P. E. (1965). Microclimate and plant disease. *Ann. Rev. Phytopathol.* **3**, 103-126.

Weaver, L. O. (1965). Diebacks and declines of hardwoods attributed to climatic changes — a review. *Arborist's News* **30**, 33-36.

Woods, F. W. (1953). Disease as a factor in the evolution of forest composition. *J. Forestry* **51**, 871-873.

Yarwood, C. E. (1959). Microclimate and infection. *In* "Plant Pathology, Problems and Progress 1908-1958" (C. S. Holton *et al.*, eds.), pp. 548-556. Univ. of Wisconsin Press, Madison, Wisconsin.

GENERAL REFERENCES

Bollard, E. G., and Matthews, R. E. F. (1966). The physiology of parasitic disease. *In* "Plant Physiology" (F. C. Steward, ed.), Vol. 4B, pp. 417-550. Academic Press, New York.

Chang, J. H. (1968). "Climate and Agriculture. An Ecological Survey." Aldine Publ. Co., Chicago, Illinois.

Fritts, H. C. (1967). Growth rings of trees: A physiological basis for their correlation with climate. *In* "Ground Level Climatology," *Publ. No.* 86, pp. 45-65. *Am. Assoc. Advance. Sci.,* Washington, D.C.

Hepting, G. H. (1962). Climate change and forest diseases. *Proc. 5th World Forestry Congr.,* Vol. 2, pp. 842-847, Aug. 29-Sept. 10, 1960, Seattle, Washington.

Massie, L. B., and Peterson, J. L. (1968). Factors affecting the initiation and development of Fusarium canker on *Sophora japonica* in relation to growth and sporulation of *Fusarium lateritium. Phytopathology* **58**, 1620-1623.

Shaw, R. H., ed. (1967). "Ground Level Climatology," *Publ. No.* 86. *Am. Assoc. Advance. Sci.,* Washington, D.C.

Skilling, D. D. (1969). The effect of temperature on ascospore release by *Scleroderris lagerbergii. Plant Disease Reptr.* **53**, 289-291.

Spurr, S. H. (1953). The vegetational significance of recent temperature changes along the Atlantic seaboard. *Am. J. Sci.* **251**, 682-688.

Taylor, J. A., ed. (1967). "Weather and Agriculture." Pergamon Press, Oxford.

Waggoner, P. E. (1968). Weather and the rise and fall of fungi. *In* "Biometeorology" (W. P. Lowry, ed.), pp. 45-66. Oregon State Univ. Press, Corvallis, Oregon.

Wallin, J. R. (1967). Ground level climate in relation to forecasting plant disease. *In* "Ground Level Climatology," *Publ. No.* 86, pp. 149-163. *Am. Assoc. Advance. Sci.,* Washington, D.C.

23

EPIDEMIOLOGY

We have given primary treatment to specific stress factors and the manner in which they influence individual trees. Historically, this has been the fundamental concern of plant pathologists. There is, however, another area of interest, comparable to the public health aspect of human medicine, which relates to disease in plant populations. The primary emphasis in this field is on the influence of a particular disease on a large number of trees. In cases of biotic disease agents, it also is concerned with the study of the population of the pathogen. Investigations of the populations of diseased plants and pathogens has uncovered unique characteristics which were not apparent from the study of diseased individuals or specific microorganisms. Knowledge concerning disease in plant populations is especially important in the study of forest tree disease. Tree pathologists are frequently concerned with large areas containing many long-lived individuals. Commonly, large numbers of trees are treated as "units," for example, plantations or stands of a specific character or age. Two of the most important concepts in the study of diseased plant populations are inoculum potential and epidemiology.

I. INOCULUM POTENTIAL

A fundamental concern of pathologists interested in the importance of a disease to a particular population of plants is an estimation of how severe the impact of the malady will be. The prediction of the severity is thought to depend in large measure on the inoculum potential. This concept has been most ably presented by Dimond and Horsfall (1960) and Waggoner (1960). Inoculum is defined as any part or fragment of a biotic disease agent capable of initiating an infection. Examples of inocula are bacterial cells, virus particles, and fungal spores or mycelial fragments. Inoculum potential has thus

been defined by Dimond and Horsfall (1960) as "the number of independent infections that are likely to occur in a given situation in a population of
susceptible healthy tissues." The unit of infection in this definition depends
on the mode of action of the pathogen. If, for example, the pathogen is systemic, then an entire infected plant is an independent infection. If the pathogen is localized, for instance, on a single leaf, then each diseased leaf represents an independent infection.

The nature of the inoculum potential is determined primarily by the
interrelationship of four factors. These include: (1) the influence of the environment on the pathogen and host (Chapter 22), (2) the susceptibility of the
host, (3) the vigor of the pathogen to establish an infection and induce disease (often termed pathogenicity or virulence), and (4) the amount of inoculum present:

$$\text{environment} + \frac{\text{host}}{\text{susceptibility}} + \frac{\text{virulence and}}{\text{inoculum quantity}} = \text{amount of disease}$$

$$\underbrace{\phantom{\text{environment} + \frac{\text{host}}{\text{susceptibility}}}}_{\text{Capacity factor}} \quad \underbrace{\phantom{\frac{\text{virulence and}}{\text{inoculum quantity}}}}_{\text{Intensity factor}} \quad \underbrace{\phantom{= \text{amount of disease}}}_{\text{Inoculum potential}}$$

Dimond and Horsfall (1960) have referred to the significance of the physical environment to disease development as the "capacity factor" and to the
virulence and inoculum quantity of the pathogen as the "intensity factor."
Quantitative estimation of the capacity factor has been difficult due to the
multiplicity of parameters and the complexity of their interaction. As we
have seen in our discussion of tree rust pathogens, however, certain environmental aspects, for example temperature and relative humidity, have been
quite accurately described.

The intensity factor is similarly complex and most importantly involves
variation in the amount of inoculum from the source of production, inter-
ception of the inoculum by the host, and virulence of the pathogen. In the
typical disease situation, inoculum amounts are reduced, and consequently
disease is reduced, as the distance from the inoculum source increases.
Examples of this situation are root rots caused by *Fomes annosus* and oak
wilts caused by *Ceratocystis fagacearum*. Occasionally, however, situations
occur in which the disease decreases in severity from the locus of primary
infection, but does not diminish entirely. An example in forest trees might be
chestnut blight caused by *Endothia parasitica*. Another infrequent happen-
stance is the case where the disease is distributed in a disjunct pattern. This
situation may occur, as in the case of dwarf mistletoe infections, where bird
vectors act to distribute the seed over very large distances. The actual trapping of inocula by the host is a poorly understood process which involves
physical configurations of the host and of the inoculum in addition to environmental factors in the immediate vicinity of plant parts. The virulence of
the inoculum is controlled by its inherent capacity to enter and degrade host

tissue and by such fortuitous circumstances as exposure to ultraviolet radiation and dessicating air currents.

As we are able to more accurately quantify the various factors comprising the inoculum potential, we will have an increasingly valuable means of predicting the course of a disease in a plant population.

II. EPIDEMIOLOGY

Epidemiology is the study of disease in populations. This study is primarily concerned with investigations of epidemics. Epidemics are extensive, temporary increases in the occurrence of a particular disease which influences, at the same time, large numbers of individuals in a given population. Plant epidemiology has been intensively studied and quantified by Van der Plank (1960, 1963, 1965).

One of the most misleading concepts relating to epidemics is that they are caused by extremely virulent pathogens which multiply rapidly and spread quickly through the host population. The rate of multiplication and spread of the pathogen is not the principle criterion for an epidemic, but rather the number of individuals infected in a particular area (Van der Plank, 1960). There is, for example, currently an epidemic of oak wilt, particularly in many of the upper midwestern states. *Ceratocystis fagacearum*, however, has relatively restricted means for spread. The main distribution is slow and is accomplished by tree-to-tree migration via root grafts. It is presumed capable of spreading by other mechanisms over greater distances but these are not yet fully appreciated. Nevertheless, the rate of disease increase is not extremely rapid. The disease is considered of epidemic character, not because of its rate of spread, but because it is influencing such a large proportion of the oak population in certain areas.

Epidemics can perhaps best be understood if they are considered as being related to a balance between appearance and disappearance of a particular pathogen. For example, a pathogen may increase, and possibly result in increased disease and epidemics, if it has a high birth rate or a low death rate (Van der Plank, 1960). Over time, phytopathologists have been primarily concerned with high birth rate epidemics and, to a certain extent, this accounts for the misconception previously mentioned. Low death rate epidemics, however, are also extremely important, especially in long-lived hosts such as trees. Pathogens which cause heartwood decay and perennial cankers and certain rust diseases may have low death rates and be capable, in certain situations, of causing low death rate epidemics.

The generalized course of an epidemic is that of the typical sigmoid curve (Fig. 48). Early in an epidemic, that is, at the bottom of the curve, the absolute rate of increase of disease is small, other things being favorable, as only a limited quantity of inoculum is available. In the middle of the curve, the

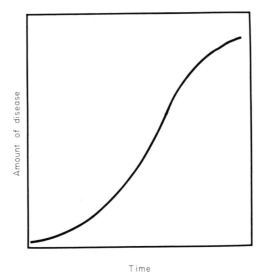

Amount of disease

Time

Fig. 48. Amount of infection existent in a plant population during the course of an epidemic. Amount of infection may represent the actual number of whole plants infected or the number of specific plant parts diseased, depending on the nature of the disease and pathogen being studied.

absolute rate may be relatively fast as restrictions imposed by limited inoculum or lack of uninfected plants or plant parts is insignificant. In the final stages of an epidemic, at the top of the curve, the rate declines as less and less host tissue remains uninfected.

The rate of increase in the amount of disease during the course of an epidemic has been designated r by Van der Plank (1963). This r is defined as the infection rate and it is, of course, also a reflection of the rate at which the population of the causal pathogen increases. The rate during the logarithmic phase of an epidemic (middle of curve, Fig. 48) is designated r_l and may be calculated using the formula:

$$r_l = \frac{1}{t_2 - t_1} \log e \frac{x_2}{x_1}$$

where x_1 and x_2 are the proportions of disease existent in a population at times t_1 and t_2, respectively. The infection rate r_l permits comparison of different epidemics and may provide much useful information in a single figure. Merrill (1967a) has analyzed several epidemics of forest tree diseases in North America using Van der Plank's formula (Table XXVI).

High values of r are seen to be associated with diseases caused by introduced pathogens. This is consistent with the theory that diseases caused by exotic agents are characteristically devastating because of a lack of inherent resistance in indigenous hosts and a potential for unrestricted pathogen development occasioned by lack of natural enemies. The relatively high values of r associated with oak wilt and elm phloem necrosis may suggest that these diseases are caused by introduced pathogens (Merrill, 1967a). Another application of the r value is in the prediction of future losses. Merrill (1967b), for example, has calculated that from 1956 to 1965, oak wilt has increased 2.4 times ($r = 0.098$ per unit per year) in Pennsylvania and 17 times ($r = 0.315$ per unit per year) in West Virginia. The proportion of the oak population diseased in 1965 was 0.000152 in Pennsylvania and 0.000341 in West Virginia. It can be calculated, therefore, if one assumes a constant rate of increase similar to the 1956–65 value, that Pennsylvania will have 1% oak infection in 50 years and that West Virginia will have 1% infection in 25 years.

TABLE XXVI

CALCULATION OF RATE OF DISEASE INCREASE PER UNIT PER YEAR (r_l) FOR SEVERAL IMPORTANT FOREST TREE DISEASES

Disease	r_l	Location
White pine blister rust	0.05	British Columbia
	0.67	Minnesota
	0.50	Maine
Dutch elm disease	1.37	Illinois
	0.50	Connecticut
	0.25	Quebec
Chestnut blight	1.42	Pennsylvania
	1.10	Virginia
	0.83	Connecticut
Elm phloem necrosis	0.46	Indiana
Oak wilt	0.10	Pennsylvania
	0.22	West Virginia
	0.22	Illinois
	0.20	Tennessee
	0.36	Arkansas
Tympanis canker (red pine)	0.08–0.15	Connecticut
Polyperus tomentosus (spruce)	0.03–0.05	Saskatchewan
Cytospora canker (spruce)	0.14	Quebec

[a]From Merrill (1967a). Reproduced by permission of the American Phytopathological Society.

Quantification of epidemic characteristics will greatly facilitate the comparison of disease importance for the establishment of research priorities, enable the prediction of losses, permit suggestion of the origin (that is exotic or native) of the causal pathogen, and aid the evaluation and justification of control efforts (Merrill, 1968).

III. EPIDEMIOLOGICAL CONSIDERATIONS IN FOREST TREE CULTURE

The cultivation of most agricultural crops involves the intensive management of large areas of a single plant species. Since this practice is unnatural and ecologically unstable, much effort must be applied to avoid the occurrence of epidemics. In forestry, however, the management is typically extensive and is concerned with a "natural" grouping of plants. In this instance, the primary disease concern is generally with native pathogens and native tree species. The coexistence of indigenous hosts and pathogens typically results in an equilibrium between the two such that only a limited number of trees are diseased by any one agent in any particular area. There may be small local and temporary outbreaks, but the general ecological patterns are those of a relatively stable community of biotic disease agents and hosts.

There are, unfortunately, at least four exceptions to this rather inocuous disease agent–host tree relationship.

a. Monospecies plantations. As forest management has become more intensive, trees have been grown on large areas in even-aged stands. If this type of growth pattern is not natural to the tree species, the situation becomes analogous to that extant in agriculture. Blister rust caused by *Cronartium ribicola* and root rot caused by *Fomes annosus* in eastern white pine and red pine, respectively, are most damaging in situations where these trees are grown in monospecific, even-aged plantations. Baxter (1967) discusses in some detail the problems peculiar to the disease aspects of plantation management.

b. Introduced pathogens. Exotic pathogens, for example, those which cause white pine blister rust, Dutch elm disease, and chestnut blight, may be particularly damaging. The absence of inherent resistance in the hosts reflects the absence of any force to naturally select those tree varieties capable of restricting infection. In addition, the development of introduced disease agents may be favored by the particular physical environment existing in their new location. They may, for example be exposed to temperature and moisture conditions even more suitable for their growth than those characteristic of their native habit. Another possible cause for the expansion of exotic disease agents concerns their natural biotic enemies. If, for example, the new environment lacks one or more of the natural enemies of a particular pathogen, the pathogen's ability to grow and flourish may be considerably enhanced.

c. Introduced hosts. In a similar manner, the movement of hosts from their native ranges may invite pathological problems. The situation in this instance is strictly analogous to that presented in Section III, *b*, above. Damage in this case, however, results when an exotic tree is moved to an area where it is susceptible to a native pathogen.

d. A native disease that expands in a native population. Occasionally, a seemingly balanced situation becomes out of balance and an epidemic may ensue. This has been documented, for example, with *Comandra* rust disease of lodgepole pine. This disease is caused by *Cronartium comandrae* which alternates between *Comandra* species (perennial herbs parasitic on plant roots) and western hard pines. The fungus is a native to this country and a relatively aggressive killer of lodgepole pine. In a very strange and unexplained manner, this pathogen caused an epidemic disease of lodgepole pine in certain western regions between 1910 and 1945 (Krebill, 1965). Hypotheses proposed to account for this expansion are: (*1*) marked increase in *Comandra* which invaded overgrazed range lands near pine forests, (*2*) altered weather conditions, or (*3*) disturbance to the intricately balanced interaction of host, parasite, and environment. *Cronartium comandrae* has recently been found to be causing serious damage to loblolly pine in localized areas of Tennessee. This damage is the consequence of a rather unusual expansion into this new area by the pathogen (Cordell and Knighten, 1969).

As forest management becomes more intensive on less land, the four special exceptions discussed above will probably become more common and significant. If this occurs, greater attention will of necessity have to be paid to pathological ramifications of managerial and silvicultural manipulations and especially to the application of more control procedures to forest tree diseases.

REFERENCES

Baxter, D. V. (1967). "Disease in Forest Plantations: Thief of Time." Cranbrook Inst. Science, Bloomfield Hills, Michigan.

Cordell, C. E., and Knighten, J. L. (1969). Comandra blister rust on young loblolly pine in eastern Tennessee. *J. Forestry* **67**, 332–333.

Dimond, A. E., and Horsfall, J. G. (1960). Prologue—inoculum and the diseased population. *In* "Plant Pathology" (J. G. Horsfall and A. E. Dimond, eds.), Vol. 3, pp. 1–22. Academic Press, New York.

Krebill, R. G. (1965). Comandra rust outbreaks in lodgepole pine. *J. Forestry* **63**, 519–522.

Merrill, W. (1967a). Analyses of some epidemics of forest tree diseases. *Phytopathology* **57**, 822 (abstr.).

Merrill, W. (1967b). The oak wilt epidemics in Pennsylvania and West Virginia: An analysis. *Phytopathology* **57**, 1206-1210.

Merrill, W. (1968). Effect of control programs on development of epidemics of Dutch elm disease. *Phytopathology* **58**, 1060 (abstr.).

Van der Plank, J. E. (1960). Analysis of epidemics. *In* "Plant Pathology" (J. G. Horsfall and A. E. Dimond, eds.), Vol. 3, pp 229-289. Academic Press, New York.

Van der Plank, J. E. (1963). "Plant Diseases." Academic Press, New York.

Van der Plank, J. E. (1965). Dynamics of epidemics of plant disease. *Science* **147**, 120-124.

Waggoner, P. E. (1960). Forecasting epidemics. *In* "Plant Pathology" (J. G. Horsfall and A. E. Dimond, eds.), Vol. 3, pp. 291-312. Academic Press, New York.

PART IV

Disease Control

24

EXCLUSION

I. GENERAL CONCEPTS OF DISEASE CONTROL

Before discussing specific control procedures, several concepts relating to control must be appreciated. The control of a plant disease refers to a *reduction* in the amount of damage a particular disease may cause. With abiotic stress factors, control may involve environmental alteration to reduce the significance of an undesirable factor. With biotic stress factors, control procedures commonly involve attempts to make the environment unsuitable for the pathogen, reduce the population size of the pathogen, or increase the resistance of the host.

Control efforts characteristically involve a partial amelioration of environmental phenomena or a partial reduction in pathogen population size. Complete removal of undesirable abiotic stresses and absolute abolition of pathogenic biotic populations is rarely desirable or necessary and is frequently impossible. Native biotic disease agents, for example, are frequently exposed to conditions which alternately favor and do not favor their development. Population sizes thus alternately expand and contract, reflecting these changing conditions (Fig. 49). The existence of pathogen populations in "peak" amounts commonly corresponds to plant losses of sufficient magnitude to warrant control efforts. In the case of native pathogens, therefore, controls are typically applied to reduce pathogen population numbers from peak amounts to more normal quantities.

Control decisions are not simple determinations. Three components are involved in the synthesis and application of these efforts:

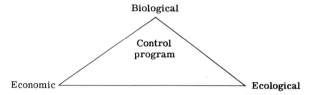

The biological component of a control program is the specific mechanism to be used to enable the creation of a more healthful environment or to reduce the size of a biotic disease agent's population. The awareness, for example, that the fungicide dichlone will kill the fungus *Venturia inaequalis* means that, "biologically," the control of the disease apple scab is possible.

The ecological consideration of control procedures may be quite broad in scope. It may, for example, refer to the importance of some minor environmental factor in the control scheme. The fact that dichlone begins to sublime at 29°C and may, as a result, disappear from foliage to which it is applied, restricts its use to the more northern apple-growing regions. Ecological ramifications also, however, relate to the "compatibility" of control efforts with other biological, sociological, and political components of the ecosystem in which the control attempt is made. The use of organochlorine sprays to control beetle vectors of *Ceratocystis ulmi* infecting elm trees in a bird sanctuary or fish hatchery is undesirable, for instance, when one realizes that birds and

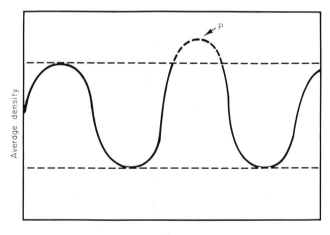

Fig. 49. Cyclic fluctuation in population size of a mythical biotic disease agent. "P" represents an abnormal peak expansion in response to some particularly favorable environmental condition(s).

fish represent endpoints of food chains and that certain species have a tendency to accumulate persistent insecticides in lethal amounts.

The economic factor of control decisions recognizes the fact that control efforts are generally applied only when their cost is less than the value gained by their implementation. While this appears to be a relatively straightforward guideline, it is in practice frequently difficult to compare cost and benefit as the benefit figures may not be readily obtained. Marty (1966), in a most interesting paper, provides a procedure for evaluating the cost of blister rust control in the eastern United States. By Marty's procedure, the estimate of the value saved is discounted and compared with the expected control cost. Immediate control is economically justified when the present worth of the value saved exceeds the cost of control.

Economic restrictions are largely responsible for making control procedures for forest tree diseases relatively uncommon, unsophisticated, and unimaginative when compared to control procedures used on agricultural crops. The reasons behind these economic constraints are many. Among the most significant are the following: the relatively low value of tree crops per unit area; the large size of trees; the extended ages attained by trees and associated long rotation times; the great sizes of the forests managed and the possible occurrence of variable topography; and the general "extensive" character of forest management relative to the "intensive" management of agricultural areas.

Historically, forest tree disease control has primarily involved minor silvicultural manipulations. Currently, however, control procedures being applied to ornamental and forest trees are more sophisticated and will continue to become more so as the demand for wood products and the amenities of standing trees increases, as forest management intensifies in reflection of a shrinking forest area, and as tree and land values escalate.

We have evidence that suggests that well-conceived control programs for forest tree diseases are effective (Hepting, 1970). Control programs have appreciably reduced the spread of oak wilt by 76% in Pennsylvania, by 50% in West Virginia, and by 42% in North Carolina-Tennessee (T. W. Jones, 1965). In the greater Chicago area, five municipalities without Dutch elm disease control programs have lost 80-94% of their elms. In the same area, however, 28 municipalities with comprehensive control programs have lost only 5-15% of their elms (Neely, 1967).

In general, procedures employed to control plant diseases may be placed in one of four categories; exclusion, eradication, protection, and resistance. All of the methods classified in each of these four groupings have not been applied to forest tree disease problems. Nevertheless, all will be briefly covered to present a reasonably comprehensive treatment of disease control techniques available, especially in awareness that many may ultimately be applied to forest disease phenomena.

II. EXCLUSION

Contained in this category are all control measures which function to prevent the entrance and establishment of a biotic disease agent into a particular area. These procedures are validly applied only when the area to which they are directed is unviolated by the pathogen. This instance is most relevant in the case of intercontinental spread of plant pathogens. Procedures applied to remove pathogens from reproductive plant parts or other plant materials are located in this category, since the primary intent of these methods is typically to exclude particular pests from areas presently lacking them. Three rather broad and somewhat unrelated control devices are considered to be the fundamental exclusion procedures: (1) the selection and treatment of propagative materials, (2) quarantines and (3) the investigation of exotic disease agents.

A. Selection and Treatment of Propagative Materials

The term propagative materials as used in this discussion refers to seeds, vegetative components used for reproductive purposes, and seedlings. Efforts to insure their freedom from pathogens are commonly made in attempts to prevent the introduction of undesirable organisms into new habitats by these materials.

The selection of propagative materials free from pathogens may appear to be a relatively simple and readily accomplished task. In the case of seedlings and cuttings, symptoms and signs may be present and facilitate culling efforts. Latent or incipient infections, however, may be very difficult to ascertain.

The selection of seed devoid of pathogens is made difficult by the absence of symptoms and the paucity of signs. Seed certification programs are widespread among the various agricultural crops. They are established by various private, state, and federal organizations whose aim it is to improve seed quality by establishing and enforcing criteria the seed must satisfy. Certification restrictions generally encompass one or more of the following; type (that is, species or variety), source, germination percentage, and insect and pathogen prevalence on or in the seed. Currently, there is no national forest tree seed certification program. There are some state and private certification efforts which are of variable character and success. Hopkins (1968) has recently described a pioneering program in the Pacific Northwest. This plan does not, however, evaluate the disease potential of the certified seed. Certainly, seed certification regulations for forest tree seed which are concerned with the occurrence of disease agents on and in the seeds and parent trees should be instrumental in permitting the selection of disease-free seed and, thereby, in excluding the introduction of pathogens into disease-free areas.

Since propagative materials are generally rather compact, they may be readily treated by various physical and chemical procedures in an attempt to kill pathogens in and on the propagative unit. Submersion of seeds or vegetative units in hot water is commonly utilized to rid plant materials of certain disease agents. Numerous chemicals are employed to kill microbes on seed exteriors. Under the plant quarantine regulations of the United States Department of Agriculture, tree seed importations are inspected and usually fumigated with methyl bromide (L. Jones and Havel, 1968). Normal fumigation dosage for imported conifer seed is 2.5 pounds of methyl bromide per 1000 cubic feet for 2.5 hours at normal air pressure and at a temperature of 80°-96°F (L. Jones et al., 1964). Unfortunately, unless careful steps are taken to insure that the seed has a relatively low moisture content (approximately 5-10%) and is adequately aerated after fumigation, the seed of many species may be damaged by the methyl bromide treatment (L. Jones and Havel, 1968; L. Jones et al., 1964).

B. Quarantines

With respect to forest tree species, quarantines represent the most important current exclusionary device. The quarantine method is predicated on two primary observations. First, there are comparatively few biotic disease agents which are cosmopolitan in distribution. In fact, several pathogens are not even distributed throughout all regions where host availability and environmental factors would permit their colonization. Second, in the absence of continuous land surfaces and continuous plant distributions, the spread of many pathogens is denied or restricted. The occurrence of mountains, deserts, and large bodies of water, for example, may make the movement of disease agents and vectors inefficient (Peace, 1962). In the presence of effective natural barriers, man assumes an important role as a vector for numerous pathogens. Laws attempting to diminish man's ability to function as a vector, directly or indirectly, are termed quarantines. General discussions of the quarantine philosophy and quarantine mechanics are available (Gram, 1960; McCubbin, 1954; Moore, 1952; Peace, 1962; Rainwater and Smith, 1966).

1. Quarantine methods.   Quarantine laws may be those adopted and imposed by the exporting or importing country. In the former, inspection of the plant materials to be released is subject primarily to the restrictions imposed by the importing country. Certain advantages accrue to quarantine inspections conducted in the exporting country *prior* to shipping. In the instance of seedlings, inspections may be initiated in the nursery and be conducted over an extended time period. Since most symptoms and signs are not continuously present, inspection over time may be more efficient in disease detection. Inspections conducted in exporting countries may also have the advantage of employing people familiar with local disease phenomena.

The majority of quarantine regulations are those imposed by countries on plant materials which are imported. Generally, these regulations are quite complex and very variously administered and enforced by the respective countries. The Food and Agriculture Organization of the United Nations has summarized many of the import regulations, with respect to trees, that currently exist (Food and Agriculture Organization, 1964).

Embargoes represent a special type of import regulation. This type of law acts to completely forbid the entrance of particular plant parts or particular varieties or species into a country. Examples of embargoes are the exclusion by New Zealand of all oak species from North America, the exclusion by England of members of the *Prunus* genus from anywhere outside Europe, and the exclusion by the United States of most foreign trees and shrubs. The Code of Federal Regulations contains a listing of the genera prohibited in the United States (U.S. Department of Agriculture, 1955). Embargoes are an extremely effective quarantine measure. They do, however, have several disadvantages. With respect to the overall trade exchange of a country, embargoes impose restrictive characteristics and may weaken bargaining positions. Historically, embargoes have frequently been used for economic and political reasons unrelated to their actual intent. In the case of certain countries, phytosanitary embargoes are not desirable. If, for example, the native flora lacks diversity, the country may be best served by not overly restricting plant imports.

2. United States quarantines.   The United States has one of the most comprehensive phytosanitary systems in existence (Agricultural Research Service, 1962). The program is administered by the Plant Quarantine Division of the Agricultural Research Service, United States Department of Agriculture. Involved in the responsibilities of the Plant Quarantine Division are: the education of importers and travelers with respect to import laws; the inspection of plant materials, including port, border, ship, aircraft, and mail inspections; fumigation and other emergency measures; and export certifications.

3. Quarantines pro and con.   Quarantine measures, while quite prevalent, have historically been relatively controversial. Proponents have offered the following arguments in their favor. Quarantine regulations have prevented the introduction of exotic pests and their financial benefits do exceed their costs. Even if not ultimately effective in excluding an undesirable pathogen, quarantines may delay introduction to such a time that the introduction can be more adequately dealt with. Quarantines represent an effective constraining influence on the traveling public. These importers are presumed to be potentially one of the most important sources of unwanted pests. The very knowledge of the general quarantine law, without awareness of specifics, is presumed to result in fewer attempts to introduce exotic plant materials. The fact that certain quarantines have notably failed is not sufficient reason to abandon the entire plan.

Opponents to quarantine legislation offer the following arguments in opposition. In view of the large number and massive size of many of the current imports, it is practically impossible to adequately sample for minute pests. Visual inspection is useless if the stage of disease development is such that symptoms or signs are not manifest. Kahn *et al.* (1967), for example, studied 1277 plant introductions imported as vegetative propagations. Sixty-two percent of these propagations were found to be virus infected, but only a small percentage exhibited symptoms. The lack of international cooperation in the creation and support of quarantine regulations has led to an inefficient and complex worldwide system. Political and special interest groups have all too frequently employed quarantine rules for purposes unrelated to phytosanitation.

C. Investigation of Exotic Disease Agents

A final, and relatively recent, exclusionary measure concerns the appreciation of currently unpossessed disease agents. These efforts are predicated on the idea that we will be best able to exclude those disease agents which we understand.

One very effective means to facilitate the acquisition of pertinent information on foreign diseases is to grow our native species in foreign lands. This procedure would presumably permit the evaluation of the impact of exotic agents on the health of native trees before the problem arises in this country. Efforts to obtain this information have been made. Spaulding (1956) has summarized the diseases of North American forest trees planted in foreign lands. Under the Agricultural Trade Development Act of 1954 (Public Law 480), numerous plantations of our native species have been established abroad (Fowells, 1966). While no epidemics or other major disease phenomena have as yet been recorded, several developing disease situations in Poland, Yugoslavia, and Uruguay are being closely examined.

A second procedure for evaluating foreign disease agents is to import them for intensive study. This effort is best made in some type of isolation laboratory (Miller, 1966). The Committee on an Isolation Laboratory of the American Phytopathological Society has recommended that a laboratory be established and that it be; (1) in an area suitable for the growth of temperate plants, (2) sufficiently remote to minimize danger of accidental distribution by migrating birds and insects, and (3) isolated from tourist routes. A suitably located island may be most practical.

II. SUMMARY

Exclusion is ideally an extremely desirable control technique for mini-mizing disease impact on vegetation. Exotic pathogens, for reasons previ-ously mentioned, are typically the most damaging of all disease agents. Ef-forts to eradicate an established disease agent are rarely successful. Exclusionary methods related to the selection and treatment of planting or reproductive materials and quarantines are comparatively effective, in some instances but, in general, are beset with numerous limitations. Perhaps the greatest potential for exclusion lies in a greater understanding of the biology of foreign disease agents. Exclusion in the past has been concerned with re-striction of intercontinental movements; exclusion in the future will assume a new dimension and be involved with interplanetary migrations (Horowitz et al., 1967; Murray et al., 1967; Sagan et al., 1968).

REFERENCES

Agricultural Research Service. (1962). A reference guide to federal plant quarantines and regulations. *U.S. Dept. Agr., Spec. Rept.* **ARS 22-76**, 1-20.

Food and Agriculture Organization of the U.N. (1964). *FAO/IUFRO Sympo-sium on Internationally Dangerous Forest Diseases and Insects,* Meeting VII-VIII, Vol. II, 20-30 July 1964, Oxford, FAO, Rome.

Fowells, H. A. (1966). Worldwide forestry research. *J. Forestry* **64**, 806-808.

Gram, E. (1960). Quarantines. *In* "Plant Pathology" (J. G. Horsfall and A. E. Dimond, eds.), Vol. 3, p. 313-356. Academic Press, New York.

Hepting, G. H. (1970). How forest disease and insect research is paying off — the case for forest pathology. *J. Forestry* **68**, 78-81.

Hopkins, H. G. (1968). Forest tree seed certification in the Pacific North-west. *J. Forestry* **66**, 400-401.

Horowitz, N. H., Sharp, R. P., and Davies, R. W. (1967). Planetary contami-nation. I. The problem and the agreements. *Science* **155**, 1501-1505.

Jones, L., Barber, J. C., and Mabry, J. E., Jr. (1964). Effect of methyl bromide fumigation on germination of longleaf, slash, and loblolly pine seed. *J. Forestry* **62**, 737-739.

Jones, L., and Havel, K. (1968). Effect of methyl bromide treatments on sev-eral species of conifer seed. *J. Forestry* **66**, 858-860.

Jones, T. W. (1965). An appraisal of oak wilt control programs in eastern United States. *Res. Paper, Central States For. Expt. Sta.,* **CS-19**, 1-24.

Kahn, R. P. *et al.* (1967). Incidence of virus detection in vegetatively propagated plant introductions under quarantine in the U.S., 1957-1967. *Plant Disease Reptr.* **51**, 715-719.

McCubbin, W. A. (1954). "The Plant Quarantine Problem." Chronica Botanica, Waltham, Massachusetts.

Marty, R. (1966). Economic guides for blister-rust control in the East. *Res. Paper, Northeast. Forest Expt. Sta.* **NE-45**, 1-14.

Miller, P. R. (1966). International usefulness of an isolation laboratory for plant pathogens, especially viruses and their vectors. *Plant Disease Reptr.* **50**, 803-805.

Moore, W. C. (1952). Principles underlying plant import and export regulations. *Plant Pathol.* **1**, 15-17.

Murray, B. C., Davies, M. E., and Eckman, P. K. (1967). Planetary contamination. II. Soviet and U.S. practices and policies. *Science* **155**, 1505-1511.

Neely, D. (1967). Dutch elm disease in Illinois cities. *Plant Disease Reptr.* **51**, 511-514.

Peace, T. R. (1962). The inter-continental spread of forest tree diseases. *Proc. 5th World Forestry Congr.,* Vol. 2, pp. 868-872, Aug. 29-Sept. 10, 1960, Seattle, Washington.

Rainwater, H. I., and Smith, C. A. (1966). Quarantines—first line of defense. *In* "Protecting our Food—Yearbook of Agriculture 1966" (J. Hayes, ed.), pp. 216-224. U.S. Govt. Printing Office, Washington, D.C.

Sagan, C., Levinthal, E. C., and Lederberg, J. (1968). Contamination of Mars. *Science* **159**, 1191-1196.

Spaulding, P. (1956). Diseases of North American forest trees planted abroad. *U.S. Dept. Agr., Agr. Handbook* **100**, 1-144.

U.S. Department of Agriculture. (1955). Rules and regulations of Plant Quarantine Branch. Title Y. *In* "The Code of Federal Regulations," Chapter III. U.S. Govt. Printing Office, Washington, D.C.

GENERAL REFERENCES

Beirne, B. P. (1967). "Pest Management." Chem. Rubber Publ. Co., Cleveland, Ohio.

Boyce, J. S. (1961). "Forest Pathology." McGraw-Hill, New York.

Glissow, H. T. (1936). Plant quarantine legislation—a review and a reform. *Phytopathology* **26**, 465-482.

Gram, E. (1955). Barriers and by-passes in plant trade. *Ann. Appl. Biol.* **42**, 76-81.

Imazeki, R. (1962). Introduced diseases with particular attention to the threat they pose forest protection in Asia. *Proc. 5th World Forestry Congr.* Vol. 2, pp. 879-882, Aug. 29-Sept. 10, 1960, Seattle, Washington.

Jones, T. W. (1963). Fumigation may end oak embargoes. *Forest Prod. J.* **13**, 564.

Kahn, R. P. *et al.* (1963). Detection of viruses in foreign plant introduction under quarantine in the United States. *Plant Disease Reptr.* **47**, 261–265.

Kilgore, W. W., and Doutt, R. L., eds. (1967). "Pest Control: Biological, Physical and Selected Chemical Methods." Academic Press, New York.

Krstic, M. M. (1962). The significance of introduced diseases from the European point of view. *Proc. 5th World Forestry Congr.* Vol. 2, pp. 873–879, Aug. 29–Sept. 10, 1960, Seattle, Washington.

Lawrence, A. O. (1963) "The Importance to Forestry of Quarantine Control," Bull. No. 17. Forests Commission of Victoria, Melbourne, Australia.

McCubbin, W. A. (1946). Preventing plant disease introduction. *Botan. Rev.* **12**, 101–139.

Moore, W. C. (1955). The development of international co-operation in crop protection. *Ann. Appl. Biol.* **42**, 67–72.

Ordish, G., and Dufour, D. (1969). Economic bases for protection against plant diseases. *Ann. Rev. Phytopathol.* **7**, 31–50.

Peace, T. R. (1962). "Pathology of Trees and Shrubs," Oxford Univ. Press, London and New York.

Pimentel, D. (1966). Complexity of ecological systems and problems in their study and management. *In* "Systems Analysis in Ecology" (K. E. F. Watt, ed.), pp. 15–35. Academic Press, New York.

Riker, A. J. (1957). The discovery of important diseases before they move from one country to another. *Phytopathology* **47**, 388–389.

Riker, A. J. (1962). Internationally dangerous tree diseases. *Proc. 5th World Forestry Congr.,* Vol. 2, pp. 890–893, Aug. 29–Sept. 10, 1960, Seattle, Washington.

Riker, A. J. (1964). Internationally dangerous tree diseases and Latin America. *J. Forestry* **62**, 229–232.

Soraci, F. A. (1957). Redefinition of the principles of plant quarantine and their relation to the current problems. *Phytopathology* **47**, 381–382.

Spaulding, P. (1958). Diseases of foreign forest trees growing in the United States. *U.S. Dept. Agr., Agr. Handbook* **139**, 1–118.

Stakman, E. C., and Harrar, J. G. (1957). "Principles of Plant Pathology" Ronald Press, New York.

Wheeler, W. H. (1957). The movement of plant pathogens. *Phytopathology* **47**, 386–388.

25

ERADICATION

Control procedures of an eradicative nature exist at the opposite end of the control spectrum, from exclusionary procedures. In the latter instance, the primary objective was to insure that a disease agent was not introduced into an uncontaminated area. In eradication efforts, however, the host is infected and the basic purpose of the control procedure is to rid the host of the disease agent. Activities associated with removing or destroying pathogens in the host, on the host, or even in the area immediately surrounding the host are considered controls of eradicative character. In general, there are four possible eradication procedures: the destruction of diseased individuals, the removal of weed or alternate hosts, therapy, and the disinfestation of the environment.

I. DESTRUCTION OF DISEASED INDIVIDUALS

In situations where many plants are growing in a relatively small area, for example, in a greenhouse or nursery bed, and when the number of diseased plants is only a relatively small percentage of the total population, culling of infected individuals is a relatively efficient and inexpensive eradication method. The procedure depends, of course, on the ability to recognize diseased plants.

Destruction of diseased trees has been widely applied to combat tree maladies. Frequently this culling operation is integrated into a regular thinning or other timber-stand improvement operation. Disease agents whose movement from tree to tree is relatively slow, for example, *Ceratocystis faga-cearum, Nectria* spp., and *Arceuthobium* spp., may be effectively contained by removing diseased hosts.

The ideal eradication effort results in the complete removal of a disease agent from an area of susceptible hosts. This objective is very rarely realized. Two instances where this ideal has been attained, however, concern tree diseases.

The classic example of a complete eradication effort is the removal of *Xanthomonas citri* from the United States (Sinclair, 1968). This virulent bacterium, which causes citrus canker, was introduced into the Gulf States from Japan in 1910 on root-stocks of Satsuma and trifoliate orange. Soon after the disease caused by *X. citri* was recognized, seven southern states and the U.S. Department of Agriculture initiated an eradication campaign. Over the ensuing years, millions of diseased trees were destroyed in active and abandoned groves, ornamental situations, and wild habitats. Quarantines and mass eradications were followed by numerous surveys to detect infected individuals. Florida, which was the primary focus of infection, has been free of citrus canker since 1927. Louisiana and Texas, which were the last two states to eradicate *X. citri*, have been free from citrus canker since 1941 and 1940, respectively.

A second, less dramatic, complete eradication effort involved the removal of *Dasyscypha willkommii* (Ascomycete) from eastern Massachusetts. This fungus, which produces a canker disease of larch species, causes serious losses to larch in Europe. In 1927, *D. willkommii* was found in two Massachusetts localities infecting European larch which had been introduced some time previously from Great Britain. All infected trees were promptly destroyed. The fungus was subsequently detected in 1935 and 1952 on European larch in the same localities and again diseased individuals were removed. The absence since 1952 of *D. willkommii* from introduced larch has led to the presumption that this organism has been eradicated.

Eradication efforts, even if they result in less than complete removal of a disease agent, may play important roles in control programs. The standard treatment for Dutch elm disease, for example, involves destroying diseased trees and parts of trees in an effort to restrict the spread of *Ceratocystis ulmi*. Actually, shortly after the introduction of *C. ulmi* in the early 1930's, intensive eradicatory programs were initiated in an attempt to completely eliminate this destructive fungus. Even though complete eradication was not obtained, the current practice of destroying diseased trees (and infected tree parts) is thought to very significantly contribute to the overall containment of *C. ulmi* (Miller et al., 1969).

One of the most notable failures of eradicatory attempts was that applied to *Endothia parasitica*, the causal agent of chestnut blight. During the course of the chestnut blight epidemic, thousands of chestnut trees were destroyed and large isolation zones were made in an effort to restrict the movement of the pathogen. All efforts met with failure, perhaps largely because of the efficient distribution of *E. parasitica* spore types and saprophytic maintenance of the fungus on several oak species.

II. REMOVAL OF ALTERNATE OR WEED HOSTS

Several disease agents and numerous insect pests require two different hosts in order to complete their life cycles. Eradication of these stress-inducing agents may be realized by destroying their alternate hosts and thus interfering with normal life-cycle processes.

An example of this type of eradicatory procedure is the destruction of currants and gooseberries (*Ribes* spp.) in an effort to control white pine blister rust caused by *Cronartium ribicola*. If suitable weather conditions prevail, basidiospores of *C. ribicola* are formed on the leaves of *Ribes* bushes. These spores, which initiate pine infection, are relatively short-lived and are not carried great distances by wind or other natural agencies. In the eastern United States, therefore, it has been found possible to control white pine blister rust by eliminating currants and gooseberries in a zone of approximately 1000 feet surrounding a pine stand. Isolation zones in the west have typically been slightly larger. In general, the goal has been to reduce the *Ribes* density to roughly 1-25 feet of live stem per acre. The self-incompatibility of currants and gooseberries results in low fruit production in sparse stands. Unfortunately, however, *Ribes* removal must be conducted on a continuing basis, as the few seeds which are produced may remain viable for extended periods in the forest litter and germinate following a disturbance, and because the plants sprout vigorously from the crown. Initially, *Ribes* removal was accomplished primarily by hand pulling or other mechanical means. More recently, in comparatively high value white pine areas, herbicides have been employed to destroy the alternate host plants.

Alternate host eradication presents little problem when one of the hosts lacks economic value or is in other ways relatively insignificant. This is clearly the instance in the white pine–*Ribes* spp. situation. In the case of *Gymnosporangium juniperi-virginianae*, however, this heteroecious fungus alternates between the cultivated apple and eastern red cedar. In this situation, both hosts are damaged by the fungus and both hosts may have economic worth in certain locations. Since effective control can be accomplished only by separating the alternate hosts by distances ranging from 1-8 miles, conflicts have been known to arise. It has been necessary for some states to pass legislation requiring the destruction of all cedars within specified distances of apple orchards.

Control by destroying "*alternate*" hosts is not restricted to heteroecious fungi. The control of many broad host spectrum disease agents may be assisted by destroying *alternative* hosts, especially if these alternative hosts are weeds or otherwise have relatively low value. The occurrence of *Macrophomina phaseoli* on weed hosts near California forest-tree nurseries has been thought undesirable as this may result in more efficient dispersal and increased soil inoculum (Ghaffar and Zentmyer, 1968). Eradication of susceptible weeds may be a necessary part of any effort to control *M. phaseoli* infection of tree seedlings in California nurseries.

III. THERAPY

Therapeutic measures applied to diseased plants have especial significance in the case of trees. The long-lived character and occasional high value of individual trees makes the consideration of therapy a relevant topic. This control technique is one of the newest employed to combat plant diseases. Presumably, as our knowledge of the biochemical nature and mechanisms of disease processes increases, we will be better able to develop and apply therapeutic methods to eradicate pathogens from infected hosts.

Therapy may be broadly divided into two subcategories. Techniques which involve surgery, environmental modification, or radiation treatment are termed physical therapy. Chemotherapy refers to the use of chemicals, either topically or systemically, in an effort to rid a host of a particular disease agent. A good review of therapeutic practices in plant disease control is available (Howard and Horsfall, 1959).

A. Physical Therapy

1. Surgery.   The removal of infected plant parts is a widely practiced control procedure in perennial plants. With relatively slow-moving localized pathogens, removal of the tissues which contain the disease agent is presumed capable of curing the diseased specimen. This practice is widely applied in treating tree diseases.

The pruning of infected branches is a widely used method of impairing the spread of dwarf mistletoe in coniferous stands in the western United States. Wilt diseases of angiosperms, for example, *Verticillium* wilt of Norway maple, is occasionally treated by pruning wilted branches. The removal of branches of pear trees several inches below the area of visible fire blight symptoms is practiced in an attempt to avoid the expansion of the causal bacterium *Erwinia amylovora*.

The removal of diseased branches infected with *Ceratocystis ulmi* has for many years been an integral component of Dutch elm disease control programs. This practice may have an ecological disadvantage, however, as Hart et al. (1967) have suggested that volatile materials released from the severed branch stubs may act to attract bark-beetle vectors.

A certain amount of physical therapy may be naturally obtained from the pruning and breakage of injured or diseased limbs and other parts by the wind and by animals. N. A. Anderson *et al.* (1967) have observed rodents feeding on the pycnia of *Peridermium stalactiforme* (Basidiomycete) formed on the canker margins of infected jack pines. In certain instances, this feeding appears to have arrested canker development and may represent an example of physical therapy unrelated to the activities of man.

2. Environmental modification. The manipulation of some physical parameter, for example, temperature or humidity, is occasionally employed to free an infected, mature host from a particular disease agent. As in the case of pest exclusion from plant materials destined for reproductive function (seeds, cuttings), heat is occasionally used to rid plants of biotic disease agents. If differential tolerance of host and disease agent to heat exists, as in certain virus diseases, then this practice may and does have practical application.

Moisture modification is also commonly practiced in physical therapy. Most disease agents require relatively high humidity environments for optimal development. Procedures acting to reduce the relative humidity of the climate of a pathogen generally inhibits the growth of the pathogen. The painting and draining of basal tree wounds, for example, acts to lower the moisture content of the wounded area and restrict the development of wood-decay fungi.

Moisture contents inside plants also are intimately associated with the development of internal pathogens. The effects of intercellular humidities, however, are complicated by their direct correlation with oxygen tension. In the range of certain moisture contents, for example, reduced humidities may favor pathogen development by permitting access to greater oxygen concentrations.

3. Radiation treatment. Numerous types of radiation have been proposed for use in treatment of plant maladies. None, however, have proved practically successful (Howard and Horsfall, 1959).

Ultraviolet radiation, because of its general adverse effect on microbial populations, has often been proposed as a therapeutic device. This radiation is extremely toxic because of its capacity to influence protein and nucleic acid structure. The shorter ultraviolet wavelengths, approximately 240 μ, are most effective. Microbial toxicity decreases as the wavelength increases up through 365 μ, the approximate upper limit of effectiveness. The inability of ultraviolet radiation to penetrate significantly beneath plant surfaces may be a primary factor in its relative therapeutic uselessness.

Infrared radiation in the 800–900 μ range has been employed to rid prepared food materials of contaminating microorganisms. It has not, however, been utilized to rid growing plants of pathogens.

Ionizing radiation has been successfully employed as a treatment for animal diseases. Several experimental applications have been attempted in the case of plant diseases. In the application of ionizing radiation to pathogenic nematodes, it has been found that relatively high doses are required for a lethal effect. The lethal range precludes the use on plants containing nematodes, as the plants would be injured at levels necessary to destroy the worms. Generally, the susceptibility of fungal disease agents has been shown to be lower than the susceptibility of the host plant to ionizing radiation. In general, however, nonselectivity, cost, and potential danger to the user have restricted the application of ionizing radiations to the treatment of diseased plants. Radiation, especially of the ionizing type, may ultimately become an effective instrument in plant disease control.

B. Chemotherapy

Chemical therapy involves the use of chemicals which, by virtue of their action on the host or pathogen, will negate the effect of a pathogen established in a host plant. Chemotherapeutants may be employed as topicals or systemics. Topical chemotherapy is the use of chemicals to destroy pathogens which injure only surface cells or localized areas of tissue. This is the older form of chemotherapy and has been used for many years to eradicate plant pathogens. Treatment of tree leaves with a fungicide to eliminate powdery mildew (caused by several Ascomycetes) is a form of topical chemotherapy. Another recent example has been reported by Wilson (1968). In this instance applications after leaf fall of the eradicant fungicide sodium pentachlorophenate to apple trees affected by European canker disease acted to suppress initiation of perithecia and conidial development by the causal agent, Nectria galligena. Systemic chemotherapy is the use of chemicals which become internally distributed within the infected plant and act to minimize or eliminate disease development.

The basic principle of chemotherapy involves selective toxicity; the chemical must be detrimental to the pathogen and innocuous to the host. This characteristic distinguishes chemotherapeutants from protectants as the latter are typically toxic to pathogens but also poorly tolerated or even toxic to the hosts (Jawetz et al., 1966).

Entomologists have successfully employed numerous systemic materials to control insect pests. Pathologists, however, have only a few compounds which have shown promise as effective chemotherapeutants.

1. Chemotherapeutants and fruit tree disease. Considerable research has been directed at finding systemic chemicals which have effectiveness against diseases of high-value fruit tree hosts. Cycloheximide acetate, cycloheximide thiosemicarbazone (Williams and Helton, 1967), and Omadine-

1484 (sodium 2-pyridinethiol, 1-oxide) (Helton and Rohrback, 1967), when used systemically, have been shown to have a suppressing influence on *Cytospora cincta* (Deuteromycete) which causes a canker disease of peach. None of these compounds acted as a systemic eradicant of *C. cincta*. Cycloheximide thiosemicarbazone and 8-quinolinol benzoate have been shown to have a comparable influence on the development of *C. cincta* in prune (Helton and Kochan, 1967b, 1968). In cherry trees artificially inoculated with *Agrobacterium tumefaciens*, cycloheximide thiosemicarbazone and cycloheximide acetate treatments appeared to have a curative influence (Helton and Williams, 1968).

    2. Chemotherapeutants and forest tree disease. The application of two antibiotics, cycloheximide and phytoactin, has been employed as a chemotherapeutic treatment for several forest tree diseases.

    Cycloheximide, whose trade name is Acti-dione, has the following structure:

Cycloheximide

This antiobiotic, which is obtained from certain strains of the actinomycete *Streptomyces griseus*, is very active against many fungi and quite ineffective against most bacteria. Fungal toxicity may result from interference with protein synthesis. Cycloheximide has been shown capable of systemic movement in northern pin oak (Phelps and Kuntz, 1965), and in eastern white pine (Phelps and Weber, 1967). When applied in fuel oil to aspen trees infected with *Hypoxylon pruinatum*, cycloheximide appeared capable of containing canker development and improving tree survival (Brown and Silverborg, 1968). *In vitro* tests have shown cycloheximide very toxic to the extremely important root rotting fungus, *Armillaria mellea* (Cheo, 1968).

    Phytoactin is obtained from an unidentified species of *Streptomyces*. It is a noncyclic polypeptide consisting of valine, α-alanine, proline, leucine or isoleucine, arginine, glycine, and serine (Lynch and Sisler, 1967). In culture the compound is toxic to many plant pathogenic fungi and bacteria. Toxicity may result from an interference with RNA synthesis. As in the case of cycloheximide, Phelps and Weber (1967) have shown that phytoactin can move systemically in eastern white pine.

Over the past several years, numerous experimental attempts have been made in an effort to control rust diseases of pines by employing aerial or basal applications of cycloheximide and phytoactin (Benedict, 1966). The evidence accumulated, occasionally somewhat controversial, has generally been interpreted as suggesting that these materials are not practically useful to eradicate rust fungi (G. W. Anderson et al., 1968; Brown and Dooling, 1968; Dimond, 1966; Leaphart and Wicker, 1968; Phelps and Weber, 1968).

3. Some new chemotherapeutants. Dimethyl sulfoxide (DMSO) is a remarkable solvent currently receiving considerable attention in human medicine. This material is derived primarily from lignin in the manufacture of paper (Leake, 1966). Helton and Kochan (1967a) employed DMSO as a solvent for several chemotherapeutants and then evaluated the abilities of the materials to influence *Cytospora* canker disease of prune. The effects of DMSO were variable. In certain instances, DMSO appeared to enhance the therapeutic effect of the fungicide, and in other cases it seemed to aggravate the disease. In experiments with young peach trees, Pine (1967) concluded that injections of DMSO had to be less than 0.5 molar concentration if permanent injury to the tree was to be avoided. This investigator also observed that DMSO appeared to have a virustatic (not viruscidal) influence on peach mosaic virus and necrotic ring spot virus.

Edginton and Barron (1967) have recently reported that the oxathiin compound (2,3-dihydro-5-carboxanilido-6-methyl-1,4-oxathiin) is a systemic in plants and extremely toxic to Basidiomycetes. In awareness of the important role these organisms play in forest tree disease, oxathiin materials may prove promising for tree disease control programs.

The possibility that certain hydrocarbons may be effective chemotherapeutants was suggested by the work of Schroth and Hildebrand (1968). An oil-water emulsion containing 1,2,3,4-tetrahydronaphthalene, diphenylmethane, dimethylnaphthalene, 2,4-xylenol, and *m*-cresol selectively destroyed gall tissue caused by *Agrobacterium tumefaciens* on almond, peach, apricot, plum, cherry, and pear and by *Pseudomonas savastanoi* on olive.

4. Future of systemic chemotherapeutants. Chemotherapeutants which act systemically have very great potential for future plant disease control efforts. Their ability to mitigate the influence of a pathogen or actually eradicate it *after* infection is a unique advantage. In general, the use of systemic compounds may result in less environmental contamination and interference with nontarget organisms, if they can be injected or otherwise introduced directly into the tree, then may accrue from broadcast spraying.

There are, however, three primary problems associated with developing practically useful chemotherapeutants; (*1*) entrance into plant, (*2*) translocation, and (3) selective toxicity. Three primary routes exist for entrance: stem, foliage, and root. Mechanical injection into the stem is commonly efficient, but generally quite costly. Entrance through the leaves typically necessitates the undesirable practice of broadcast spray application and involves inefficient downward movement. Materials designed to enter through the roots may be relatively inexpensively applied but are, unfortunately, subject to numerous subtractive influences. Compounds may, for example, be unduly diluted by the time they reach the root due to adsorption by soil particles, chemical alteration by physical soil factors, and biological degradation.

Translocation of systemic chemicals is much less efficient in plants than in animals. Lacking a circulatory system, plants generally only poorly distribute chemicals uniformly to all organs. The upward translocation system operates appreciably more effectively than the downward or lateral systems. Application of a chemotherapeutant to the root may result in reasonable distribution throughout the crown of a tree. Foliar applications, in contrast, may result in little downward distribution. Of necessity, of course, chemotherapeutants must be innocuous to the host. In addition, the character of the systemic should be such that host metabolism does not function to reduce its microbial toxicity.

Finding and developing chemicals which avoid the above problems and which are relatively inexpensive and have relatively low mammalian and avian toxicity has been a slow process. Continued effort is justified, nevertheless, in view of the advantages systemic chemotherapeutants offer.

IV. DISINFESTATION OF THE ENVIRONMENT

The final control procedure considered to be eradicatory in nature is the destruction of all pathogens in a given area. This method is not commonly employed and generally is restricted to greenhouse or nursery situations. Generally, the technique involves the use of a relatively potent biocide to rid soil or some other medium of all potentially dangerous biotic agents. Domsch (1964) has reviewed the area of soil fungicides.

The use of this procedure is sufficiently drastic and poorly understood to potentially result in unanticipated and undesirable consequences. The use of broad spectrum materials in nematode eradication, for example, may not restrict the ultimate development of damaging nematode populations (Harrison, 1967).

V. SUMMARY

Eradication via the removal of infected individuals and destruction of alternate hosts has been relatively widely applied in the control of numerous forest tree disorders. The development of efficient therapeutic techniques has very great potential for treating tree diseases. The availability of low-cost, nontoxic systemic chemotherapeutants will be a primary objective of future tree disease control research.

REFERENCES

Anderson, G. W., Anderson, R. L., French, D. W., and Flink, P. R. (1968). Antibiotic treatments to prevent stem rusts on jack pine seedlings in nursery seedbeds. *Plant Disease Reptr.* **52**, 538-541.

Anderson, N. A., French, D. W., and Anderson, R. L. (1967). The stalactiform rust on jack pine. *J. Forestry* **65**, 398-402.

Benedict, W. V. (1966). Experience with antibiotics to control white pine blister rust. *J. Forestry* **64**, 382-384.

Brown, D. H., and Dooling, O. J. (1968). Helicopter application of phytoactin to whitebark pine. *Phytopathology* **58**, 1045 (abstr.).

Brown, D. H., and Silverborg, S. B. (1968). Chemical treatment of *Hypoxylon* cankers on aspen. *Phytopathology* **58**, 1045 (abstr.).

Cheo, P. C. (1968). Control of *Armillaria mellea* with systemic chemicals. *Plant Disease Reptr.* **52**, 639-651.

Dimond, A. E. (1966). Effectiveness of antibiotics against forest tree rusts. *J. Forestry* **64**, 379-382.

Domsch, K. H. (1964). Soil fungicides. *Ann. Rev. Phytopathol.* **2**, 293-320.

Edginton, L. V., and Barron, G. L. (1967). Fungitoxic spectrum of oxathiin compounds. *Phytopathology* **57**, 1256-1257.

Ghaffar, A., and Zentmyer, G. A. (1968). *Macrophomina phaseoli* on some new weed hosts in California. *Plant Disease Reptr.* **52**, 223.

Harrison, M. B. (1967). Influence of nematocidal treatments on nematode populations. *Phytopathology* **57**, 650-652.

Hart, J. H., Wallner, W. E., Caris, M. R., and Dennis, G. K. (1967). Increase in Dutch elm disease associated with summer trimming. *Plant Disease Reptr.* **51**, 476-479.

Helton, A. W., and Kochan, W. J. (1967a). Chemotherapeutic effects of cycloheximide thiosemicarbazone, phytoactin, and 8-quinolinol benzoate, with and without dimethyl sulfoxide and pruning, on the Cytospora canker disease of trees. *Plant Disease Reptr.* **51**, 340-344.

Helton, A. W., and Kochan, W. J. (1967b). First and second year effects on Cytospora canker disease of "Italian" prune trees sprayed with four concentrations of cycloheximide thiosemicarbazone. *Plant Disease Reptr.* **51**, 655-658.

Helton, A. W., and Kochan, W. J. (1968). Systemic-chemical paints for the control of Cytospora canker disease in prune trees. *Plant Disease Reptr.* **52**, 154-157.

Helton, A. W., and Rohrbach, K. G. (1967). Chemotherapy of Cytospora canker disease in peach trees. *Phytopathology* **57**, 442–446.

Helton, A. W., and Williams, R. W. (1968). Control of aerial crown-gall disease in cherry trees with spray-applied systemic fungicides. *Phytopathology* **58**, 782–787.

Howard, F. L., and Horsfall, J. G. (1959). Therapy. *In* "Plant Pathology" (J. G. Horsfall and A. E. Dimond, eds.), Vol. 1, pp. 563–604. Academic Press, New York.

Jawetz, E., Melnick, J. L., and Adelberg, E. A. (1966). "Review of Medical Microbiology." Lange Med. Publ., Los Altos, California.

Leake, C. D. (1966). Dimethyl sulfoxide. *Science* **152**, 1646–1649.

Leaphart, C. D., and Wicker, E. F. (1968). The ineffectiveness of cyclohex-imide and phytoactin as chemical controls of the blister rust disease. *Plant Disease Reptr.* **52**, 6–10.

Lynch, J. P., and Sisler, H. D. (1967). Mechanism of action of phytoactin in *Saccharomyces pastorianus. Phytopathology* **57**, 367–373.

Miller, H. C., Silverborg, S. B., and Campana, R. J. (1969). Dutch elm disease: Relation of spread and intensification to control by sanitation in Syracuse, New York. *Plant Disease Reptr.* **53**, 551–555.

Phelps, W. R., and Kuntz, J. E. (1965). Translocation and persistence of cyclo-heximide and oligomycin in northern pin oaks. *Forest Sci.* **11**, 353–359.

Phelps, W. R., and Weber, R. (1967). Translocation and persistence of cyclo-heximide and phytoactin in eastern white pine. *Forest Sci.* **13**, 90–94.

Phelps, W. R., and Weber, R. (1968). Antibiotics do not control blister rust in eastern white pine seedlings. *Res. Note, North Central Forest Expt. Sta.,* **NC-52**, 1–3.

Pine, T. S. (1967). Reactions of peach trees and peach tree viruses to treatment with dimethyl sulfoxide and other chemicals. *Phytopathology* **57**, 671–673.

Schroth, M. N., and Hildebrand, D. C. (1968). A chemotherapeutic treatment for selectively eradicating crown gall and olive knot neoplasms. *Phytopathology* **58**, 848–854.

Sinclair, J. B. (1968). Eradication of citrus canker from Louisiana. *Plant Disease Reptr.* **52**, 667–670.

Williams, R. E., and Helton, A. W. (1967). Prevention and cure of Cytospora canker disease of peach trees with systemic chemicals. *Plant Disease Reptr.* **51**, 834–838.

Wilson, E. E. (1968). Control of European canker of apple by eradicative and protective fungicides. *Plant Disease Reptr.* **52**, 277–231.

GENERAL REFERENCES

Baker, K. F., and Fuller, W. H. (1969). Soil treatment by microwave energy to destroy plant pathogens. *Phytopathology* **59**, 193-197.

Benedict, W. G. (1969). Effect of aureofungin on Dutch elm disease. *Phytopathology* **59**, 516-517.

Brown, D. H. (1969). Aerial application of antibiotic solutions to whitebark pine infected with *Cronartium ribicola*. *Plant Disease Reptr.* **53**, 487-489.

Harvey, A. E. (1967). Effect of phytoactin treatment on mycorrhizal-root associations in western white pine. *Plant Disease Reptr.* **51**, 1012-1013.

Howe, R. G. (1965) Application of biocides in forest nurseries. *Proc. Nursery Soil Improvement Sessions,* pp. 57-63, Jan. 25-28, 1965, *Syracuse Univ., Syracuse, N.Y.*

Mathie, D. E. (1968). Uptake and binding of oxathiin systemic fungicides by resistant and sensitive fungi. *Phytopathology* **58**, 1464-1469.

Nyland, G. (1969). Heat therapy of virus diseases of perennial plants. *Ann. Rev. Phytopathol.* **7**, 331-354.

Offord, H. R. (1962). New approaches to forest disease control by chemicals. *Proc. 5th World Forestry Cong.* Vol. 2, pp. 882-887, Aug. 29-Sept. 10, 1960, Seattle, Washington.

Phelps, W. R., and Weber, R. (1969). An evaluation of chemotherapeutants for control of blister rust cankers in eastern white pine. *Plant Disease Reptr.* **53**, 514-517.

Pramer, D. (1961). Eradicant and therapeutic materials for disease control. Antibiotics. *In* "Recent Advances in Botany," p. 452-456. Vol. I, IX Inter. Bot. Cong., Montreal 1959, Univ. of Toronto Press, Toronto.

Ram, C. S. V. (1969). Systemic control of *Exobasidium vexans* on tea with 1,4-oxathiin derivatives. *Phytopathology* **59**, 125-128.

Rich, S., ed. (1963). Perspectives of biochemical plant pathology. *Conn. Agr. Exptl. Sta. New Haven, Bull.* **663**, 1-191.

Roberts, B. R., and Stipes, R. J. (1969). Response of American elm seedlings to treatment with captan and cycloheximide. *Forest Sci.* **15**, 97-91.

Schmid, W. E. (1968). On the effects of DMSO in cation transport by excised barley roots. *Am. J. Botany* **55**, 757-761.

Schreiber, L. R. (1969). A method for the injection of chemicals into trees. *Plant Disease Reptr.* **53**, 764-765.

Stakman, E. C., and Harrar, J. G. (1967). "Plant Pathology," Ronald Press, New York.

White, D. P. (1965). Biocides in forest nursery management. *Proc. Nursery Soil Improvement Sessions,* pp. 51-56, Jan. 25-28, 1965, *Syracuse Univ., Syracuse, N.Y.*

26

PROTECTION

Protective control procedures are those which are employed when a stress factor cannot be excluded or eradicated from an area containing vulnerable plants. Protection is employed only when the plants are uninfluenced (abiotic stress factors) or uninfected (biotic disease agents) but where the possibility of undesirable consequences exists. Protection may be achieved, in the case of biotic disease agents, by directly controlling the agent or indirectly by controlling a necessary vector.

Four primary control practices are considered capable of providing protection from disease; environmental modification, silvicultural practices, biological protection, and chemical protection.

I. ENVIRONMENTAL MODIFICATION

As in eradication, environmental modification is employed as a protective device to control certain plant stress factors. In fruit tree orchards, for example, large fans are occasionally employed to circulate the air and preclude the development of freezing air temperatures. Portable heaters are also employed in these orchards for a similar purpose.

Environmental modification is, however, not widely applicable to forest trees. Examples, nevertheless, can be found in greenhouse and nursery situations. In these, efforts to regulate the amount of moisture and light in the seedling environment are frequently employed primarily to avoid injury or infection. In certain high-value mature tree stands, for example, seed orchards, some environmental modifications, similar to those employed in fruit tree orchards, may be justified.

II. SILVICULTURAL PRACTICES

The use of cultural practices to protect plants from injury and infection may be relatively inexpensive and has been widely employed to control tree diseases.

A. Selection of Planting Site

When the opportunity exists to select an area in which trees are to be grown, pathological considerations should be taken into account. Meaningful thought employed on the pathological consequences of a planting site is quite inexpensive and may result in significant savings at a later point in the rotation.

In the case of abiotic stress factors, numerous examples might be mentioned. Low-temperature stress is easily avoided. We recognize, for example, that frost injury is more frequent in certain topographic situations; for example, valleys, depressions, and northern slopes. These areas should be avoided when planting species susceptible to low-temperature damage.

Wind stress is another abiotic factor whose influence may be mitigated by appropriate site selection. Trousdell (1965) studied the damage occasioned by hurricane Donna to recently thinned loblolly pine stands in the coastal plain of Virginia and North Carolina. Trees that were wind thrown, broken, or displaced were considered damaged. Damage was more severe on soils having moderately coarse textured profiles than on soils with finer textured profiles. The most severely damaged stands were those located on soils which contained a restrictive layer which presumably retarded root development. In the establishment of comparatively high-value tree stands, for example, seed orchards or production areas, it would be well to avoid soils which would contribute to a lack of wind firmness. Planting species especially susceptible to wind injury in regions of frequent wind-storm occurrence or generally exposed situations is equally undesirable.

Losses due to biotic agents can also be avoided or lessened by careful planting site selection. Van Arsdel's research (Chapter 22) suggests, for example, that areas in southern Wisconsin where the cool fall temperatures are interrupted by warm periods are more desirable for white pine establishment than more continually cool locations. The latter sites have a higher incidence of *Cronartium ribicola* infections.

In the southeastern United States, the incidence of root disease in conifers caused by *Fomes annosus* has been slower to develop in plantations established on land previously supporting hardwoods than on land previously cropped to conifers. The advantage of establishing a pine plantation on ex-hardwood sites presumably involves the exposure of the pines to less *F. annosus* inoculum.

B. Selection of Silvicultural Method

Once a stand has been established, or in managing an older forest, the silvicultural manipulations employed may significantly influence disease development.

An example of the consideration of silvicultural methods used in forest regeneration and tree stresses has been given by Tryon (1966). This silviculturist considered the influence of uneven-aged (selection or group selection) and even-aged (clear-cut or shelterwood) regeneration methods on abiotic and biotic stresses of tree species of the eastern United States. The author concluded that the influence of frost, glaze, drought, and heat injury to a developing stand could be reduced by the appropriate selection of a regeneration technique (Table XXVII).

Selection cutting in an uneven-aged stand was suggested as most desirable to minimize frost, drought, and heat injury presumably due to avoidance of the creation of cold microsites and undue exposure to drying and heating forces, respectively. The reasons for selecting a clear-cut even-aged system to reproduce trees under glaze stress are less clear, especially in view of the suggestion that reproduction under snow stress is unaffected by regeneration method.

With regard to biotic agents, Tryon considered oak wilt, wood decay, dampingoff, blister rust, and root rot caused by *Fomes annosus* all amenable to reduction by the selection of the proper regeneration method (Table XXVIII). Clear cutting even-aged stands was deemed optimal for minimizing the effects of all of the above except blister rust. Clear cutting would presum-

TABLE XXVII

SUGGESTED METHODS OF OBTAINING NATURAL REGENERATION IN FOREST STANDS TO MINIMIZE DAMAGE BY ABIOTIC STRESS FACTORS[a,b]

Disease or agent	No apparent difference	Uneven aged		Even aged		Comments
		Selection	Group selection	Clear cut	Shelter wood	
Frost		1st	2nd			Groups < 1/4 acre
Glaze				1st		
Drought						Or even aged with heavy
(as oak decline)	2nd	1st				thinning near maturity
Heat injury						
(hardwood seedlings)	2nd	1st			2nd	
Snow	1st					Not serious with hardwoods
Wind	1st					
Lightning	1st					

[a]From Tryon (1966). Reproduced by permission of the author.

[b]1st = preferred method; 2nd = second choice.

TABLE XXVIII

SUGGESTED METHODS OF OBTAINING NATURAL REGENERATION
IN FOREST STANDS TO MINIMIZE DAMAGE BY BIOTIC STRESS
FACTORS[a,b]

Disease or organism	No apparent difference	Uneven aged		Even aged		Comments
		Selection	Group selection	Clear cut	Shelter wood	
Oak wilt	2nd			1st		
Heartrots				1st	2nd	Avoid skidding and felling damage
Seedling diseases of hardwoods, such as damping off				1st	2nd	Limited knowledge
White pine blister rust	2nd				1st	To reduce *Ribes* abundance
Fomes annosus	2nd			1st		With additional direct control
Black knot	1st	2nd	2nd			Favor mixed stands, could reduce cherry abundance (selection)
Dutch elm disease	1st	2nd				Favor mixed stands, could reduce elm abundance (selection)
Strumella canker	1st			2nd		
Nectria canker	1st					
Chestnut blight	1st					
Beech bark disease	1st					

[a]From Tryon (1966). Reproduced by permission of the author.
[b]1st = preferred method; 2nd = second choice.

ably reduce the amount of residual inoculum of *Ceratocystis fagacearum* and *Fomes annosus* and thereby reduce the possibility of oak wilt and root rot in the new stand. Wood decay of crop trees would be lessened as no infection courts due to harvest activities would be created. Dampingoff might be minimized since a generally drier environment for seedlings would exist and possibly because developing seedlings would be more vigorous in the presence of more light. The suggestion that the damage resulting from *Cronartium ribicola* infection may be minimized by employing a shelterwood even-aged system may be predicated on the apparent intolerance of many eastern *Ribes* spp.

The selection of specific silvicultural techniques in the management of forest areas, like rotation length determination, is based on a multitude of biological and economic factors. Nevertheless, consideration of the pathological consequences of silvicultural practices should be made. This effort is one of the most inexpensive disease control mechanisms and may provide significant tree disease protection.

III. BIOLOGICAL PROTECTION

The protection of plants from undesirable consequences "biologically" is possible where the stress factor is living. Biotic agents themselves typically have a multitude of natural enemies, antagonists, or competitors. The manipulation of one or more of these interfering organisms to the detriment of a biotic stress agent has generally, but not exclusively, constituted biological control.

Entomologists have been particularly successful in taking advantage of these naturally occurring relationships to reduce insect impact on certain crop plants. Recently, a French wasp *Dendrosoter protuberans* was introduced into this country. In order to obtain their food, the larvae of this wasp parasitize the larvae of elm bark beetles. Tests are currently being made to evaluate the capacity of *D. protuberans* to reduce the population of bark beetles as a possible means to reduce the distribution of *Ceratocystis ulmi.*

Pathologists, in general, have enjoyed somewhat less success in pitting one biological system against another than have entomologists. Darpoux (1960), however, has reviewed the numerous biological constraints imposed on plant pathogens by other organisms. The possibility that some of these constraints may be able to be incorporated into practical control programs is very real.

Timonin (1966), in a study of the rhizosphere populations of healthy and diseased lodgepole pine seedlings, found that the rhizospheres of the latter contained a denser microbial population than the former. More significantly, perhaps, was the observation that the incidence of spore-forming bacteria antagonistic to *Fusarium culmorum* and *Rhizoctonia solani* was approximately six times greater in the rhizospheres of healthy seedlings. Much more information would be required to permit the suggestion that the bacteria were performing a protective function.

Fomes annosus, which is a vigorous colonizer of coniferous heartwood, has only limited ability to compete effectively with many associated fungi. The inability of *F. annosus* to become established on stump surfaces several weeks old, for example, is presumed due to the intense competition provided on these surfaces by other fungi previously established. Meredith (1959, 1960) observed that the fungus *Peniophora gigantea* (Basidiomycete) was a vigorous competitor of *F. annosus.* Rishbeth (1961, 1963) found that inoculation of Scotch and Austrian pine stumps with spores of *P. gigantea* prevented establishment of *F. annosus.* Other investigators have also presented evidence indicating the ability of *P. gigantea* to suppress the development of *F. annosus* in field and laboratory observations (Curl and Arnold 1964; Gremmen, 1963; Hodges, 1964; Negruckij, 1963).

Other microorganisms which have been shown to have some inhibitory influence on the growth of *F. annosus* are *Trichoderma* spp. (Boyce, 1963;

Negruckij, 1963; Persson-Hüppel, 1963) and *Streptomyces griseus* (Gundersen, 1961, 1962). There is little doubt that these and other natural antagonists play an important role in limiting the growth of *F. annosus* in nature. The artificial manipulation of these competitors for *F. annosus* control, however, currently has only limited application because of the equipment, skills, and costs required for their handling.

Numerous other potentially significant biological control mechanisms, for example, the importance of *Tuberculina maxima* (Basidiomycete) as a hyperparasite of *Cronartium ribicola* in western white pine cankers (Dimond, 1966) or the importance of mycorrhizal fungi in protecting mycorrhizal roots (Zak, 1964) should be mentioned. The attractiveness and potential of biological control procedures, however, are not equalled by their practicality. To date, for example, no very useful biological control system has been developed and applied to the treatment of any forest tree disease or any other plant disease. Presumably, the failure to realize practical biological control schemes stems, in large measure, from the fact that most biological systems are well buffered. "Buffering," in this sense, means that these systems have gradually evolved a certain stability and that they are quite resistant to any radical changes. Unfortunately, biological control procedures frequently involve radical change; for example, the introduction of an exotic organism or the unnatural increase in the size of a native population. All too often changes of this type are made with incomplete research and information on, for example, the influence of environmental stresses or native enemies on an introduced organism or undesirable side effects of increasing indiginous populations of undetrimental organisms to unnatural and possibly detrimental levels. The desirability of biological protection, on the other hand, especially when compared to chemical protection, more than justifies continued research on the former.

IV. CHEMICAL PROTECTION

The use of chemicals to protect plants from biotic stress agents is widespread in agricultural practice. In efforts to control disease agents, nematocides, bactericides, and fungicides have been applied to plants or to the environments in which plants grow. Of the pesticides employed in plant disease control, fungicides are the most extensively employed. Agriculturists in the United States use approximately $100 million worth of fungicides per year (Rich, 1966). The use of chemical protectants in forest tree disease control has not been great. The employment of these materials in certain phases of forest tree culture, however, is increasing. The fungicide ferbam, for example, is applied to developing pine strobili in slash pine seed orchards to protect them from *Cronartium strobilinum*, the causal agent of southern cone rust (Matthews, 1964). In all probability, the use of chemicals to facilitate forest tree disease control will become more extensive as the value of trees increases.

Fungicides, as used in this discussion, are chemicals which are capable of killing fungi and which are applied to plants to protect them from fungal pathogens. The materials are typically applied to the outer surfaces of the plant parts to be protected. In this position, the fungicides act as a barrier to infection. Since most fungicides are toxic to higher plants as well as fungi, it is necessary that their application is restricted to cutinized epidermal surfaces. A large body of literature exists on fungicides. Their ability to kill fungi has been detailed (Horsfall, 1945, 1956; McCallan and Miller 1963; Sisler and Cox, 1960; Sisler, 1963); their chemistry has been discussed (Rich, 1960; Spencer, 1963); and their application, use, and environmental interactions reviewed (Torgeson, 1967).

In an effort to present a general impression of the character of fungicides, representative major groups will be briefly discussed.

A. Inorganic Fungicides

1. *Metals.* Metallic compounds, generally less toxic than most organic fungicides, are the most popular inorganic fungal poisons. The decending order of fungitoxicity for metal cations is: Silver (Ag), mercury (Hg), copper (Cu), cadmium (Cd), chromium (Cr), nickel (Ni), lead (Pb), cobalt (Co), zinc (Zn), iron (Fe), and calcium (Ca) (Horsfall, 1956). Metals may act as toxins by virtue of their ability to combine with metabolites, enzymes, and/or proteins. This binding, or chelation, presumably removes the bound compound from its normal metabolic pathway or causes abnormal behavior within the pathway.

2. *Nonmetals.* Historically, sulfur has been, and presently is, a principal inorganic fungicide. The ancient Greeks appreciated the pesticidal qualities of sulfur. During the eighteenth century, copper sulfate was used as a fungicide. In the mid-1800's the French botanist, Millardet, fostered the widespread use of Bordeaux mixture, copper sulfate and lime, in the vineyards of France. The basis of the toxic action of sulfur on microbial systems is unknown. Evidence has been presented which suggests that sulfur may function to cause abnormal metabolism by acting as a hydrogen acceptor or as a strong oxidizing agent.

Other nonmetallic, inorganic fungicides include halogenated compounds, formaldehyde (organic), and ammonia. Calcium hypochlorite (CaOCl) and sodium hypochlorite (NaOCl) are two widely employed halogen fungicides. These materials are efficient germicides because of their extreme oxidizing power in solution and perhaps their ability to halogenate microbial metabolites. Formaldehyde (HCHO) has the capacity to combine readily with amino acids and thereby denature proteins. Fumigation with ammonia may result in severe internal pH changes in exposed fungi as the gas is highly soluble in water and forms NH_4OH (Rich, 1960).

B. Organic Fungicides

1. Dithiocarbamates and related compounds. These materials are all derivatives of dithiocarbamic acid:

Thiram   Nabam

Other fungicides in this class include; ferbam, maneb, zineb, ziram, and Thioneb. The precise mechanism of toxicity of these compounds is unclear but may involve the chelation of required heavy metals or interference with enzymes or proteins.

2. Heterocyclic nitrogen compounds. This is a relatively large group of fungicides which possess widely different toxic mechanisms. Examples include; aminopyridine, cycloheximide, Dyrene, glyodin, pyridine-thione compounds, and captan. Captan, whose toxic mechanism is imperfectly understood, has the following structure:

Captan

3. Quinones. These materials are potent fungicides and bactericides. Tetrabromobenzoquinone, chloranil, and dichlone are among the most widely used. The structures of the latter two are as follows:

Chloranil   Dichlone

The most likely toxic mechanisms of quinone materials are binding the quinone nucleus to SH or NH_2 groups in the fungus cell or disturbing the fungal electron transport system.

4. Derivatives of phenol.   Derivatives of carbolic acid are relatively nonspecific protoplasmic poisons and extensively employed as germicidal agents. Some of the more common fungicides include: chlorodimethyl-phenoxyethanol, methylparaben, propylparaben, *o*-phenylphenol, sodium *o*-phenylphenate, trichlorophenol, tetrachlorophenol, and dichlorophene.

Dichlorophene

These four organic classes, in addition to the inorganic compounds discussed, are the most extensively employed fungicides in agricultural crop protection. A large number of additional chemicals are also utilized in protective efforts. Names, structural formulae, physical properties, toxicities, and uses of most of these compounds may be obtained in Frear (1965) or Thomson (1967).

C. The Pesticide Problem

A discussion of the use of chemicals to protect plants from disease agents would be incomplete without viewing this use in the larger context. Pesticides are chemical agents used to kill any living organism which is free living or has a free living stage in its life history (Moore, 1967). In addition to fungicides; acaricides, insecticides, nematocides, herbicides, molluscicides, repellents, algaecides, and rodenticides are typically included in the pesticide group. Even though the use of pesticides is frequently justified in a biological (that is, ability to kill target organism) and economic sense, their use is commonly unjustified or their consequences unknown in an ecological sense. This latter fact is important because pecticides do not operate on pests alone but rather on ecosystems in which pests are present.

Like the ecosystems in which pesticides are employed, the pesticide problem has many facets and is extremely complex. The biological, economic, and ecological aspects of the problem have been reviewed in *National Academy of Sciences — National Research Council* (1966), Headley and Lewis (1967), Moore (1967), and Rudd (1964). Two primary aspects of the problem are (*1*) some pesticides kill nontarget organisms and (*2*) some pesticides are recalcitrant.

Pesticides are generally nonspecific poisons. Their placement into the environment, therefore, may result in the death of organisms not intended to be killed. Numerous examples of this phenomenon have been cited, as for example, Dustman and Stickel (1966).

The documentation of the killing of nontarget organisms by pesticides used in controlling tree disease agents is not extensive. The reduction of soil animals, especially earthworms, however, by the repeated applications of copper fungicides in English apple orchards has been cited by Raw (1962). Severe bird mortality following the use of DDT in a Dutch elm disease control effort has been documented by Wurster et al. (1965).

If a pesticide is toxic to mammals, its influence on man as well as on other organisms must be considered. An imperfect estimate of mammalian toxicity is provided by the "mean lethal dose" (LD_{50}). This figure, commonly available for most pesticides, is based on the influence of the chemical on some small laboratory mammal. Its influence on man is presumed to approximate that of its influence on these animals. Toxicity data are usually presented as the number of milligrams of a chemical per kilogram of body weight which, when taken orally, will cause mortality. Relative toxicities of various pesticides may be obtained by use of a standard toxicity rating (Table XXIX).

TABLE XXIX

TOXICITY RATING[a,b]

	Probable lethal dose (human)	
Toxicity rating or class	mg/per kg	For a 70-kg man (150 lb)
6 "Super toxic"	Less than 5	A taste (less than 7 drops)
5 Extremely toxic	5-50	Between 7 drops and 1 teaspoonful
4 Very toxic	50-500	Between 1 tsp and 1 ounce
3 Moderately toxic	500-5 (gm/kg)	Between 1 oz and 1 pint (or 1 lb)
2 Slightly toxic	5-15 (gm/kg)	Between 1 pt and 1 quart
1 Practically nontoxic	Above 15 (gm/kg)	More than 1 quart

[a]From Gleason et al. (1969). Reproduced by permission of Williams and Wilkins Co.

[b]Modified from H. C. Hodge and J. H. Sterner (Amer. Indust. Hygiene Assoc. Quar. 10:4, 1949) whose original table was designed for industrial chemicals, not consumer compounds.

Pesticides, once introduced into the environment, are subject to loss by various factors. Included among these factors, for example, are volatilization, leaching, biodegradation, and alteration by various physical factors. Those chemicals which are unaffected or little affected by these factors are said to be persistent or recalcitrant. Examples of these materials include the organochlorine insecticides (Nash and Woodson, 1967), certain fungicides which produce stable copper and sulfur residues (Mellanby, 1967), and mercury and other heavy-metal fungicides (Hunt, 1966).

Two undesirable consequences of persistence are: (1) it frequently results in dispersal of the chemicals to sites far removed from their place of application (Moore, 1967), and (2) organisms which exist at high trophic levels in food chains may tend to accumulate the chemicals in injurious amounts (Woodwell et al., 1967).

In general, fungicides have not been at the center of pesticide controversies. Several factors probably contribute to this situation. Most fungicides are chemicals toxic to plants and generally innocuous to man and other animals (Rich, 1966). Many fungicides, especially the organic ones, for example, dithiocarbamates (Kunze, 1966), are not persistent in the environment. The use of fungicides is frequently confined to "emergency" situations only, that is, instances where conditions of the environment and other fortuitous circumstances interact to create a potential disease hazard.

If the use of pesticides is viewed in the full ecologic perspective, and objectively, the application of some materials to control plant pests is wise and the use of other compounds is unwise. Of all the arguments which have been presented for and against pesticides, none has been or could be as adequately defended as the argument for more research and information on the total influence of pesticides in complete ecosystems.

V. SUMMARY

Silvicultural practices have been the most widely employed protective devices used in forest tree disease control. Continued and expanded use of pathological criteria in planting site and silvicultural method selection is highly desirable. The use of biological protective schemes, while attractive because of their specificity, have frequently been shown to be impractical in field situations. The use of chemicals to protect forest trees from disease agents has not been prevalent in the past. Expanding use of chemical controls, however, may be expected as tree and land values increase. The use of chemicals should be restricted to "crisis" periods, and they should not be used indescriminately even then. Users of fungicides, bactericides, nematocides, and herbicides should make an effort to avail themselves of whatever information may be available on the overall influence of the materials in the ecosystems to which they will be introduced. The use of compounds which may significantly influence nontarget organisms, persist for extended periods in the environment, or result in other known undesirable consequences should be avoided.

REFERENCES

Boyce, J. S., Jr. (1963). Growth of *Fomes annosus* into slash pine stumps after top inoculation. *Plant Disease Reptr.* **47**, 218-221.

Curl, E. A., and Arnold, M. M. (1964). Influence of forest organic matter and microbial interactions on growth of *Fomes annosus. Phytopathology* **54**, 1486-1487.

Darpoux, H. (1960). Biological interference with epidemics. *In* "Plant Pathology" (J. G. Horsfall and A. E. Dimond, eds.), Vol. 3, pp. 521-565. Academic Press, New York.

Dimond, A. E. (1966). Effectiveness of antibiotics against forest tree rusts: A summary of present status. *J. Forestry* **64**, 379-382.

Dustman, E. H., and Stickel, L. F. (1966). Pesticide residues in the ecosystem. *In* "Pesticides and Their Effects on Soils and Water," Spec. Publ. No. 8, pp. 109-121. *Soil Sci. Soc. Am.*, Madison, Wisconsin.

Frear, D. E. H. (1965). "Pesticide Index." Coll. Sci. Publ., State College, Pennsylvania.

Gleason, M. N., Gosselin, R. E., Hodge, H. C., and Smith, R. P. (1969). "Clinical Toxicology of Commercial Products. Acute Poisoning (Home and Farm)." Williams & Wilkins, Baltimore, Maryland.

Gremmen, J. (1963). Biological control of *Fomes annosus* by *Peniophora gigantea. Ned. Bosbouw Tijdschr.* **35**, 356-367; *Forestry Abstr.* **25**, 266-267 (1964).

Gundersen, K. (1961). Cycloheximide, the active substance in *Streptomyces griseus* antagonism against *Fomes annosus. Acta Horti Gotoburg.* **25**, 1-24; *Biol. Abstr.* **40**, 1907 (1962).

Gundersen, K. (1962). Induced resistance in *Fomes annosus* to the antibiotic cycloheximide. *Acta Horti Gotoburg.* **25**, 1-31; *Biol. Abstr.* **40**, 1907 (1962).

Headley, J. C., and Lewis, J. N. (1967). "The Pesticide Problem: An Economic Approach to Public Policy." Johns Hopkins Press, Baltimore, Maryland.

Hodges, C. S. (1964). The effect of competition by *Peniophora gigantea* on the growth of *Fomes annosus* in stumps and roots. *Phytopathology* **54**, 623.

Horsfall, J. G. (1945). "Fungicides and Their Action." Chronica Botanica, Waltham, Massachusetts.

Horsfall, J. G. (1956). "Principles of Fungicidal Action." Chronica Botanica, Waltham, Massachusetts.

Hunt, E. G. (1966). Biological magnification of pesticides. *Natl. Acad. Sci. — Natl. Res. Council, Publ.* **1402**, 251-262.

Kunze, G. W. (1966). Pesticides and clay minerals. *In* "Pesticides and Their Effects on Soils and Water," *Spec. Publ. No. 8, Soil Sci. Soc. Am.*, pp. 49-70. Madison, Wisconsin.

McCallan, S. E. A., and Miller, L. P. (1963). Uptake of fungitoxicants by spores. *Conn. Agr. Expt. Sta., Bull.* **663**, 137-148.

Matthews, F. R. (1964). Some aspects of the biology and the control of southern cone rust. *J. Forestry* **62**, 881-884.

Mellanby, K. (1967). "Pesticides and Pollution." Collins, St. James's Place, London.

Meredith, D. S. (1959). The infection of pine stumps by *Fomes annosus* and other fungi. *Ann. Botany (London)* [N.S.] **23**, 455-476.

Meredith, D. S. (1960). Further observations on fungi inhabiting pine stumps. *Ann. Botany (London)* [N.S.] **24**, 63-78.

Moore, N. W. (1967). A synopsis of the pesticide problem. *Advan. Ecol. Res.* **4**, 75-129.

Nash, R. G., and Woolson, E. A. (1967). Persistence of chlorinated hydrocarbon insecticides in soils. *Science* **157**, 924-926.

National Academy of Sciences — National Research Council. (1966). "Scientific Aspects of Pest Control — A Symposium," *Publ. No. 1402. Natl. Acad. Sci. — Natl. Res. Council,* Washington, D.C.

Negruckij, S. F. (1963). The use of fungal antagonists for control of *Fomes annosus. Mikrobiologia* **32**, 632-635; *Forestry Abstr.* **26**, 96 (1965).

Persson-Hüppel, A. (1963). The influence of temperature on the antagonistic effect of *Trichoderma viridi* Fr. on *Fomes annosus* (Fr.). *Cke. Stud Forest Suecica* **4**, 1-13; *Biol. Abstr.* **46**, 1421 (1965).

Raw, F. (1962). Studies of earthworm populations in orchards. *Ann. Appl. Biol.* **50**, 389-404.

Rich, S. (1960). Fungicidal chemistry. *In* "Plant Pathology" (J. G. Horsfall and A. E. Dimond, eds.), Vol. 2, pp. 553-602. Academic Press, New York.

Rich, S. (1966). Chemistry of fungicides. *In* "Pesticides and Their Effects on Soils and Water," *Spec. Publ. No. 8*, pp. 44-48. *Soil Sci. Soc. Am.*, Madison, Wisconsin.

Rishbeth, J. (1961). Inoculation of pine stumps against infection by *Fomes annosus. Nature* **191**, 826-827.

Rishbeth, J. (1963). Stump protection against *Fomes annosus*. III. Inoculation with *Peniophora gigantea. Ann. Appl. Biol.* **52**, 63-77.

Rudd, R. L. (1964). "Pesticides and the Living Landscape." Univ. of Wisconsin Press, Madison, Wisconsin.

Sisler, H. D. (1963). Fungitoxic mechanisms. *Conn. Agr. Expt. Sta., New Haven, Bull.* **663**, 116-133.

Sisler, H. D., and Cox, C. E. (1960). Physiology of fungitoxicity. *In* "Plant Pathology" (J. G. Horsfall and A. E. Dimond, eds.), Vol. 2, pp. 507–552. Academic Press, New York.

Spencer, E. Y. (1963). Structure and activity relations among fungicides. *Conn. Agr. Expt. Sta., New Haven, Bull.* **663**, 95–112.

Thomson, W. T. (1967). "Agricultural Chemicals," Book IV. Fungicides. Thomson Publ., Davis, California.

Timonin, M. I. (1966). Rhizosphere effect of healthy and diseased lodgepole pine seedlings. *Can. J. Microbiol.* **12**, 531–537.

Torgeson, D. C., ed. (1967). "Fungicides," Vol. 1. Academic Press, New York.

Trousdell, K. B. (1965). Damage to recently thinned loblolly pine stands by hurricane Donna. *J. Forestry* **63**, 96–100.

Tryon, E. H. (1966). Implications of even-aged management on protection. *44th Ann. Winter Meeting, Allegheny Sect., Soc. Am. Foresters, Philadelphia, Pa., Feb. 10, 1966.*

Woodwell, G. M., Wurster, C. F., Jr., and Isaacson, P. A. (1967). DDT residues in an East coast estuary: A case of biological concentration of a persistent insecticide. *Science* **156**, 821–824.

Wurster, D. H., Wurster, C. F., and Strickland, W. H. (1965). Bird mortality following DDT spray for Dutch elm disease. *Ecology* **46**, 488–499.

Zak, B. (1964). Role of mycorrhizae in root disease. *Ann. Rev. Phytopathol.* **2**, 377–392.

GENERAL REFERENCES

Allen, M. W. (1960). Nematocides. *In* "Plant Pathology" (J. G. Horsfall and A. E. Dimond, eds.), Vol. 2, pp. 603–638. Academic Press, New York.

Barker, K. R. (1964). On the disease reduction and reproduction of the nematode *Aphelenchus avenae* on isolates of *Rhizoctonia solani. Plant Disease Reptr.* **48**, 428–432.

Barras, S. J. (1969). *Penicillium implicatum* antagonistic to *Ceratocystis minor* and *C. ips. Phytopathology* **59**, 520.

Benedict, W. V., and Baker, W. L. (1963). Pesticides in forestry — a review of current practices. *J. Forestry* **61**, 340–344.

Carson, R. (1962). "Silent Spring." Houghton, Boston, Massachusetts.

Casida, J. E., and Fukunaga, K. (1968). Pesticides: Metabolism, degradation and mode of action. *Science* **60**, 445–450.

Chang, I-pin, and Kommedahl, T. (1968). Biological control of seedling blight of corn by coating kernels with antagonistic microorganisms. *Phytopathology* **58**, 1395–1401.

Cornelius, R. B. (1965). Where are we going in forest pest control. *J. Forestry* **63**, 661–664.

Evans, E. (1968). "Plant Diseases and Their Chemical Control." Blackwell, Oxford.

Frear, D. E. H. (1967). "Pesticide Handbook—Entoma." Coll. Sci. Publ., State College, Pennsylvania.

Gould, R. F., ed. (1966). "Organic Pesticides in the Environment," *Advan. Chem. Ser. No. 60, Am. Chem. Soc.,* Washington, D.C.

Graham, F., Jr. (1967). The uncertain defenders. *Audubon* **69**, (3)28-37.

Houston, D. R., and Eno, H. G. (1969). Use of soil fumigants to control spread of *Fomes annosus. Res. Paper, Northeast. Forest Expt. Sta.* **NE-123**, 1-23.

Jukes, T. H. (1963). People and pesticides. *Am. Scientist* **51**, 355-361.

Kimmey, J. W. (1969). Inactivation of lethal-type blister rust cankers on western white pine. *J. Forestry* **67**, 296-299.

Lukens, R. J. (1969). Fungitoxic action of nonmetallic organic fungicides. *In* "Biodeterioration of Materials," Elsevier Publ. Com. Ltd., Essex, England, pp. 487-497.

McClellan, W. D. (1966). Common names for pesticides. *Plant Disease Reptr.* **50**, 725-729.

Marx, D. H. (1969). The influence of ectotrophic mycorrhizal fungi on the resistance of pine roots to pathogenic infections. II. Production, identification, and biological activity of antibiotics produced by *Leucopaxillus cerealis* var. *piceina. Phytopathology* **59**, 411-417.

Marx, D. H., and Davey, C. B. (1969). The influence of ectotrophic mycorrhizal fungi on the resistance of pine roots to pathogenic infections. III. Resistance of aseptically formed mycorrhizae to infection by *Phytophthora cinnamomi. Phytopathology* **59**, 549-558.

Marx, D. H., and Davey, C. B. (1969). The influence of ectotrophic mycorrhizal fungi on the resistance of pine roots to pathogenic infections. IV. Resistance of naturally occurring mycorrhizae to infections by *Phytophthora cinnamomi. Phytopathology* **59**, 559-565.

Marx, D. H., and Bryan, W. C. (1969). Effect of soil bacteria on the mode of infection of pine roots by *Phytophthora cinnamomi. Phytopathology* **59**, 614-619.

Parris, G. K. (1969). Control of the brown-spot-disease on loblolly pine in Mississippi by spraying. *Phytopathology* **59**, 116 (abstr.).

Soil Science Society of America, Inc. (1966). "Pesticides and Their Effects on Soil and Water," *Spec. Publ. No. 8. Soil Sci. Soc. Am.,* Madison, Wisconsin.

Subcommittee on Reorganization of the Senate. Committee on Government Operations. (1966). "Pesticides and Public Policy," Rept. No. 1379. U.S. Govt. Printing Office, Washington, D.C.

Thomson, W. T. (1967). "Agricultural Chemicals," Book I. Insecticides, Acaracides, and Ovicides. Thomson Publ., Davis, California.

Thomson, W. T. (1967). "Agricultural Chemicals," Book II. Herbicides. Thomson Publ., Davis, California.

Thomson, W. T. (1967). "Agricultural Chemicals," Book III. Miscellaneous Chemicals. Fumigants, Growth Regulators, Repellents, Rodenticides. Thomson Publ., Davis, California.

Torgeson, D. C., ed. (1969). "Fungicides," Vol. 2. Academic Press, New York.

Wester, H. V. (1968). Spraying and other controls for diseases and insects that attack trees and shrubs. Tree Preservation Bull. No. 6. Natl. Park Ser., Washington, D.C.

Whitten, J. L. (1966). "That We May Live." Van Nostrand, Princeton, New Jersey.

Woodwell, G. M., Malcolm, W. M., and Whittaker, R. H. (1966). A-bombs, bugbombs, and us. *Brookhaven Natl. Lab.* **BNL 9842**.

27

RESISTANCE

The term resistance refers to those control procedures which involve the concepts of immunity, resistance, or tolerance of plants to disease agents. A plant is called immune when it appears free of disease symptoms in the presence of a disease agent under all environmental conditions. It is generally presumed that no growth of the parasite is supported. Resistance involves the inherent ability of a plant to avoid or restrict entrance or subsequent development of a pathogen when environmental conditions are suitable for infection. Tolerance concerns the ability of certain plants to persist in a reasonably healthful condition even in the presence of a certain amount of infection. The conditions of immunity and tolerance are relatively uncommon occurrences and therefore quite unimportant in a control sense. The phenomenon of resistance, however, is fairly prevalent. Actually, disease resistance is a general aspect of plant character and most plants are resistant to most diseases.

In agricultural practice, the use of resistant varieties to control plant diseases has proved to be the most efficient and economical control procedure.

I. MECHANISMS OF RESISTANCE
The means by which plants resist infection by pathogens are extremely varied. A reasonably comprehensive discussion has been presented by Wood (1967). In an effort to provide an impression of the variation several examples will be discussed. For convenience, resistance mechanisms may be divided into physical and chemical types present prior to infection (passive) or which develop following infection (induced).

A. Physical
Physical resistance mechanisms are morphological and anatomical phenomena which reduce susceptibility to damage by disease agents.

1. Passive.   Resistance in this instance is dependent on structures in existence prior to infection.

Quantitative and qualitative characteristics of the cuticle have been shown to influence disease resistance. Differences in waxes and cutin acids of young and old lime (*Citrus aurantifolia*) leaves have been correlated with resistance to infection by *Gloeosporium limetticola* (Deuteromycete) (Roberts and Martin, 1963). Eglinton and Hamilton (1967) have recently detailed the chemistry of leaf waxes.

The size and distribution of stomates and lenticels are important factors in many disease phenomena. The narrowness of the stomatal opening in mandarin orange (*Citrus nobilis*), for example, may impair the entrance of the canker-inducing bacterium *Pseudomonas citri* (Wood, 1967).

Internal structural differences are also significant in resistance. In general, the greater the amount of suberization and lignification which have occurred in a cell wall, the greater is the resistance of this wall to colonization by most pathogens.

2. Induced.   This section is concerned with those structures significant in resistance which are not present before the plant is infected.

A rather general phenomenon of plants invaded by microbial pathogens, or injured abiotically, is the process of "wound healing." The primary result of this process, which may be mediated by wound hormones, is the development of a relatively impermeable barrier between damaged and undamaged cells. Certain varieties of plum, for example, when infected by *Stereum purpureum* (Basidiomycete) will form large quantities of gum in the wood that act to restrict the movement of the fungus.

There is some evidence to suggest that tyloses, which form in response to infection by vascular pathogens (for example, *Verticillium* spp. and *Ceratocystis* spp. in trees), may contribute to resistance. The action of tyloses and gel plugs (masses of jellylike material) may be to physically restrict the movement of the inducing microbe.

Differential susceptibility of white pine trees to infection by *Cronartium ribicola* may be related to the formation of cork (Struckmeyer and Riker, 1951). In resistant white pines, penetration of the stem by the fungus occasions the development of a cambium which produces a cork barrier and inhibits deep penetration by the fungus.

B. Chemical

All physical resistance mechanisms do, of course, have chemical bases. Chemical resistance mechanisms as discussed in this section, however, refer to those instances where chemicals, either preformed or induced, play *direct* roles in reducing disease phenomena.

1. Passive.   The compounds which naturally exist in uninfected plants and which may play important roles in resistance to disease agents are extremely varied. These materials may operate outside the plant, for example, in leaf or root exudates, or inside the plant.

Buxton (1957, 1962) has presented evidence that suggests that materials released from the roots of pea and banana plants are effective in determining varietal resistance. In both these instances, root exudate materials from resistant varieties allowed less spore germination of soil pathogens than root exudates from susceptible varieties. *Ginkgo biloba* is an extremely interesting tree and a plant curiosity because it is a relic species (Major, 1967). It is also of phytopathological interest because it has comparatively few disease agents. Johnston and Sproston (1965) have shown that chloroform-soluble materials from gingko leaf cuticle are capable of reducing spore germination and germ tube development of certain leaf pathogens.

The greatest research effort on chemicals significant in resistance has been made on preformed compounds effective inside host plants. Resistance roles have been claimed for certain phenolics, alkaloids, glycosides, amino acids, proteins, carbohydrates, volatile hydrocarbons, and others.

Simple phenols, polyphenols, and quinones (oxidation products of phenols) have been implicated in disease resistance mechanisms of a multitude of plants (Biehn *et al.*, 1968; Wood, 1967). Toxic extractible substances deposited during the formation of heartwood are presumed the principal source of decay resistance in wood. Most of these extractible substances are phenols (Scheffer and Cowling, 1966). More than 50 phenolic substances were detected in the needles and bark of *Pinus monticola* resistant and susceptible to *Cronartium ribicola* infection (Hanover, 1966). No qualitative differences, however, were found between resistant and susceptible trees. Chestnut species resistant to *Endothia parasitica*, for example, Chinese and Japanese varieties, have higher contents of water-soluble tannins than American chestnut (Wood, 1967). These tannins may be involved in disease resistance.

Glycosides, combinations of certain hydroxy compounds with a sugar, may be present in ash bark. Jung and Hubbes (1965) have indicated that glycosides from the bark of white, green, black, and European ashes are inhibitory to the *in vitro* growth of *Bacillus cereus*.

Volatile components of ponderosa pine oleoresin have been shown by Cobb *et al.* (1968) to inhibit the *in vitro* growth of certain fungal pathogens. Heptane was found most inhibitory and was considered fungistatic to *Fomes annosus* and *Ceratocystis pilifera*.

2. *Induced.*   A great deal of evidence has been accumulated indicating that numerous pathogens, after they enter host plants, induce the formation of compounds which have microbial toxicity. Examples of induced toxins include; ipomeamarone, chlorogenic acid, *iso*-chlorogenic acid, umbelliferon, ipomeanine, scopoletin, and batatic acid (Wood, 1967). More re-

cently, materials discovered having the characteristics of those mentioned above have been termed phytoalexins.

Phytoalexins have been defined as "antibiotics which are produced as a result of an interaction of two metabolic systems, host and parasite, and which inhibit the growth of microorganisms pathogenic to plants" (Cruickshank, 1963). Several constraints are involved in the phytoalexin concept. Phytoalexins are formed only when living host cells come in contact with living pathogen cells. The inhibitory substances produced are chemicals and are nonspecific in their fungal toxicity. Different fungal species may, however, be differentially influenced by them. The basic phytoalexin response is similar in resistant and susceptible hosts, but the rate of formation is presumed faster in resistant plants (Cruickshank, 1963).

A well-studied phytoalexin is pisatin (3-hydroxy-7-methoxy-4′,5′-methylene-dioxychromano-coumarin) from peas.

Pisatin

This fungitoxic material is produced in stems, leaves, and pods of pea following infection by *Sclerotinia fructicola* (Ascomycete).

In loblolly pine, a "reaction zone" formed between sound sapwood and sapwood infected by *Fomes annosus* has been described by Shain (1967). Pinosylvin and pinosylvin monomethylether were extractable from this reaction zone and may be phytoalexins.

Pinosylvin

II. CONTROL THROUGH DISEASE RESISTANCE

There are essentially two basic techniques which permit the incorporation of resistant varieties in control programs. The first is selection and the second is breeding or artificial efforts, for example, mutagenic agent application, to create resistant plants.

A. Selection

Use of natural varieties which possess resistance to a particular disease may be a very efficient and inexpensive means of control. It does, however, involve a search in order to locate and select the desirable individuals.

Over the past several decades, extensive efforts have been made to locate a native American chestnut resistant to *Endothia parasitica*. Thousands of persons have responded to U.S. Department of Agriculture requests to supply them with information concerning apparently resistant chestnuts. Even though most responses have been useless, more than 500 promising trees, larger than 8 inches in diameter, have been located since 1957. Unfortunately, however, exposure of these trees, or vegetative material from these trees, to *E. parasitica* inoculum has resulted in infection.

The most logical area to screen for naturally occurring resistance is in the region where the pathogen is endemic. In the case of *Endothia parasitica* the area of endemism is Asia. During the latter 1930's, the U.S. Department of Agriculture established asiatic chestnut plantations in eight eastern states. The plots contained approximately 25 strains including: Chinese, Japanese, Henry, and sequin species. Over the years, a Chinese chestnut variety from Nanking has shown desirable attributes such as disease resistance, good growth and form, and medium-sized, good quality fruit (Diller and Clapper, 1965).

B. Breeding

This procedure involves the artificial incorporation of the gene(s) for resistance into a plant species by hybridization or subjection to mutagenic agents.

In the chestnut breeding program of the U.S. Department of Agriculture, the most promising hybrid has been the Clapper chestnut. This tree represents a cross between an American and Chinese chestnut backcrossed with the American parent (Little and Diller, 1964). The chestnut breeding program of the Connecticut Agricultural Experiment Station has produced a Japanese × American hybrid of relatively promising character.

The hybrid produced by crossing longleaf and slash pines may prove useful in reducing the influence of two significant southeastern pine disease phenomena. The brown spot needle blight caused by *Scirrhia acicola* (Ascomycete) on longleaf pine seedlings impairs the regeneration of this species on many southern sites. Slash pine, on the other hand, is highly resistant to brown spot disease. Unfortunately, however, slash pine is very susceptible to a southern fusiform rust caused by *Cronartium fusiforme* (Basidiomycete). Interestingly enough, when these two species were crossed, the progeny were found resistant to infection by both *S. acicola* and *C. fusiforme*. In addition, at age 7 years, the hybrids appeared to possess other desirable characters, for example, good branching habit and growth rate (Derr, 1966).

C. Genetic Character of Disease Resistance

Resistance to disease is regulated by the same genetic principles which control the inheritance of other plant traits, such as physiological, anatomical, and morphological characteristics. As such, two kinds of resistance inheritance patterns may be recognized.

If resistance is controlled by a single gene pair, the resistance is variously termed single, major gene, or monogenic, true, or qualitative resistance. Generally, species with this type of resistance are only able to resist infection by certain varieties or races of a particular pathogen. Typically, discrete classes of resistant and susceptible species can be established in progenies from crosses between qualitatively resistant and susceptible parents (Tomiyama, 1963).

If resistance is dependent on the additive influence of two or more genes, it is termed polygenic or quantitative resistance. Species characterized by this type of resistance are usually not as highly resistant as those with qualitative resistance and have their resistance rather easily influenced by changes in environmental conditions. They are less liable, however, to lose their resistant nature if a new variety or race of the pathogen appears. In the case of quantitative resistance, the establishment of discontinuous resistant and susceptible classes within segregating progenies is impossible (Tomiyama, 1963). Examples of tree species with quantitative resistance might include eastern white pine and American elm to infection by *Cronartium ribicola* and *Ceratocystis ulmi*, respectively.

III. SUMMARY

Resistance mechanisms in plants are extremely diverse. The inheritance of the patterns responsible for these mechanisms may be via a single gene pair or multiple gene pairs.

One of the greatest problems associated with incorporating resistance into control programs is the possibility that the pathogen will alter its genetic constitution and circumvent the plants defense. Pathogens undergo genetic change via mutation, sexual recombination, and parasexuality. From this standpoint quantitative resistance is presumed superior to qualitative resistance. If resistance is controlled by a single gene, a relatively minor alteration on the part of the pathogen may be sufficient to permit the pathogen to parasitize a host. Quantitative resistance on the other hand, may involve such numerous and divergent resistance mechanisms that only major changes on the part of the pathogen may permit significant parasitism.

The application of genetics to forest trees is a continually expanding and developing field. Development of new tree varieties, however, is not a rapid process. Nevertheless, since increasing efforts are being directed at creating new strains, it is not unreasonable to suppose that greater disease control may be achieved by utilizing inherent resistance. Criteria for disease resistance are being incorporated into an enlarging number of tree breeding and selection programs.

REFERENCES

Biehn, W. L., Kue, J., and Williams, E. B. (1968). Accumulation of phenols in resistant plant-fungi interactions. *Phytopathology* **58**, 1255-1260.

Buxton, E. W. (1957). Differential rhizosphere effects of three pea cultivars on physiologic races of *Fusarium oxysporium* L. *pisi. Brit. Mycol. Soc. Trans.* **40**, 305-316.

Buxton, E. W. (1962). Root exudates from banana and their relationships to strains of the *Fusarium* causing Panama wilt. *Ann. Appl. Biol.* **50**, 269-282.

Cobb, F. W., Jr., Krstic, M., Zavarin, E., and Barber, H. V., Jr. (1968). Inhibitory effects of volatile oleoresin components on *Fomes annosus* and four *Ceratocystis* species. *Phytopathology* **58**, 1327-1335.

Cruickshank, I. A. M. (1963). Phytoalexins. *Ann. Rev. Phytopathol.* **1**, 351-374.

Derr, H. J. (1966). Longleaf x slash hybrids at age 7: Survival, growth and disease susceptibility. *J. Forestry* **64**, 236-239.

Diller, J. D., and Clapper, R. B. (1965). A progress report on attempts to bring back the chestnut tree in the eastern United States, 1954-1964. *J. Forestry* **63**, 186-188.

Eglinton, G., and Hamilton, R. J. (1967). Leaf epicuticular waxes. *Science* **156**, 1322-1335.

Hanover, J. W. (1966). A comparison of phenolic constituents of *Pinus monticola* resistant and susceptible to *Cronartium ribicola. Physiol. Plantarum* **19**, 554-562.

Johnston, H. W., and Sproston, T. (1965). The inhibition of fungus infection pegs in *Ginkgo biloba. Phytopathology* **55**, 225-227.

Jung, J., and Hubbes, M. (1965). Growth inhibition of *Bacillus cereus in vitro* by glycosidal substances extracted from bark of Fraxinus. *Can. J. Botany* **43**, 469-474.

Little, E. L., Jr., and Diller, J. D. (1964). Clapper chestnut, a hybrid forest tree. *J. Forestry* **62**, 109-110.

Major, R. T. (1967). The ginkgo, the most ancient living tree. *Science* **157**, 1270-1273.

Roberts, M. F., and Martin, J. T. (1963). Withertip disease of limes (*Citrus aurantifolia*) in Zanzibar. *Ann. Appl. Biol.* **51**, 411-413.

Scheffer, T. C., and Cowling, E. B. (1966). Natural resistance of wood to microbial deterioration. *Ann. Rev. Phytopathol.* **4**, 147-170.

Shain, L. (1967). Resistance of sapwood in stems of loblolly pine to infection by *Fomes annosus*. *Phytopathology* **57**, 1043-1045.

Struckmeyer, E. B., and Riker, A. J. (1951). Wound-periderm formation in white-pine resistant to blister rust. *Phytopathology* **41**, 276-281.

Tomiyama, K. (1963). Physiology and biochemistry of disease resistance of plants. *Ann. Rev. Phytopathol.* **1**, 295-324.

Wood, R. K. S. (1967). "Physiological Plant Pathology." Blackwell, Oxford.

GENERAL REFERENCES

Allard, R. W. (1960). "Principles of Plant Breeding." Wiley, New York.

Bollard, E. G., and Matthews, R. E. F. (1966). The physiology of parasitic disease. *In* "Plant Physiology" (F. C. Steward, ed.), Vol. 4, pp. 417-550. Academic Press, New York.

Diller, J. D., and Clapper, R. B. (1969). Asiatic and hybrid chestnut trees in the eastern United States. *J. Forestry* **67**, 328-331.

Gerhold, H. D., Schreiner, E. J., McDermott, R. E., and Winieski, J. A., eds. (1966). "Breeding Pest-Resistant Trees." Pergamon Press, Oxford.

Hare, R. C. (1966). Physiology of resistance to fungal diseases in plants. *Botan. Rev.* **32**, 95-137.

Hattemer, H. H. (1967). Genetic mechanisms allowing an equilibrium between a parasitic fungus and a forest species. *14th I.U.F.R.O. Congr.,* Vol. III, Sect. 22, pp. 414-425, München, 1967.

Keyes, C. R. (1969). Effect of pinene on mycelial growth of representative wood-inhabiting fungi. *Phytopathology* **59**, 400 (abstr.).

Kinloch, B. B., and Stonecypher, R. W. (1969). Genetic variation in susceptibility to fusiform rust in seedlings from a wild population of loblolly pine. *Phytopathology* **59**, 1246-1255.

Kosuge, T. (1969). The role of phenolics in host response to infection. *Ann. Rev. Phytopathol.* **7**, 195-222.

Van der Plank, J. E. (1968). "Disease Resistance in Plants." Academic Press, New York.

Wood, F. A. (1966). The current status of basic knowledge of forest tree disease resistance research. *In* "Breeding Pest-Resistant Trees" (H. D. Gerhold *et al.*, eds.), pp. 293-300. Pergamon Press, Oxford.

SUBJECT INDEX

A

Abies, 133, 212
  balsamea, 59
  concolor, 59
  grandis, 10
Acer, 10, 110, 133, 212
  macrocarpa, 110
  negundo, 39, 95, 110
  platanoides, 39, 95, 110
  pseudoplatanus, 110
  rubrum, 95, 110
  saccharinum, 39
  saccharum, 11, 39, 59, 95
Acervulus, 147, 148, 195
Acti-dione, *see* Cycloheximide
Actinomycetes, 209, 215
Aeciospores, 176, 180, 181, 183, 233, 236
Aecium, 177, 180, 181, 183, 238
Agaricaceae, 165
Agaricales, 147, 148
Agaricus, 148
  campestris bisporus, 147
Agrobacterium, 120, 128, 209
  tumefaciens, 131–132, 266, 267
Ailanthus glandulosa, 39
Air pollution, 2, 51–60
  nonphotochemically produced gases, 52–56
  particulate matter, 52
  photochemically produced gases, 56–60
Aldehydes, 56, 59
Alder, black, 14
Almond, 221, 267
Amanita, 215
Aminopyridine, 279

Ammonia, 9, 22, 56, 278
Anthocyanescence, 44
Anthracnose, 195
Antibodies, 112–113
Antigens, 112–113
Aphelenchoides, 89
Aphelenchus avenae, 89
Aphids, 105, 109, 110
Aplanospores, 152
Apothecium, 142, 143, 195
Apple, 221, 262, 265, 281
  scab, 251
Appressorium, 156, 157, 211
Apricot, 267
Arceuthobium, 221, 222, 260
  americanum, 224
Armillaria, 148
  mellea, 32, 147, 155, 266
Arthrobacter, 209
Arthrobotrys oligospora, 88
Arthrospores, 152
Ascocarp, 141
Ascomycetes, 140–144, 147, 148, 164, 169, 186, 193, 197, 200
  Euascomycetes, 142–144, 148
  Hemiascomycetes, 141–142, 148
Ascospores, 141, 142, 190, 191, 195, 197, 202, 204
Ascus, 141–143, 195
Ash, 14, 27, 73, 190, 238, 290
  Arizona, 111
  black, 112, 290
  canker, 129
  dieback, 112, 193, 234
  European, 40, 111, 290
  flowering, 111

297